Basic Child Psychiatry
Fifth Edition

Philip Barker

MB, BS, FRCP(Ed), FRCPsych, FRCP(C), DPM, DCH

Professor of Psychiatry and Paediatrics,
University of Calgary,
Psychiatrist, Alberta Children's Hospital

D0620369

Blackwell Scientific Publications
OXFORD LONDON EDINBURGH
BOSTON MELBOURNE

Blackwell Scientific Publications
Editorial Offices:
Osney Mead, Oxford OX2 0EL
25 John Street, London WC1N 2BL
23 Ainslie Place, Edinburgh EH3 6AJ
3 Cambridge Center, Suite 208,
    Cambridge, Massachusetts 02142, USA
54 University Street, Carlton
    Victoria 3053, Australia

First published in Great Britain by
Crosby Lockwood Staples 1971
Reprinted 1973
Second edition published by Granada
Publishing Limited
in Crosby Lockwood Staples 1976
Reprinted 1977
Third edition 1979
Reprinted by Granada Publishing Ltd 1981
Fourth edition published by Granada
Publishing Ltd 1983
Reprinted 1984 (ISBN 0-246-11944-6)
Reprinted by Collins Professional and
Technical Books 1986
Fifth edition published by
Blackwell Scientific Publications 1988
Reprinted 1990

Set by DP Photosetting, Aylesbury, Bucks
Printed and bound in Great Britain by
Billing & Sons Ltd, Worcester

DISTRIBUTORS
Marston Book Services Ltd
PO Box 87
Oxford OX2 0DT
(*Orders*: Tel. 0865 791155
    Fax: 0865 791927
    Telex: 837515)
USA
Year Book Medical Publishers
200 North LaSalle Street
Chicago, Ilinois 60601
(*Orders:* Tel. (312) 726-9733)

Canada
The C.V. Mosby Company
5240 Finch Avenue East,
Scarborough, Ontario
(*Orders*: Tel. (416) 298-1588)

Australia
Blackwell Scientific Publications
(Australia) Pty Ltd
54 University Steet
Carlton, Victoria 3053
(*Orders*: Tel. (03) 347 0300)

British Library
Cataloguing in Publication Data

Barker, Philip, *1929—*
    Basic child psychiatry.—5th ed.
    1. Children, Psychiatry
    I. Title
    618.92'89

ISBN 0-632-02063-6
ISBN 0-632-01923-9 Pbk

Library of Congress
Cataloging-in-Publication Data

Barker, Philip.
    Basic child psychiatry.

    Bibliography: p.
    Includes index.
    1. Child psychiatry. I. Title [DNLM: 1.
Child Psychiatry. WS 350 B255b]
RJ499.B27 1988   618.92'89   87—3508
ISBN 0-632-02063-6
ISBN 0-632-01923-9 (pbk.)

To Heather, Edmund, Lorna, Alice, Brenda, Janok and Susan, who
have taught me so much about child development and family life.

Contents

Foreword

Michael Rutter, FRS, Professor of Child Psychiatry, Institute of Psychiatry and Honorary Director, MRC Child Psychiatry Unit

Child psychiatry constitutes one of the most exciting branches of psychiatry in which to work. In part this stems from the challenge of seeking to alleviate the disorders that interfere with the developmental process in the growing child. In part, too, it derives from the opportunity to participate in an area of clinical work where, despite marked limits to our powers of effective prevention and intervention, there continues to be substantial growth in an understanding of the nature and causes of disorder, accompanied by increases in therapeutic efficacy. Yet many newcomers to child psychiatry feel quite uncertain of their bearings at first. Trained as medical doctors, they find themselves working in an interdisciplinary arena where psychologists and social workers possess many of the relevant clinical skills, so that trainee child psychiatrists wonder what their own role should be. Being used, for the most part, to having responsibility just to their individual patient, they are faced with children referred by someone else and whose problems often present in the context of family difficulties. Who is the patient? What is just a hiccup in the normal developmental process, what are social, rather than medical problems and what are 'proper' diseases? Novices look both to their clinical teachers and to introductory text books to provide guidance on how they should proceed.

The latter face the difficult task of steering a course between the Scylla of muddledom deriving from an attempt to present all the complexities involved and the Charybdis of unwarranted certainty based on a theory that fails to fit all the facts or a procrustean attempt to force all children's disorders into a series of neat diagnostic pigeon-holes. They want the reassurance of being told just what to do in the practical situations they face in their everyday clinical practice, but also they need to gain an appreciation of where the subject has come from and where it is going to. Medicine does not stand still and it is of no help to be presented with a set of *obiter dicta* that pose as 'facts' and which in the future will prove to be mistaken as new empirical data become available. Inevitably, a high proportion of what students learn today will be overtaken by advances that take place during the some four decades of their professional lifetime. It is essential that trainees acquire a critical frame of mind that will allow them to evaluate research claims as they appear in the future. Of course, that is too much to expect of any introductory text but, still, a good one should at least give a flavour of what is involved and should provide pointers as to where the details of evidence are to be found and where competing views are compared, contrasted, and debated. At the same time, safe and effective clinical practice rests on a confidence that one knows what one's doing and on a secure grasp of the available concepts and factual knowledge.

The fifth edition of Philip Barker's *Basic Child Psychiatry* admirably meets these competing needs. Both the 'art' and 'science' of the subject are present in good measure. It is eclectic in the best sense of an awareness of the real contributions that stem from diverse fields, whilst avoiding the sterile indecisiveness of trying to be all things to all people. It is non-doctrinaire but it is appropriately didactically practical when that is called for. This is shown well, for example, in the clear account in Chapter 3 of how to set about assessing children and their families with a sensitivity to their needs and a hypothesis-testing approach to how these needs should be met. Of course, not all experts will agree with the details of each aspect described, but readers are shown a workable approach based on a wealth of experience, as well as a knowledge of the (rather limited) research findings. This smooth integration of clinical experience and empirical research perhaps provides the hallmark of the book. In the past, psychiatry has sometimes suffered from needless and fruitless battles between those who wish to present personal views as dogma and those who cast doubt on everything unless proved to the hilt. Philip Barker has no truck with that dispute. It is clear that we have to act now on the basis of what we know – and that knowledge is clearly and unambiguously presented. Equally, we must be aware of the areas of doubt and dispute and these too are noted in the context of the relevant research findings.

Most of all this is a very readable book written in an easy and interesting style that conveys much of Philip Barker's own enthusiasm and commitment. The references, although plentiful, do not interfere with the flow of presentation and they are refreshingly up to date. It does not seek to be encyclopaedic; larger text books are available for those who want to go into the subject in greater depth. Nevertheless, a surprising amount of ground is covered in what is still a comfortably sized volume. It presents an excellent introduction to child psychiatry.

Introduction

The changes that have occurred in the field of child psychiatry since the first, slim edition of this book appeared in 1971 are remarkable. There has been a veritable explosion of research in the field and our knowledge of the psychiatric disorders that may afflict children has grown enormously.

Many conditions that were unknown, or were given scant attention, in 1971 are now the focus of the attention of workers in the field. Examples are the 'fragile X syndrome'; the cognitive difficulties of children with other sex chromosome abnormalities; sleep apnoea; the 'brain fag' or 'school anxiety' syndrome seen in African children; the neuropsychiatric syndromes seen in children with acquired immune deficiency syndrome; and major depressive disorders which are now being more generally recognized in children. The physical, sexual and emotional abuse of children, while certainly not new, have increasingly come to the notice of psychiatrists and our paediatric colleagues; and the field of infant psychiatry has developed from almost nothing to become a major branch of child psychiatry. Sadly, drug and alcohol abuse exact a grim and seemingly increasing toll on our young people, stunting or distorting their psychological and emotional development, and sometimes bringing these processes to a permanent stop through death.

New classifications of child psychiatric disorders have been proposed and used, particularly multiaxial ones. Indeed as this edition was being prepared the revised version of the third edition of the American Psychiatric Association's Diagnostic and Statistical Manual (DSM-III-R) appeared. This differs in various ways from its predecessor, DSM-III, and when discussing the American Psychiatric Associations' recommendations I have used it rather than DSM-III. Research has also broadened and deepened our knowledge in many other areas, including the epidemiology of child psychiatric disorders, the processes of bonding that occur between parents and their children, infantile autism and the role of the school in promoting the development of children.

Treatment methods, too, have developed. Perhaps the most significant advance in the last two decades has been the widespread adoption of family therapy techniques in child psychiatry, but behaviour therapy methods have been greatly refined and our knowledge of child psychopharmacology has increased. The place of residential treatment has been scrutinized and redefined. This is the first edition of this book to include a section on hypnotherapy, something which was probably overdue. Another important concept introduced, if tentatively, in this edition is that of 'state-dependent learning'. I believe this offers a new and helpful way of looking at many psychiatric problems. I shall be surprised if it does not merit much more attention when the time comes for the sixth edition.

Although much remains to be learned about the treatment of child psychiatric disorders, we can now offer the children who are brought to us, and their families, much more than we could in 1971.

All this is very gratifying to those of us working in the field but it's hard on the writers of basic texts. There is so much more to cover that the task of condensing existing knowledge into a reasonably brief space is magnified. Inevitably this edition is somewhat longer than previous ones. A major difference is the great increase in the number of references to the literature. As more and more information, much of which can only be mentioned cursorily in an introductory book, becomes available it is necessary to tell those who want to learn more how they can do so. The references, I hope, will help.

In view of the extensive advances in the field, I thought it necessary on this occasion to subject *Basic Child Psychiatry* to a radical revision. I was assisted in doing so by the University of Calgary, which granted me sabbatical leave for this, and other, purposes. This edition has twenty chapters, three more than the fourth edition. Four of them are new, however, since the chapter on psychological tests has been incorporated into the one on assessing children. Psychological tests are dealt with more briefly, not because I consider them any less important, but because the field of testing, like child psychiatry itself, has grown so much. Excellent texts on psychology and psychological tests are available and it is to them that those wanting information should turn. Their authors know much more about these tests than I do. I have therefore confined myself to setting out the role of tests in the assessment of children. I have outlined how they may help, and have indicated how we can work with our psychologist colleagues to make best use of the tests which can assist us in so many ways.

The chapter on 'psychotic disorders' in the previous edition has been split into two. One deals with 'pervasive developmental disorders', as autism and related conditions are now best called, the other with schizophrenia and other psychoses. Juvenile schizophrenia is at least two-thirds as prevalent as autism, yet has received much less attention in most child psychiatry books, including previous editions of this one. I have therefore given it more emphasis this time.

Encopresis and enuresis have been separated from the hyperkinetic or 'attention-deficit' disorders. Previously all were covered in one chapter but there seemed little logic in that. There is a new chapter on affective disorders, principally depression, and one on legal aspects of child psychiatry.

Despite its title, this is a book about children and adolescents. Except where the context indicates otherwise, you should read 'child or adolescent' for 'child'. To write 'child or adolescent' every time would be tedious for author and reader. The term 'child', of course, also covers infants.

In recent years children with psychiatric problems have increasingly been studied, understood and treated in the context of their families. Frequently the child's problems are so much part and parcel of a dysfunctional family system that the two cannot be separated in any logical way. It is often impossible to say which came first and for therapeutic purposes it may not matter. Treatment addressed to the family system problems is often the main need. I was therefore faced, in preparing this edition, with deciding how extensively I should deal with family therapy concepts and techniques. In 1986, however, a second, expanded edition of the companion book *Basic Family Therapy* (published in the UK by Blackwell Scientific Publications and in New York by Oxford University Press) appeared. I have therefore covered only briefly the assessment of families and family therapy generally. Readers wishing to know more should consult *Basic Family Therapy* or one of the other books on the subject. I do not believe that one introductory book can do justice to both child psychiatry and family therapy.

Despite the many changes in this edition, its purpose remains the same as that of previous ones, namely to provide the newcomer to the field with the basic facts of the subject and information about where to learn more. Many of the references have been selected because they contain, or consist of, reviews of particular aspects of the field. They will lead the interested reader to many other sources of information.

The case histories are all from my own practice. I have changed names and other details which might serve to identify the children or their families in order to ensure their anonymity.

The striking advances in child psychiatry which have occurred since this book first appeared have been due to the efforts of many researchers and clinicians worldwide. Outstanding among these have been Professor Michael Rutter and his colleagues at the Institute of Psychiatry, University of London. They have contributed enormously to our knowledge of child psychiatric epidemiology and of a vast range of clinical and theoretical problems. I am therefore delighted that Professor Rutter has honoured me by writing the Foreword to this new edition of *Basic Child Psychiatry*.

Philip Barker
Calgary, 1988

Acknowledgments

Many teachers, colleagues and patients have helped me acquire the information I have tried to pass on in this book and it is impossible to acknowledge them all. I owe a special debt of gratitude to Philip Connell, who taught me the basics of child psychiatry. My colleagues in the Mental Health Programme of Alberta Children's Hospital have, in recent years, also taught me much and I am especially grateful to Paul Oliphant, the psychologist colleague who read and commented helpfully on the section on psychological tests. Mark Lauderdale reviewed a draft of the section on hypnotherapy and made several helpful suggestions.

Much of this edition was written while I was on sabbatical leave at the John A. Burns School of Medicine, University of Hawaii at Manoa. Jack McDermott and his colleagues were most hospitable to me during this time, and William Bolman kindly read and commented helpfully on a section of the book. Ikuku Uesato, the librarian at the Kapiolani Women's and Children's Medical Centre was patient, diligent and courteous in obtaining reference material for me and I am greatly indebted to her for her help. I am also deeply grateful to Barbara Hatt, librarian at Alberta Children's Hospital, and her assistant, Elisabeth Nielson. They operate a library service which is second to none in my experience. Without their help, and that of Ikuku Uesato, I would not have been able to provide as extensive a guide to further reading as is contained in the references.

My wife, Heather and daughter, Lorna, read drafts of much of the book. Their comments have helped me make my meaning clearer and express myself in more economical language; without their input the book would have read less well. My son, Edmund, has performed a similar function; he has also commented from the perspective of a young physician better informed than I of developments in other fields of medicine.

Richard Miles, my publisher, has been as helpful and supportive to me in the preparation of this edition as he was in the preparation of the third and fourth editions of the book, and of both editions of *Basic Family Therapy*. It has been a privilege in the past to work with him and his colleagues at Collins Professional and Technical Books. I am delighted that he and his staff have moved to Blackwell Scientific Publications, the publisher of this edition, so that I have been able to continue working with them.

Author's note

Throughout this book it has been necessary to make repeated references to the two widely used systems of classifying psychiatric disorders, the International Classification of Diseases, ninth edition (ICD-9) and the revised version of the third edition of the American Psychiatric Association's Diagnostic and Statistical Manual (DSM-III-R). Occasional reference to the original version (DSM-III) was also necessary. It seemed a needless use of space to refer to the sources of these publications by inserting '(World Health Organization, 1977a)' and '(American Psychiatric Association, 1980 or 1987)', respectively, each time these publications were mentioned. I have therefore confined myself to using the abbreviations 'ICD-9' 'DSM-III' and 'DSM-III-R'. The respective references are cited in the list at the end of the text.

Chapter 1

Normal Child and Family Development

In order to deal effectively with disturbed young people we must understand the normal process of development from helpless infant to independent adult. When emotional, social and intellectual functioning are assessed, the range of normal for the child's age and social setting have to be taken into account. What *is* normal is best learned through contact with developing children and their families. It is important also to understand the family life cycle, since many of the problems with which children present prove to be related to difficulties their families are having in passing from one stage of this cycle to the next.

Among the many theories of child development are the psycho-analytic approach of Sigmund Freud (1905), Erik Erikson's psychoso-cial approach (1965, 1968) and the work of Jean Piaget. The latter was summarized by Beard (1969) and more fully described by Flavell (1963); recently Hobson (1985) has provided an excellent brief critical review of Piaget's work. Important contributions to the study of children's development were also made by Anna Freud (1966) and by Melanie Klein (1948).

More recently research has focussed on the process of 'bonding' between children, particularly infants, and their parents. John Bowlby has provided a good, concise account of this process (1977), as well as longer works on attachment and related processes (1969, 1979). Learning theory has also contributed to our understanding of how children develop. Its contribution is discussed by Maccoby and Martin, (1983).

This chapter can only provide a brief overview of child, adolescent and family development. Readers without first-hand experience with children of different ages should seek such experience, as well as consulting some of the many available texts on child development. Normal family functioning and family development are discussed in *Basic Family Therapy* (Barker, 1986). Fuller accounts of family development are those of Duvall and Miller (1985) and McGoldrick and Carter (1982).

The first year of life

Following birth, infants are totally dependent on those caring for them. Their responses vary however and, in turn, influence the behaviour of their care-givers – normally the parents. During the last twenty-five years the behaviour and temperaments of infants have been much studied. The New York Longitudinal Study, initiated in 1956, consisted of a detailed study of a cohort of infants who were eventually followed into adult life (Thomas and Chess, 1977; Chess and Thomas, 1984). It revealed marked differences in behaviour and temperamental style between infants. Nine behavioural traits were defined; these are listed and described in Chapter 2. The course of events during infancy and subsequently depends in part on the 'fit' between the child's behavioural style and the parents' temperaments and ways of reacting.

The first year of life has been called the 'oral stage' by psychoanalysts because the baby's main satisfactions seem to arise from feeding and sucking. The importance of these activities may nevertheless have been over-emphasized. They are not, for example, primarily involved in the formation of emotional attachments. Erikson (1965) calls this period that of 'basic trust versus basic mistrust'. This is the first of his 'eight stages of man'. A healthy outcome results when the child experiences the world, during this period, as nurturing, reliable and trustworthy. Children who have such experiences develop the capacity for satisfying intimate relationships. Those who lack warm, nurturing experiences may show impaired capacity for intimacy.

Motor functions develop rapidly during the first year. By about one year the child is walking. There are also big developments in social behaviour. By three weeks the child smiles at people's faces. At first this is a reflex response – the 'endogenous smile' – but by 2 to 3 months of age children smile selectively at their mothers – the 'social smile'. By 6 months they have learned to distinguish familiar from unfamiliar people, smiling selectively at the former. Then, by about eight months, signs of fear and anxiety ('stranger anxiety') appear in the presence of unfamiliar people, especially if there is no parent present and in unfamiliar situations. Soon afterwards 'separation anxiety' appears. This is anxiety upon separation from the mother, especially if in an unfamiliar place or with unfamiliar people. It is a sign that the child has developed a close relationship with the mother. For this to occur it is necessary for the child to have been cared for regularly and consistently by the same person (mother or mother-substitute). The process whereby this relationship develops is called 'bonding'.

Attachment behaviour in early childhood is characterized by the attainment or maintenance of physical proximity by the child to the object of the attachment (Bowlby, 1977). When this is happening, the child is said to have bonded to the person concerned. The process seems to be a biological phenomenon, characteristic of many primate species. Attachment theory conceives of this behaviour as being in a class at least as important as feeding and sexual behaviour, but distinct and different. Features of attachment behaviour in the first year are crying, calling, stranger anxiety and separation anxiety, all of which tend to bring about proximity to the attachment figure. The theory states that an infant's attachment results primarily from the availability of a familiar figure. The more social interaction there is with that figure, the more likely it is the subject will become attached to that person. The process does not depend on gratification of needs. Indeed, in monkeys, attachment can occur to a soft, cuddly dummy as well as to a live mother monkey (Harlow, 1958).

By the end of the first year the child should have a close, secure relationship with the mother (or mother-substitute), and an ordered pattern of feeding and sleeping should have been established. Attachment to other family members, such as the father and siblings occurs too, depending on the amount of interaction there is with such people.

Fixed, rigid feeding schedules are no longer usual in western countries (they never were in most of the rest of the world). Semi-solid foods tend to be introduced earlier, sometimes at two or three months, than they were in the past. Perhaps for this reason, weaning seldom seems to cause difficulty. In many parts of the world, especially the underdeveloped ones, breast feeding is continued well into the second year, even beyond. This is much to be desired when alternative sources of nutrition for children are scarce. It also has the advantage of helping space children more widely, since nursing mothers do not usually ovulate and so do not become pregnant.

Intellectual development proceeds rapidly in the first year. Piaget called this year, and the following one, the 'sensorimotor period'. Children learn certain basic things about their relationship to the environment. They discover that objects exist apart from themselves, and continue to exist when they no longer perceive them. They also learn simple cause-and-effect relationships. They gain an understanding of spatial relationships, and acquire some idea of how one thing can symbolize another. All these processes involve action by the child, and depend on current sensory input and motor activity.

The second year

At about the beginning of the second year children start to walk and so become able actively to explore their environments. They also start to talk. More demands are made of them, particularly over bowel and bladder training and limiting their exploratory behaviour. The period covering the second and third years has been called the 'anal stage' by psychoanalysts, because of the supposed importance of the processes whereby bowel and bladder control are achieved. Yet many other developments are occurring and there is little evidence that eliminatory functions and toilet training are the crucial issues they were once thought to be.

Erikson (1965) considers the main issue of the second year to be that of 'autonomy versus shame and doubt'. The child should develop a sense of being in control of his or her self, combined with pleasant, self-confident feelings. These features stand in contrast with feelings of shame and doubt about oneself – feelings which characterize many young people who present with psychiatric problems. During this period children normally obtain pleasure from gradually gaining control of bowel and bladder functions, and of their bodies generally. Erikson does not relate anal activity and defecation to sexual gratification, as classical psychoanalytic theory does.

The successful performance of the developmental tasks of the second year requires a warm, secure relationship between child and parents. In such contexts children want to please their parents, and will be made anxious by parental disapproval. They learn to inhibit or release their behaviour accordingly. This applies not only to bowel and bladder training (which may not commence until the second year or later), but to behaviour generally. Learning theory helps us understand this process. Although biological readiness is necessary for particular learning processes to occur, the principles of operant and respondent conditioning (see Chapter 19) govern their operation. Attachment behaviour should be well established by the second year (Bowlby, 1977). It contrasts with exploratory behaviour, which becomes possible once the child can walk. From a secure base the child can move into the environment to explore it, returning to mother when frightened or tired. As the child grows, the time and distance spent away from the mother without discomfort steadily increase.

Nevertheless some exploratory behaviour has to be limited. Children must learn not to play with fire, run out into the roadway, drop crockery on the floor and so on. There is usually resistance to the imposition of limits, often expressed as temper tantrums. These commmonly start in the second year and are a normal reaction when a child's wishes are not gratified. They can cause concern to an inexperienced parent, when a previously well-behaved child suddenly starts displaying tantrum behaviour such as screaming, kicking and waving the arms about. Normally, however, tantrums are a transient feature of the toddler period, and they die away as the child learns to accept the behavioural restraints imposed by parents and others. This process is greatly helped by a secure loving relationship between child and parents.

The development of speech and its comprehension considerably refines the process of communication between child and parents. Speech and language development are discussed further in Chapter 10.

The second year sees the end of Piaget's period of sensori-motor intelligence. Next comes the period of 'concrete operations of classes, relations and numbers'. This starts about mid-way through the second year, as the acquisition of verbal language commences, and extends up to about eleven or twelve years of age. The concrete operations stage has a number of substages, which will be discussed in the following section.

During the second year, children continue to see themselves as the centre of their world and remain closely dependent on their parents.

The pre-school period (ages two to five)

During this period there is:

- Further development of intellectual functions, especially a rapid increase in the complexity of language used and understood.
- A big advance in socialization, as the child learns to live as a member of the family group.
- Rapid progress in the development of the child's sexual identity. Psychoanalysts have called this the 'genital stage', because of the importance they attribute to sexual development at this time.
- Identification with the parents, and the resulting development of the motivation to do certain things, or be a certain kind of person.
- The beginning of conscience formation.
- The establishment of a pattern of 'defence mechanisms' to deal with anxiety and guilt.
- The development of patterns of behaviour towards those outside the family.

Erikson considers this period to be that in which the issue of 'initiative versus guilt' is normally resolved. A successful outcome is a child who feels able to do many exciting, even almost magical, things as opposed to feeling frightened and guilty about taking the initiative. Children who fail to achieve this may believe that if they don't do what others wish, those people will be angry with them or even destroy them. Ideally children should emerge from this period of development confident in their abilities, but with their impulses under adequate control.

The establishment of a child's sex role starts with the acquisition of the general idea that people are divided into male and female categories. This is fostered by the different appearance, clothing and behaviour of the sexes. The child then comes to feel a member of one or other group. This is brought about partly through the child becoming aware of the anatomical differences between the sexes, and partly because of the operation of inborn biological factors. The parents are normally the child's main models of the male and female roles. Sex play, often with undressing or sexual exploration, is common at this time (Newson and Newson, 1968), as is interest in the genitals of siblings and playmates. As sexual awareness develops, the boy or girl is faced with the problem of his or her position *vis-à-vis* the parents. Psychoanalysts emphasize the importance of the rivalry the child may feel with the parent of the same sex for the affection of the other parent. This is the famous 'oedipal stage' of development. The conflict is resolved, according to psychoanalytic theory, by identification with the parent of the same sex.

While the appropriate sex role is being adopted most children experience some uncertainty and curiosity on the subject. Fear of loss of male characteristics ('castration fears') in the boy and concern about the lack of male genitals in the girl, may cause transient anxiety. Psychoanalysts have emphasized the roles such worries may play in causing emotional problems but less stress is placed on them now that psychoanalytic theories of development hold less exclusive sway. Masturbation is so common in this period, especially in boys, as to be a normal phenomenon. If sensibly handled it usually lessens in frequency or ceases; if it continues the child usually learns to avoid indulging in it at socially inappropriate times.

The development of conscience is closely related to the process of identification with the parents. The child comes to feel that certain types of attitudes and actions are right and others are wrong, and so feels guilty about those in the 'wrong' category. Children are usually unaware, at the conscious level, of the cause of the consequent anxiety, namely their internalization of their parents' standards. In children lacking stable relationships with parent figures, the process of conscience formation is impaired. Conscience, and the capacity to feel guilty, tend to be poorly developed in children brought up in large impersonal institutions. The same applies also to many of those who have moved frequently from one set of parent figures to another during their early years.

Defence mechanisms are means whereby people cope with feelings of anxiety which might otherwise be intolerable. Anxiety, a normal feature of our emotional lives, may arise from an act or threat from outside (as with 'stranger anxiety', mentioned above), from the lack of familiar or expected objects or experiences, or from the operation of conscience. It may also be communicated, as from an anxious parent with whom a child is closely identified.

Anxiety may be directly expressed, but during the pre-school period children learn 'defences' (also called 'defence mechanisms' or 'mental mechanisms') which are used to deal both with normal anxieties, and with the abnormal ones associated with psychiatric disorders. A basic defence mechanism is 'repression', the consigning to the unconscious of ideas not acceptable (because too threatening, anxiety-producing or otherwise intolerable) at the conscious level. The repressed ideas or feelings may, however, continue to influence the person's behaviour and emotional state. They may be expressed in dreams, during hypnosis or in the course of psychoanalysis.

The repressed ideas may be denied at the conscious level, and actions or attitudes arising from them may be 'rationalized' – that is, an alternative, consciously acceptable explanation may be given. Thus a boy who is asked to do some shopping may say he is too tired or is frightened of the shopkeeper, but his reluctance might actually be due to repressed (and so unconscious) anxiety about what will happen to his mother while he is away, or to a fear that she may play with his brother towards whom he feels (again, perhaps, unconsciously) jealous. 'Compensation' is an attempt to make up for unconsciously felt inferiority; 'reaction formation' is a more extreme form of compensation; the individual behaves in ways which are the opposite of those which the unconscious feelings would dictate if they were directly expressed. For example, the individual who unconsciously wishes someone dead may consciously feel and show special solicitude and concern for that person.

'Displacement' and 'projection' involve the transfer of feelings from one to another, more acceptable, object. Thus the child who hates his father may repress this and consciously express much of the hate towards, for example, his teacher. Projection is the attribution of one's disclaimed characteristics on to another person. So the person tempted by the desire to steal (and feeling guilty about it) may repress this and unjustly attribute to others the propensity to steal.

'Obsessional' ideas are apparently irrational but nevertheless intrude into consciousness. They have their origin in unconscious anxiety or guilt, and represent a 'magical' way of dealing with the anxiety or guilt. Though perceived as illogical, and resisted by the subject, they nevertheless continue to intrude themselves into consciousness. 'Compulsions' are actions arising from such thoughts. Examples of common compulsive behaviours are avoiding the cracks in paving stones and touching lamp standards as they are passed. Such actions are means of dealing with the normal anxieties of this period. In the same way anxiety or guilt arising in any situation may be dealt with in this way; the mechanisms themselves are normal processes which operate in all of us.

Fantasy is important in children's mental lives. Children in the pre-school period usually have rich and vivid fantasy lives. In fantasy they can temporarily substitute for the real world one in which desires and wishes can be fulfilled, regardless of reality. Young children's fantasy lives are often expressed in play with other children and with dolls and toys. Despite their apparent involvement in such play, they normally remain able to distinguish fantasy from reality. Persistent inability to do so is a sign of deviant development. Children lacking siblings or friends to play with may invent imaginary playmates with names and detailed descriptions. They may carry on long conversations with such 'friends'. One boy, an only child, always insisted that a place be set at table for his 'friend'. This ceased, however, soon after he started attending nursery school at age 4.

Fantasy ideas and play help young children understand the world of which they are gradually becoming aware. Relationships such as mother-child, father-child, sibling-sibling, teacher-pupil and patient-nurse can be enacted and explored. The knowledge that it is all fantasy makes this safe and less anxiety-provoking than in real life. Children develop their own inner lives, partly corresponding to reality, partly comprising fantasy, and the world can be distorted to meet their current emotional needs. As development proceeds, fantasy becomes less prominent, though most adults resort to it from time to time.

The term 'transitional object' was coined by Winnicott (1965). Such an object – which is sometimes called a 'cuddly', and sometimes a 'security blanket' – may be any item to which a child develops an enduring attachment and which appears to give comfort and reas-surance in stressful situations; it must not be part of the child's body, nor an object (such as a pacifier) provided by the parents for oral gratification (Busch et al., 1973). It may be a piece of blanket or other material, a teddy bear or a toy of some sort. It is treated by the child as an object of special value. It may be cuddled or sucked and the child may want to take it everywhere, but especially to bed at bedtime. It is believed that it temporarily takes the place of the mother to whom the child has been attached and is a substitute for her in stressful situations. Transitional objects are used mainly by children aged two to five. It seems that institutionalized children do not use them (Provence and Lipton, 1962). Litt (1981) found that transitional objects were significantly more common in a group of private patients than in a group of black lower-middle and lower income patients attending a clinic. Their use seemed to bear some relationship to the nature of the child-rearing practices used in their families.

Shafii (1986) gave a questionnaire to 233 students aged 13 and 14, of whom 130 responded. 87 per cent of the girls and 71 per cent of the boys reported having had a transitional object at some time, and it is remarkable that 21 per cent of the girls and 12 per cent of the boys reported still using them. Based partly on consultation with their families, the girls reported first using their transitional objects between 6 months and one year of age, the boys between 2 and 5 years. Most of the children abandoned their use between 5 and 7 years.

'Transitional phenomena' such as rituals, songs, stories and particular movements, have been described as serving functions similar to those of transitional objects (Hong, 1978).

The pre-school period is one of increasing socialization. By the end of it the business of learning to live in a group of three – the other two being the parents – should have been mastered. Progress should also have been made in coming to terms with any siblings, though some degree of rivalry is normal at this stage.

In many societies organized pre-school experiences are provided in nursery schools, play groups and kindergartens. These offer children further opportunities to learn social skills, and can provide gentle introductions to the outside world.

Temper tantrums often continue in the 2- to 5-year age range, but lessen in intensity. They have usually died out by the time the child starts school.

Attachment behaviour continues to be readily activated until about the end of the third year of life. After that time it is less easily elicited, though it is apparently a property of normal human beings throughout life (Bowlby, 1977).

The pre-school period comprises the first part of Piaget's 'period of concrete operations'. This is subdivided, the first section (about 18 months to 7 years) being a 'pre-operational period'. This is again subdivided into 'pre-conceptual stage' (up to about the age of 4), and an 'intuitive stage'. In the pre-conceptual stage children become increasingly able to represent one thing by another, so that they can use language symbols and can represent things by drawing them. But they cannot yet form true concepts nor properly understand that an item belongs to a class of objects. Between ages 4 and 5 this substage gives way to the intuitive substage, the main features of which are described in the next section.

During this period the child still feels at the centre of the world, and tends to consider inanimate objects as having feelings and opinions.

Middle childhood (ages 5 or 6 to 10)

By the start of this period the child should have a clear conception of his or her position in the family group, and also a well defined identity as a boy or girl. Psychoanalysts have named it the 'latency period', supposing psychosexual development to be relatively quiescent. This view was questioned by Rutter (1971) who pointed out that in many non-western cultures sex play and lovemaking have been found to be common in this period; similar findings have emerged from research in the USA. In western society there may be greater concealment of sexual interests and activities, but they are nevertheless present. Masturbation in boys is common in middle childhood, but less so in girls. Heterosexual play also increases. Broderick and Rowe (1968) studied 1029 boys and girls in the age range 10–12 and found clear evidence of a set of stages which most adolescents go through on their way to 'social heterosexual maturation'. The term 'middle childhood' is probably better than 'latency'.

Erikson (1965) called this period the stage of 'industry versus inferiority'. Children gain satisfaction from doing the things which are taught, in one way or another, in all cultures at this stage. Children also learn the 'fundamentals of technology' (which of course differ from culture to culture), and come to enjoy the personal satisfaction, the recognition from others and the chance to relate to other people which result. The main danger is that the child will develop instead a sense of inadequacy and inferiority. This happens when children despair of their skills and capabilities, or of their status among their peers. The development of self-esteem is thus a central issue; because of its importance it is discussed more fully in a later section.

While in most societies the formal teaching of children occurs mainly in school, children also learn in more informal ways at home, in other social situations, and in organizations such as Cub Scouts, Brownies, and religious and other youth groups. The child now has an opportunity to learn to cope with more complex and less supportive environments than the family group, and to meet the challenge of mastering the skills of reading, writing and dealing with mathematical concepts. The teacher becomes an important person. Children's attitudes towards learning depend largely on their relationships with their teachers, though parents' attitudes are important too. Ideally parents and teachers cooperate in presenting children with information and values, each complementing what the other is doing.

During this period children form ideas about their capacities and limitations, and they work out patterns of social behaviour which may be in various degrees active or passive, leader or follower, outgoing or inturning. Temperamental characteristics continue to be important determinants of the child's behaviour, and it is a mistake to attribute everything to the manner of the child's upbringing.

During middle childhood there is further development of the use of defence mechanisms to deal with anxiety and guilt. This parallels the development of the conscience. Children come to have their own individual patterns of psychological defences, depending in part on constitutional factors and in part on environmental, especially family ones. Standards of social behaviour are further refined and ideas of right and wrong elaborated. The personality attributes a child has acquired by the end of this period tend to persist into adult life.

Piaget describes the period from about 4 ½ to 7 years as the 'intuitive substage'. Children can give reasons for their actions and beliefs, but their thinking remains 'pre-operational' – that is, it depends on immediate perceptions rather than on the mental representation of concepts. This often results in the attribution of causation to something which just happens to occur at the same time as the event concerned, and to frequent changes of opinion. The young child's attitude also remains egocentric. Life and feelings are still attributed to inanimate objects, and relationships between classes are not well understood.

This stage is followed at about age 7 by the 'subperiod of concrete operations'. This continues until the onset of adolescence which marks the start of the 'period of formal operations'. The main changes in the concrete operational period are that children can internalize the properties of objects and their thinking becomes less egocentric. This capacity to internalize means that objects can be put in order, or classified by size, shape or colour, without being physically compared with each other. The child can now, as it were, arrange them mentally and thus come up with answers more rapidly. The other principal change affects play and activities with others. Previously children have played on their own or in company with others; now we see the start of cooperative play. Piaget considered this to be related to the increased capacity to perceive relationships. Beard (1969) warns that at this stage thinking is still largely intuitive, however, and that the development of individuals is often more piecemeal than Piaget suggested. Children's verbal fluency may conceal the fact that they have not yet grasped concepts such as weight or numerical relationships – as when they know their multiplication tables by rote, but do not understand what they signify.

Adolescence

The onset of menstruation in the girl and of seminal emissions in the boy mark the onset of puberty and thus the start of adolescence. Puberty arrives most often between 11 and 13 in girls, and between 13 and 17 in boys, but the range of normal is wider. The biological changes are spread over a longer period. In both sexes the pattern of production of sex hormones starts to change between the ages of 8 and 10. The physical changes, including a marked growth spurt, the growth of the genitals and of hair in certain parts of the body, and breast development in girls, are spread over several years. The period tends to be longer in boys (4 to 5 years) than in girls (usually 3 to 4).

Erikson (1965) considered the main issue to be dealt with during adolescence to be that of 'identity versus role confusion'. With the end of childhood proper, the youth must now achieve a view of his or her own identity and individual characteristics. The young adult emerging from adolescence should know who he or she is, and be confident in making this identity known to the world. This personal identity becomes the basis for the individual's relationships. Those who have failed to negotiate this period successfully do not know who they are or where they want to go in life. Identity formation has of course started much earlier in childhood, but the process intensifies during adolescence and should have been largely completed by the end of the teen years.

The Group for the Advancement of Psychiatry (1968), discussing normal adolescence, defined four main developmental tasks. These are:

- changing from being nurtured and cared for to being able to nurture and care for others;
- learning to work and acquiring the skills to become materially self-supporting;
- accepting and becoming proficient in the adult sexual role, and coping with heterosexual relationships;
- moving out of the family of origin to form a new family of procreation.

Adolescence sees a marked increase in heterosexual interests and activity. The early adolescent usually first makes tentative and unselfconfident approaches to the opposite sex. By late adolescence the individual should be able to enter into relationships involving tender affection as well as sexual feelings. In due course the person becomes able to enter into deeper and more lasting heterosexual relationships. Thus it becomes possible for the third and fourth of the above developmental tasks to be accomplished.

The ways in which adolescents' developing sexual feelings are expressed depend on sociocultural standards and family rules and restrictions. Masturbation is almost universal in boys, less common in girls. In many societies dating and kissing start in the early teen years, and a mid-70s British study indicated that by age seventeen, 50 per cent of boys and 39 per cent of girls had had sexual intercourse (Farrell and Kellahar, 1978).

Peer group relationships are important in the lives of most adolescents, most of whom make friends easily. Deep and sometimes lasting relationships commonly develop, especially among girls. As well as having individual friendships, adolescents often belong to groups. These support the members in the sometimes anxiety-provoking task of moving out of the family group to become autonomous adults. With group support young people may do things they could not manage unaided. Groups may be as small as two or three, but they may run to ten, twenty or even more. An adolescent may belong to more than one group. The influence of such groups is often beneficial, but it may not be so, as in the case of delinquent gangs.

Relationships with parents gradually change in the adolescent period. The nature of these changes has been reviewed by Rutter and his colleagues (1976), using especially the results of an epidemiological study in the Isle of Wight. It is clear from this research and other studies that parent-child alienation is not common, certainly at age 14, the age group studied in the Isle of Wight. It may be a little commoner in late adolescence, but most adolescents trust their parents, share many of their values and accept the need for parental restrictions and controls on their behaviour. The process of moving out of the family group thus proceeds smoothly and gradually in most instances. Research in both Britain and North America suggests that alienation, breakdown and overt rebellion are more characteristic of that small segment of the teenage population referred for psychiatric care.

The same review (Rutter *et al.*, 1976) used the Isle of Wight findings to discover whether 'inner turmoil' is characteristic of adolescence, as some believe. There was some support for this notion in that more than one-fifth of the 14- and 15-year-olds they studied reported feeling miserable and depressed and a similar proportion reported sleep difficulties. In psychiatric interviews with a sample of adolescents from the general population studied, nearly one-half reported some misery or depression, though only 1 in 8 actually looked sad to the psychiatrist. Self-depreciation was less common than reported, misery occurred in about 20 per cent. Only about 7 per cent of either sex had entertained suicidal ideas. There is thus some evidence of what might be called emotional turmoil, but in some cases it was quite mild and just over half those studied showed none at all.

Piaget called adolescence the period of 'formal operations'. Thinking becomes more flexible. The main features are:

- the ability to accept assumptions for the sake of argument and to make hypotheses and set up propositions to test them;
- the ability to look for general properties and laws in symbolic, especially verbal, material and so to invent imaginary systems and conceive things beyond what is tangible, finite and familiar;
- becoming aware of one's own thinking, and using it to justify the judgments one makes;
- becoming able to deal with such complex ideas as proportionality and correlation.

The Group for the Advancement of Psychiatry (1968) summarized the resolution of adolescence as comprising:

- the attainment of separation and independence from parents;
- the establishment of a sexual identity;
- the commitment to work;
- the development of a personal moral system;
- the capacity for lasting relationships, and for both tender and genital sexual love in heterosexual relationships;
- a return to the parents in a new relationship based on a relative equality.

The ease with which these developmental challenges are met depends largely on the young person's relationship with his or her parents. Developments earlier in childhood are crucial: the more secure these have been, the easier the handing over of responsibility will be. Despite widely differing sociocultural norms, it seems that the handover of responsibility by parents to their adolescent offspring usually goes smoothly. Serious difficulties are the exception, not the rule.

The development of self-esteem

The acquisition of a sense of self-worth is a major developmental task of childhood. It is a continuing process which starts in infancy, and continues thoughout childhood and adolescence; indeed it does not stop when a person enters adulthood. Since there is no absolute standard by which an individual's worth can be judged, for practical purposes we are what we believe we are, and this depends very much on our childhood experiences.

Cotton (1983) reviewed the process whereby self-esteem develops. It starts in infancy with 'relationships with empathic others', and the child's emerging capacity to accomplish tasks successfully. The 'basic trust' described by Erikson (1965) develops in the context of an empathic parent-child relationship, ideally one in which the parents' and the child's temperamental characteristics are well matched. The development of the toddler's self-esteem continues to depend on parental attitudes, opinions and behaviour, combined with the child's experience of mastery of the environment.

As toddlers learn to walk, explore their environment, play, throw things, talk and engage in all sorts of social interactions, they look to their parents and other adults for their reactions. In healthy families these are affirming and supportive, even when limits have to be set on the child's behaviour. Realistic expectations should also be set by the parents.

Similar processes continue in middle childhood, except that children's social circles widen, and their self-esteem comes to be influenced by a wider range of people. How much effect the attitudes and expressed opinions of others have also depends upon how highly such people are valued by the child. A mother's reaction can be expected to have a more telling effect than a stranger's. Important, too, are children's successes and failures. Those with handicaps may compare themselves unfavourably with others, so that it may be more difficult for them to obtain that sense of mastery over their environment that is an important ingredient of self-esteem.

Coopersmith (1967), on the basis of a study of preadolescent, white and 'normal' (that is, free of symptoms of stress or emotional disorder) boys, concluded that high self-esteem is likely to develop in conditions of:

- 'total or nearly total acceptance of the children by their parents';
- 'clearly defined and enforced limits';
- respect and latitude for the individual's action, within defined limits.

As the years pass, children's feelings about their worth and capabilities increasingly become internalized. That is, they are less dependent upon the immediate response of the environment. By adolescence their self-images have become a part of their personality structures, or what Erikson (1968) calls their 'ego-identity', though they are still subject to modification. Changing a person's self-image, however, becomes a bigger task as the years succeed one another.

Development in adulthood

Erikson (1965) describes three more 'ages of man'. These cover the stages of development through which children's parents and grandparents are going. The first is that of 'intimacy versus isolation'. The young adult, having completed her or his search for identity, is now ready for intimacy with others, in close relationships including sexual union. Failure at this stage results in isolation. Instead of developing close relationships the person may isolate, or even destroy, forces and people that appear threatening in some way.

The next stage is that of 'generativity versus stagnation'. The essence of generativity is the establishing and guiding of the next generation. This is achieved not only, nor even necessarily, by parenthood, though for many people becoming parents is a central feature of the process. Failure to achieve generativity leads to a sense of stagnation and personal impoverishment.

The final stage is that of 'ego integrity versus despair'. Ego integrity is the mature integration of one's life's experiences, people and things taken care of, triumphs and disappointments accepted. It is the feeling of things accomplished, and life lived satisfactorily. Failure to achieve ego integrity results in despair, a characteristic of which is fear of death due to the feeling that time is now too short to live another life.

Family development

The way children develop is greatly influenced by their social setting. This is normally a family unit of some sort. In many societies it has traditionally been an extended family network, with important roles being played by grandparents, aunts and uncles, siblings, cousins and other family members. As societies became industrialized the 'nuclear family', consisting of two parents and their children, assumed greater importance. This trend continued as people became more mobile and no longer lived in the same village, town or even country all their lives. But the stresses of nuclear family life, especially without extended family support, led to frequent family breakdowns. Increasingly, too, nuclear families have come to contain only one parent, usually the mother. Consequently we now have many types of family. Traditional two-parent families, each containing only the children of the two parents, are now a minority.

Although families vary greatly in their composition and nature, nearly every child grows up in a family group of some sort. The way this functions needs to change as the children who are born or adopted into it mature and eventually leave. The development of children is intimately tied to the development and functioning of the family groups in which they grow up. An understanding of family functioning and development is thus necessary if child development and its problems are to be understood.

Family development has been divided into stages in various ways. The following is that suggested by McGoldrick and Carter (1982).

The unattached young adult is the first stage. This is a person who is between families. Such an individual should have achieved separation from his or her family of origin, a sense of self differentiated from the family of origin, the capacity to develop intimate relations with peers, and a suitable place in the workforce.

The joining of families through marriage, which nowadays may not be legally formalized, comes next. This involves commitment of the two partners to each other, with the formation of a new marital system. At the same time the appropriate adjustments must be made in the couple's relationships with extended family and friends.

The family with young children is the third stage. The arrival of the first child necessitates great changes in the family system. To the marital system is added a new parental system. The new generation must be accepted into the family and there is further change in the family's relationships with the extended family. The grandparents may assume significant and important roles in relation to the children.

The family with adolescents is Stage 4. This stage sees a gradual but substantial change in parent-child relationships, with the children becoming increasingly independent; for a time the adolescent children may move in and out of the family, the boundaries of which become more flexible. At the same time the parents turn their attention again to marital as opposed to parental issues, and perhaps also to career issues; some women who have stayed at home to rear their children may return to the workforce, or seek new social activities.

Launching children and moving on comes next. This is almost a new stage, since until quite recently most parents were engaged in raising their children throughout their active adult lives. The low birth rate and the longer life span have now changed this, and the many years a couple may live after their children have departed represent a challenge and can lead to difficulties. During this period various family members may enter or leave the family. While the younger generation leaves, the parents' parents may become frail or ill, and thus dependent on *their* children. A new relationship develops with the children who have left home, one based on adult-to-adult equality. Then, as the children marry and have children, the role of grandparent develops. During this stage the family may have to deal with illness or deaths in the older generations.

The family in later life is the sixth and final stage in McGoldrick and

Carter's (1982) scheme. The parental generation has become the grandparental generation, and the grandparents may be on their own. They may need to acquire new interests and a new social circle. The middle generation comes to play a more central role in the affairs of the family, perhaps looking after the older one, rather than the reverse. It should also make room for and use the wisdom and experience of the older generation. This is also a time when illness and death in the older generation are common.

The above scheme is but one way of conceptualizing and simplifying a complex process. Moreover, many things may happen to modify or interrupt the smooth development of family groups. These include separation and divorce, remarriage, serious illness or death in family members, the late arrival of a child, the separation of parents because of vocational demands or imprisonment, financial disaster, the loss of the family home by fire or foreclosure, and the many other vicissitudes families may experience.

Families are particularly liable to get into difficulties when faced with the transition from one phase of the family life cycle to the next. Barnhill and Longo (1978) defined nine 'transition points', based on Duvall and Miller's (1985) eight stages of family development. They suggested that families are especially subject to stress when one of the transitions has not been successfully managed. These issues are considered further in Chapter 2 of *Basic Family Therapy* (Barker, 1986).

The healthy family is a flexible social system which adapts to the ever-changing needs of its members. It should facilitate the development of its members, whose behaviours and patterns of interaction in turn continually influence it. In assessing and treating the psychiatric problems of children these processes should ever be borne in mind.

Normal families and their development are discussed more fully in *Basic Family Therapy* (Barker, 1986). Other relevant books are *Marriage and Family Development* (Duvall and Miller, 1985), and *The Family Life Cycle* (Carter and McGoldrick, 1980). A book edited by Froma Walsh (1982) discusses normal families in their various forms.

Chapter 2

Causes, Classification and Prevalence of Child Psychiatric Disorders

The causes of child psychiatric disorders

Few child psychiatric disorders have single, clear-cut causes. We are usually dealing with complex reactions to a variety of factors in developing personalities, rather than with 'disease entities' like appendicitis or measles. Four groups of factors may contribute:

- constitutional factors;
- physical disease and injury;
- temperamental factors;
- environmental, including family, factors.

Sometimes 'psychological' factors, such as unconscious conflicts, or perceptual and other cognitive problems, are added but these are the result of combinations of factors in the above groups.

(1) Constitutional factors

Constitutional factors are those with which a child is born. We must consider:

- genetic factors;
- the effects of chromosome abnormalities;
- the consequences of intra-uterine damage;
- the results of birth injury.

Genetic factors

Few child psychiatric disorders are due to specific genetic factors, though such factors are responsible for certain forms of mental retardation, the commonest being phenylketonuria (PKU). This is an inborn error of metabolism which, if untreated, leads to severe mental retardation. It is inherited as a Mendelian recessive trait. That is to say a single gene is involved, and at the site (or 'locus' in the jargon of geneticists) of that gene there will be one of two alternative alleles which we may call P and p. The disease is only evident in the homozygote (PP), though heterozygotes (Pp) may be detected by their abnormal responses to the administration of phenylalanine, the amino acid which individuals with PKU do not metabolize normally. Homozygotes (pp) metabolize phenylalanine normally.

The above is an example of 'monogenic' inheritance. More important in child psychiatry is 'polygenic' inheritance. This is the process whereby a characteristic is coded for by two or more genes, located at two or more loci which, acting additively, increase the likelihood that a particular trait will be manifest. In many cases environmental factors also play a part in determining whether the trait appears, and when they do inheritance is said to be 'multifactorial'. Polygenic influences, combined with environmental factors, appear to play significant roles in causing many child psychiatric disorders, and also in determining intelligence levels.

Twin and adoption studies can each tell us how much polygenic factors contribute to the appearance of particular traits. Monozygotic (MZ) twins have identical genes, so that if genetic causes were wholly responsible for a trait the correlation beween MZ twins for that trait would be 1.0. For intelligence the correlation is 0.86 for MZ twins reared together, and 0.72 for MZ twins reared apart (McGuffin and Gottesman 1985; Bouchard and McGue 1981). This indicates that while polygenic factors are important, environmental ones play their part too.

Dizygotic (DZ) twins have approximately 50 per cent of their genes in common, so we would expect a correlation of 0.5 between such twins if genetic factors were solely responsible for intelligence. According to the sources quoted above, the correlation is actually 0.60, the 10 point difference presumably being due to the common environment of twins reared together (no figures are quoted for DZ twins reared apart).

Full siblings also share 50 per cent of their genes. Reared together, the correlation between intelligence levels (in a total of 25,473 sibling pairs) was 0.47; but in 203 sibling pairs reared apart, the correlation was only 0.24, further evidence of the role of non-genetic factors. The interaction of genetic and other factors is similarly evident when populations of half-siblings and cousins are studied.

The term 'heritability' is used to describe the degree to which a trait is attributable to genetic factors (Falconer, 1981). It consists of the variance due to genetic factors divided by the total variance observed in the subjects. It is only meaningful when applied to populations, since certain individuals may have particularly unfavourable (or favourable) environmental experiences. The former might cause a great lowering of intelligence (if that were the trait being studied), regardless of the person's genetically determined potential.

To what traits, other than intelligence, do polygenic factors contribute? It seems that personality and temperament are to some extent genetically influenced (Goldsmith, 1983), and McGuffin and Gottesman (1985) cite evidence that genetic factors contribute to reading disabilities, enuresis, sleepwalking, travel sickness, nail biting and thumb sucking. Polygenic factors may also contribute to infantile autism, childhood schizophrenia and the hyperkinetic syndrome. *The Heredity of Behavior Disorders in Adults and Children* (Vandenberg *et al.*, 1986), reviews research on the genetics of infantile autism, specific reading disability, hyperactivity, conduct disorders, stuttering, eating disorders, sleep disorders, enuresis, encopresis and tics. It is clear that much further research is needed before the role of heredity in these conditions is fully understood.

Chromosome abnormalities

Observable abnormalities of the chromosomes may cause physical abnormalities, sometimes severe or even fatal, they may affect intelligence and they may contribute to other psychological problems. In trisomy 21, or Down's syndrome (formerly known as mongolism, and discussed further in Chapter 16), affected individuals have three of the chromosomes numbered 21, instead of the normal two. The other known abnormalities of the autosomes (the non-sex chromosomes) are of little practical importance in child psychiatry. Many are incompatible with life and lead to abortion or stillbirths.

Sex chromosome abnormalities generally have less drastic effects. Girls with Turner's syndrome have only one X chromosome instead of the normal two, and a total of 45 chromosomes instead of 46 (45,XO). Nielson and Silbeson (1981), in Denmark, found that one girl in about 4000 had this condition. These girls tend to have difficulty dealing with spatial information, in the 'organization of disparate elements into synthetic wholes' and in perceiving, visualizing and remembering spatial configurations (Walzer, 1985). Consequently they have depressed performance IQ scores (see Chapter 3), and trouble acquiring mathematical and scientific skills. Though they tend to be small and immature as children, most do not show evidence of psychiatric disorder.

Girls with extra X chromosomes tend to be mentally retarded, mildly so in the case of the triple X condition (47,XXX), but more severely so in those rare cases in which there are more than three X chromosomes. 47,XXX girls find the auditory processing of information difficult, and they have impaired receptive and expressive language difficulties, especially the latter. These deficits can lead to poor academic performance (Walzer, 1985). Thus an extra X chromosome apparently leads to poor verbal skills and the lack of an X chromosome adversely affects non-verbal skills.

In Klinefelter's syndrome the individual, phenotypically a male but often with some feminine characteristics, has the chromosome complement 47,XXY. This condition also has been found to be associated with impaired development of language, particularly expressive language. This is the case in about half of these boys. Auditory processing, auditory memory, language, reading and spelling may all be affected (Walzer, 1985). Otherwise children with Klinefelter's syndrome probably do not have a higher incidence of psychiatric disorders than children generally. Adolescents with Klinefelter's syndrome have, however, been reported to have more behaviour problems, as well as having learning difficulties (Ratcliffe *et al.*, 1982).

A fuller review of research on the cognitive difficulties of children with extra X chromosomes is that of Walzer (1985).

About one in every 1000 boys born has a 47,XYY chromosome complement. Such boys tend to be taller than the average for their age, and there is some evidence of an association between aggressive and antisocial behaviour, and also delayed speech development, and the presence of the extra Y chromosome (Nielson and Christensen, 1974; Ratcliffe, 1982). Nevertheless, most 'XYY' individuals show no evidence of psychiatric abnormality, and an extra Y chromosome is present in only a very small proportion of children with behaviour problems.

In the 'fragile X' syndrome, or 'X-linked mental retardation' (Jacobs *et al.*, 1983), an abnormal X chromosome is present; on it there is a 'fragile site', which is visible as a constriction near one end of the chromosome. The chromosome may break at this point. Affected individuals are mentally retarded, and have language impairment. Expressive language is affected more than receptive language. Boys with this condition typically have large testes and ears and are generally more severely retarded than girls with a fragile X chromosome. The latter may be normal or mildly retarded, presumably because they have one normal X chromosome.

The fragile X condition may also be associated with autism. Gillberg and Wahlstrom (1985) found 8 out of 40 autistic boys (20 per cent) to have it, and Fisch *et al.* (1986) report its presence in 18 of 144 autistic children (12.5 per cent). But Wright *et al.* (1986) found only one case in 40 autistic children. Further study of autistic children's chromosomes is clearly needed.

Intrauterine damage or disease

The fetus may be adversely affected in various ways during the pregnancy. Infections such as rubella, toxoplasmosis, syphilis and acquired immune deficiency syndrome (AIDS), all of which may affect the developing nervous system, may be transferred from the mother to the fetus. Fetal damage or retarded development may also be caused by placental insufficiency, other causes of impaired oxygen supply, and the abuse of drugs by the mother during the pregnancy. The 'fetal alcohol syndrome' may follow severe alcohol abuse during pregnancy. It comprises growth deficiency, mental retardation, short palpebral fissure, a thin upper lip and abnormalities of the nose, eyes, ears and heart (Little and Streissgath, 1981). It may affect 0.4 to 3.1 per 1000 live-born children. Among the children of alcoholic mothers its incidence is much higher, estimates ranging from 24 to 690 per 1000, depending on the severity of the mother's alcohol abuse (Cooper, 1987). Heavy smoking by the mother during pregnancy is associated with lowered birth weight and poorer adjustment of the children at age 7 (Davie *et al.*, 1972). Smoking, drug abuse and alcoholism are, however, often associated with other parental personality problems and family difficulties and it can be hard to differentiate their respective effects.

Premature birth and injury at birth

These may contribute to abnormal development, and to behavioural and other difficulties later in childhood. Children who are small for their gestational ages at birth also tend later to be less developmentally advanced. They also show behavioural differences when compared to children with normal birth weights (Parkinson *et al.*, 1986).

Hack *et al.* (1979) found that 82 per cent of surviving babies weighing between 1000 and 1500 grams at birth were developing normally two years later, but the other 18 per cent had serious neurological or intellectual impairment, or both. Driscoll *et al.* (1982) reported on 45 infants who weighed 1000 grams or less at birth and were admitted to a neonatal intensive care nursery. 28 had died. Of the 23 followed up 19 (83 per cent) were neurologically normal, but the overall complication rate, including mental retardation, was 30 per cent. Small babies are therefore still at risk, even though their outlook is better than it used to be.

Many of the adverse influences mentioned above act by causing a lowering of intelligence. While mental retardation, especially when severe, is a serious condition in its own right, many individuals whose intellectual functioning has been affected by the factors we have considered lead full lives and show no evidence of psychiatric abnormality. There is also some evidence that very bright children may not fare as well as children of more modest abilities (Robinson, 1981), though how often intellectual giftedness leads to emotional problems is unclear.

(2) Physical disease and injury

Brain disease or damage may produce impairment of intelligence, loss of particular motor or sensory functions, epilepsy or (probably) specific forms of abnormal behaviour like motor overactivity. It can also have less specific effects; in the Isle of Wight epidemiological studies, children with definite evidence of brain damage were found to have psychiatric disorders five times as often as the general child population, and three times as commonly as children with chronic physical handicaps not involving the brain (Rutter, Graham et al., 1970).

Brain damage may be caused by injury, infections (abscesses and the various forms of encephalitis), metabolic disorders, tumours, degenerative disorders of unknown cause and severe malnutrition in early life. Since malnutrition is usually associated with other adverse social circumstances, however, it can be hard to distinguish its effects on behaviour and intelligence from those of other stresses (Cravioto and Arrieta, 1983). 'Non-accidental injury' (see Chapter 18) may also cause brain injury. It, too, may be accompanied by poor nutrition, psychological neglect, or both (Scott, 1977).

Head injuries are common in childhood (Shaffer, 1985a) and many brain injured children are later found to have behavioural or emotional problems. This is partly because children who already have such problems are more likely to suffer head injuries (Brown et al., 1981). Head injuries are also more likely to occur in the children of poorly functioning families, since such families will tend to be less effective in safeguarding them from injury. There is, however, evidence that, even when allowance is made for these factors, severe head injury with prolonged coma is often followed by psychiatric sequelae (Brown et al., 1981; Rutter et al., 1980). The sequelae vary and are non-specific, apart from disinhibited and socially inappropriate behaviour, which may be especially common in these children.

Shaffer (1985a) provides an excellent overview of the effects of brain damage. Neurological disorders associated with abnormal mental states are discussed further in Chapter 6.

Physical diseases not directly affecting the brain can have psychological repercussions. They may act through the physical handicap they impose, or the anxiety or guilt they stimulate in child, parents or the whole family. Much can be done to help children with such severe handicaps as cerebral palsy or blindness lead full lives; they need not develop emotional problems as complications of their physical ones. For this to be achieved, special skill and patience are needed in those caring for and educating them. Many other chronic conditions, for instance diabetes, asthma, congenital heart disease and the various forms of dwarfism may cause emotional problems, through their physically handicapping effects, the restrictions they impose on the child's social life, the anxiety and fears of death they may cause, and their effects on the attitudes of family, friends and teachers.

Injuries, especially serious ones like severe burns, can have similar effects. They may give rise to guilt feelings in the parents and in the children, any or all of whom may blame themselves for the injury. Anger, withdrawal and depression may develop. But many years ago Woodward and Jackson (1961) showed, in studies of burned children, that much depends on the way child and family are handled during treatment.

(3) Temperamental factors

Children's temperaments vary. Each child's unique combination of temperamental characteristics plays its part in determining whether that child develops a psychiatric disorder under any particular circumstances. Children's temperaments have been studied by Alexander Thomas and Stella Chess as a part of the New York Longitudinal Study (NYLS) of 133 children from infancy into adult life. Their book *Origins and Evolution of Behavior Disorders from Infancy to Early Adult Life* (Chess and Thomas, 1984) summarizes 25 years' research.

Nine categories of temperament were identified from data relating to 22 of the NYLS infants, as follows:

(1) Activity level: the motor component present in a given child's functioning and the diurnal proportion of active and inactive periods.
(2) Rhythmicity (regularity): the predictability and/or unpredictability) in time of any biological function.
(3) Approach or withdrawal: the nature of the initial response to a new stimulus, be it a food, toy, place, person, etc. Approach responses are positive, whether displayed by mood expression (smiling, verbalizations, etc.) or motor activity (swallowing a new food, reaching for a new toy, active play, etc.). Withdrawal reactions are negative, whether displayed by mood expression (crying, fussing, grimacing, verbalizations, etc.) or motor activity

(moving away, spitting new food out, pushing a new toy away, etc.).

(4)   Adaptability: responses to new or altered situations. One is not concerned with the nature of the initial responses, but with the ease with which they are modified in desired directions.

(5)   Threshold of responsiveness: the intensity level of stimulation that is necessary to evoke a discernible response, irrespective of the specific form the response may take, or the sensory modality affected.

(6)   Intensity of reaction: the energy level of response, irrespective of its quality or direction.

(7)   Quality of mood: the amount of pleasant, joyful and friendly behaviour; as contrasted with unpleasant, crying and unfriendly behaviour.

(8)   Distractibility: the effectiveness of extraneous environmental stimuli in interfering with or altering the direction of the ongoing behaviour.

(9)   Attention span and persistence: two categories which are related. Attention span concerns the length of time a particular activity is pursued by the child. Persistence refers to the continuation of an activity direction in the face of obstacles to its continuation *(reproduced from Chess and Thomas, 1984, pages 42-43, quoted with kind permission of Brunner/Mazel Inc., the publishers).*

Analysis of the data obtained in the study revealed three main 'temperamental constellations'. The infants in the first group, comprising about 40 per cent of the NYLS sample, were characterized by:

- regularity;
- positive approach responses to new stimuli;
- high adaptability to change;
- mild or moderate mood intensity which is preponderantly positive.

These were called 'easy children'. They quickly fall into regular sleep and feeding schedules, and take readily to new foods, strangers, new schools and the rules of new games, as well as accepting frustration without much fuss.

By contrast the 'difficult child' – about 10 per cent of the sample – shows:

- irregularity in biological functions;
- negative withdrawal responses to new stimuli;
- non-adaptability or slow adaptability to change;
- intense mood expressions which are frequently negative.

These children sleep and demand food irregularly, and adjust with difficulty to new foods, routines, people and situations. They cry and laugh loudly, are easily frustrated and often have tantrums.

The third group – about 15 per cent – show:

- negative responses of mild intensity to new stimuli, with slow adaptability after repeated contact;
- mild intensity of reactions generally;
- less irregularity of biological functioning than the 'difficult' children.

These children were categorized as 'slow-to-warm-up'.

The other 35 per cent were children who did not fit into any of these categories, but had instead various other combinations of temperamental traits.

The above descriptions are simply of 'behavioural styles'. The nine categories and their variations, and the three commonly met with constellations, are the temperamental equivalents of the variations in body build, or eye or hair colour, observed in any population. How children with different temperamental styles fare depends also upon other factors, especially environmental ones.

Although temperament seems to be in part genetically determined (Torgerson, 1981), environmental factors have their effects too. Cameron (1977) found associations between temperamental changes over time and parental characteristics. One cluster of parental characteristics, described as 'parental disapproval, intolerance and rejection', was associated, by the second year, with daughters who were less persistent and less active in their reactions than the majority; and also with change in the daughters' temperaments over a 2-3 year period towards less adaptability and less positive mood.

A study of preterm infants at 3, 6 and 12 months of age, (Washington *et al.*, 1986) found that there were significantly more 'difficult' children in the sample than in a comparable series of full term infants. This constellation of traits was not related to the severity of perinatal or postnatal complications, but to features of the mother-child interaction. Thus the nature of this interaction, in this study also, appeared to have important effects on the developing temperaments of the infants.

(4) Environmental factors

A child's environment comprises the family group in which she or he is growing up, and the wider social setting in which the family is living. Physical features of the environment may play their parts too. For example, there is some evidence that certain children experience affective symptoms, such as depression, irritability, school difficulties and sleep changes, during the winter months, and that these clear up during the summer. It is has been suggested that treatment with a bright light environment alleviates the symptoms (Rosenthal *et al.*, 1986).

While the importance of the physical environment is by no means established, that of the family setting is well established. The family should provide a sheltered training ground in which the child learns to live as a member of a society. Families are miniature societies in which children make their first attempts at adapting to others, and in which they learn patterns of social behaviour which tend to persist throughout life.

The family should facilitate development from infantile dependence to adult independence. As children grow up they should be expected progressively to assume more self-control and responsibility for their actions. At each age neither too little nor too much should be done for them. If too much is done, the process of growing up and becoming independent may be retarded; if too little, the child's level of anxiety may become intolerably great and psychiatric disorder may develop.

Poor early adjustment to family life is often followed by poor adjustment in society at large. Attitudes towards parents may become generalized, and later be applied to a wider circle of people. As a background for the transfer of responsibility from parents to child, a secure and stable family setting, with reasonably consistent and constant parent figures is important. This does not mean that there must never be disagreements or arguments, or that members of the family will not sometimes become angry with each other. On the contrary, it is necessary that children be exposed to a range of emotions and situations as they will be in adult life. The repression by parents of all their negative emotions would provide their children with a poor preparation for the realities of life in the adult world.

Children who are deprived of a stable family group in which to grow up suffer a serious handicap. Changes of family or caretakers, as when children are repeatedly placed in and out of the care of child welfare agencies, or are moved frequently from one foster home or place of care to another, can be damaging. Some children survive such experiences well, probably because of innate personality strengths and certain positive features of their environment, such as a continuing healthy relationship with a stable adult figure. Most, however, grow up burdened by such problems as feelings of insecurity, lack of self-esteem, unresolved anger, and difficulty in entering into trusting, loving relationships with people.

'General systems theory' (von Bertalanffy, 1948) deals in a general way with interactions between parts, and the rules which govern such interactions. Its ideas have been found useful by family therapists striving to understand the processes going on in families and other social groups. Systems thinking involves looking upon the family as a unit which is more than the sum of its parts and has it own unwritten rules and customary ways of functioning. Its parts are its members; these are dynamically interrelated and interdependent. Their behaviour cannot be understood in isolation from the system as a whole. The system is 'open', that is to say it is in constant interaction with forces in the wider sociocultural setting. It usually belongs to several 'suprasystems', such as the extended family, the neighbourhood network, the village, the tribe and so on.

Families also contain subsystems, such as the marital, parental and child subsystems. Individuals can, and often do, belong to more than one system, for example to systems at school or at work as well as to their family system.

Every system has a boundary. Certain things can pass readily through the boundary, while others cannot pass so readily, or perhaps not at all. System boundaries may be rigid and well defined, or weak and blurred. The more rigid the boundary, the harder communication of feelings and ideas across it; the weaker it is, the easier the communication across it. Minuchin's (1974) term for situations in which there are rigid boundaries is 'disengagement', while he describes the other extreme as 'enmeshment'. He conceives of these two terms as representing the two ends of a continuum. While families falling at either end may function well, healthy families tend to be nearer the middle.

All systems are governed by 'rules'. These are really established, habitual patterns of functioning. In families the members are not consciously aware of most of the rules governing their behaviour. These have grown up over time rather than being deliberately planned and implemented. Nevertheless they influence powerfully the behaviour of the family members.

Disturbed behaviour in a family member is often found to be associated with a 'dysfunctional' family system. That is to say the family's rules and way of functioning depend upon one or more members having symptoms or being disabled in some way. The system is then not operating, as it should, to realise each member's potential for healthy development and a constructive life.

Haley (1976) pointed out that central to many family problems is a malfunctioning hierarchy. To take a simple example, consider a three-member family in which there is over-involvement of one parent and child, let us say mother and son, to the exclusion of the other parent. This can lead to various problems for the son who may become overdependent on his mother, and in time may come to be so immature and anxious that he develops school refusal (see Chapter 5). Instead of the parental couple helping the boy to grow up, one of them is keeping him a baby while the other is uninvolved in the family. The uninvolved parent may instead have an intense involvement in work or in a relationship outside the family. Another possible outcome is obesity in the son. As an aspect of enmeshment of mother and son, the former overfeeds the latter, whose weight then becomes another of her concerns; fruitless attempts at dieting may then perpetuate the dysfunctional over-involvement. In such a case therapy might aim to bring the parents closer together, both as a marital couple and as a parental subsystem, while lessening the enmeshment of mother and son. We may represent this process as follows:

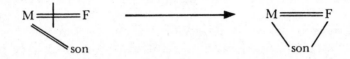

Many other and more complex dysfunctional family patterns are possible. They may involve three generations or even four; and extended family members, or non-family members, may be involved too. Dysfunctional systems are often found elsewhere, for example in schools, places of work and neighbourhood groups.

The study of family systems has led to the identification of a variety of idiosyncratic roles which family members, often children, may play. These include the roles of 'scapegoat', upon whom the family's problems and difficulties may be projected, sick member, crazy member, 'parental child', and 'family angel'. Being cast in such a role may have serious implications for a child's development. The functioning of family systems, and the problems that may arise in them, are discussed more fully in *Basic Family Therapy* (Barker, 1986).

Other specific factors may contribute to the development of emotional and behavioural problems in children. These include parental, especially maternal, depression (Wolkind, 1981), prolonged institutional care (Wolkind, 1974; Tizard and Hodges, 1978), and loss of a parent by death or divorce – though in the case of divorce the family strife which has often existed for years previously may be more important than the actual loss of one parent (Hetherington *et al.*, 1982; Wallerstein and Kelly, 1980).

Wallerstein (1983) discusses the tasks faced by children whose parents have been divorced, and it seems that their adjustment depends largely on how well they have mastered these tasks. The tasks are:

- acknowledging the marital disruption;
- regaining a sense of direction and freedom to pursue customary activities;
- dealing with loss and feelings of rejection;
- forgiving the parents;
- accepting the permanence of the divorce and relinquishing longings for the restoration of the predivorce family.

In the divorce-prone society in which we live nowadays many children present who are having difficuties in surmounting various of these tasks.

A major influence on most children is the school. Just how much schools can affect their pupils emerged in a study of secondary schools in London (Rutter *et al.*, 1979; Rutter, 1980a). The investigators first studied a large group of children before they were admitted to their secondary schools. The extent to which they were at risk of developing the problems with which the research was concerned was determined, and their academic progress and behaviour were then monitored in the secondary schools. Big variations in outcome were found when the various secondary schools were compared. These held up after the differences in the types of children admitted were taken into account. Much proved to depend on the characteristics of the schools as social institutions. Factors favourably influencing behaviour and attainments were:

(1) a reasonable balance between intellectually able and less able children;
(2) the ample use of rewards, praise, and appreciation by teachers;
(3) a pleasant, comfortable and attractive school environment;
(4) plenty of opportunity for children to be responsible for and participate in the running of the school;
(5) an appropriate emphasis on academic matters;
(6) good models of behaviour provided by teachers;
(7) the use of appropriate group management skills in classrooms;
(8) firm leadership in the school, combined with a decision-making process involving all staff and leading to a cohesive approach in which staff members support each other.

The wider social environment is also important. Psychiatric disorders are commoner, in both adults and children, in inner city areas than in rural areas and small towns. Rutter (1981) reviewed the relationship between city life and psychiatric disorder, and concluded that the reported differences in prevalence rates are real. Inner city areas are not homogeneous, however, and even within them prevalence rates vary.

The higher urban rates of psychiatric disorder apply to boys and girls, men and women, and to crime, delinquency, depression and emotional disorders. It seems that various aspects of the ecology of cities, including the schools, contribute to the causation of these disorders. While some of the factors, such as those operating in schools, affect children directly, many have their effects through the families. The greatest effect seems to be on 'early onset, chronic disorders in children which are associated with severe family pathology'.

Drugs, both those prescribed for medical conditions, and those used illicitly, may cause or contribute to psychiatric problems. Thus some children react to phenobarbitone, an anticonvulsant used for the treatment of epilepsy, with both behavioural and emotional problems; and theophylline, which is widely used in the treatment of asthma, can adversely affect both behaviour and performance in school (Rachelefsky *et al.*, 1986). Recent decades have also seen increasing use of alcohol and street drugs by young people.

(5) Other considerations

'Goodness of fit'

We have seen that child psychiatric problems are usually due to a combination of factors in the child and factors in the environment. Chess and Thomas (1984) emphasize the importance of the goodness, or poorness, of fit between child and environment. In Chapter 22 of their book they give examples of children from the NYLS in whom there were various degrees of goodness of fit, and describe how these affected the children's development. They make it clear that there is no 'optimal' temperamental style that ideally all children should display, nor is there one ideal environment for children's development.

The validity of the goodness of fit model was strikingly demonstrated in a study by de Vries (reported by Chess and Thomas, 1984, pages 289–90), who studied 47 infants, aged 2–4 months, of the Masai tribe in Kenya. Ratings of temperament were obtained as a severe drought was beginning, and the 10 infants with the most easy temperaments, and the 10 with the most difficult, were identified. Five months later de Vries returned to the area, and was able to discover what had happened to 7 of the 'easy' babies and 6 of the 'difficult' ones, the other families having moved to escape the drought. Five of the easy babies had died, but all 6 of the difficult ones had survived. The adaptive value of any particular temperamental style clearly depends on the fit between it and environmental circumstances.

The etiology of most psychiatric disorders is multifactorial, the child, the environment and the relationship between child and environment all being involved. If we stop searching or thinking when we come across the first contributing factor, we are likely to make many mistakes. One of the merits of systems thinking, as Marmor (1983) has pointed out, is that it can serve as a safeguard against considering the causation of psychiatric disorders in linear terms; linear thinking leads to the attribution of responsibility to one particular factor, whether biological, psychological or sociological.

Self-esteem

Although self-esteem is not easy to define, it is an important factor in determining people's behaviour, how they relate to others, and whether they develop psychiatric disorders. We have seen, in Chapter 1, that the acquisition of good feelings of self-worth is one of the major developmental tasks of childhood. Positive self-esteem develops as the child has the experience of mastering the environment in ways which provide feelings of satisfaction and appropriate, affirming feedback from the environment. 'Unfavourable experiences with social functioning and task mastery, together with confusing, contradictory, and inappropriate environmental feedback, will, on the other hand, foster the development of negative self-esteem' (Chess and Thomas, 1984, page 280).

Mack and Ablon (1983), in their preface to the book *The Development of Self-Esteem in Childhood*, point out that:

'The quest for a sense of personal worth, so critical to small children, remains of central importance for human beings throughout their lives. It motivates much of our activity in seeking personal attachments and meaningful work ... Nothing is more important for the maintenance of well-being. Conversely, no experience is more obviously distressing, or more intimately linked to emotional disturbances of many kinds and, in psychiatry, to various types of psychopathology, than is a diminished sense of worth or a low opinion of oneself.' (Mack and Ablon, 1983, page xiii.)

A poor measure of self-esteem is a central problem of many disturbed children. It can be self-perpetuating and even self-reinforcing: as children act out their feelings of being bad people, others in their environments may react by making critical remarks or even labelling them as 'bad'. So while we must look carefully at the background factors which have led to the present situation, we must also consider children's current views of themselves. We should strive to understand how these are being reinforced, or modified, by their

environments, in order to devise suitable treatment plans. Coopersmith points out that:

> '... in children domination, rejection, and severe punishment result
> in lowered self-esteem. Under such conditions [children] have fewer
> experiences of love and success and tend to become generally
> submissive and withdrawn (although occasionally veering to the
> opposite extreme of aggression and domination). Children reared
> under such crippling circumstances are unlikely to be realistic and
> effective in their everyday functioning and are more likely to
> manifest deviant behaviour patterns.' (Coopersmith, 1967, page 4.)

Classification of psychiatric disorders in children and adolescents

No entirely satisfactory classification of child psychiatric disorders
exists, but the two multiaxial schemes currently used are
improvements on what went before. The third edition of the
American Psychiatric Association's *Diagnostic and Statistical Manual*
appeared in 1980 (American Psychiatric Association, 1980) and a
revised version (DSM-III-R) was published in 1987 (American Psychiatric Association, 1987). Rutter, Shaffer and Sturge (1975) devised a
scheme based, in four of its five axes, on the ninth edition of the
International Classification of Diseases (ICD-9) (World Health Organization,
1977a).

Both these schemes lay down the parameters, or axes, which must
be considered when a disorder is being classified. They recognize that
there are a number of different classes of information which should be
considered separately. For example a child may have a certain clinical
psychiatric syndrome, such as a conduct disorder, and may also be
delayed in one particular area of development, for example language
development. In each of the schemes there are therefore separate axes
for these two classes of information.

Again, clinical psychiatric syndrome and level of intellectual
functioning are different concepts. Thus infantile autism, for example,
may occur in individuals of any level of intelligence. Rutter and his
colleagues have therefore provided an axis for intellectual level,
separate from that which deals with clinical psychiatric syndromes.
DSM-III-R does not provide a separate axis for level of intellectual
functioning but places mental retardation among the developmental
disorders included in Axis II.

The selection of axes is an arbitrary matter. It depends largely on the
purpose for which the classification scheme is to be used. It would be
easy to think of possible axes which neither scheme uses, for example

temperamental style, or the quality of the subject's relationships. There is no theoretical reason why such axes should not be included, if there were reason to believe that they would serve a useful clinical or research purpose.

ICD-9 and its multiaxial modification (Rutter, Shaffer and Sturge, 1975)

This classification is designed to cover all ages, but in the following summary, the categories in Axis One most likely to be used for childhood and adolescent disorders appear in **heavy type**. Any item may however be used for a child or adolescent.

Categories derived from ICD-9
    Axis One (Clinical Psychiatric Syndrome)
    Psychoses (290-299)
        Senile and Presenile Organic Psychotic Conditions
        Alcoholic Psychoses
        Drug Induced Psychoses
        Transient Organic Conditions
        Other Organic Psychotic Conditions (Chronic)
        Schizophrenic Psychoses
        Affective Psychoses
        Paranoid States
        Other Non-organic Psychoses
        Psychoses Specific to Childhood
    Neurotic Disorders, Personality Disorders and Other Non-Psychotic Mental Disorders
        Neurotic Disorders
        Personality or Character Disorders
        Sexual Deviations and Disorders
        Alcohol Dependence
        Drug Dependence
        Non-Dependent Abuse of Drugs
        Physical Conditions Arising from Mental Factors
        Special Symptoms or Syndromes not Elsewhere Classified
        Acute Reaction to Stress
        Adjustment Reaction
        Specific Non-Psychotic Disorders following Brain Damage
        Depressive Disorders not Elsewhere Classified
        Disturbance of Conduct not Elsewhere Classified
        Disturbance of Emotions Specific to Childhood and Adolescence
        Hyperkinetic Syndrome of Childhood

Psychic Factors Associated with Diseases Classified Elsewhere
Axis Two (Specific Delays in Development)
No Specific Delay
Specific Reading Retardation
Specific Arithmetical Retardation
Other Specific Learning Difficulty
Developmental Speech/Language Disorder
Specific Motor Retardation
Mixed Developmental Disorder
Other Specified
Unspecified
Axis Three (Intellectual Level)
Normal Variation
Mild Mental Retardation
Moderate Mental Retardation
Severe Mental Retardation
Profound Mental Retardation
Unspecified Mental Retardation
Intellectual Level Unknown
Axis Four (Medical Conditions)
This includes all remaining codes in ICD-9

Items not Derived from ICD-9
Axis Five (Abnormal Psychosocial Situations)
No significant distortion or inadequacy of the psychosocial environment
Mental disturbance in other family members
Discordant intra-familial relationships
Lack of warmth in intra-familial relationships
Familial over-involvement
Inadequate or inconsistent parental control
Inadequate social, linguistic or perceptual stimulation
Inadequate living conditions
Inadequate or distorted intra-familial communication
Anomalous family situation
Stresses or disturbance in school or work environment
Migration or social transplantation
Natural disaster
Other intra-familial psychosocial stress
Other extra-familial psychosocial stress
Persecution or adverse discrimination
Other psychosocial disturbance in society in general
Other (Specified)
Psychosocial situation unknown

ICD-9 contains descriptions of the items in the first three axes, and Rutter, Shaffer and Sturge (1975) define the items in the fifth axis. The reliability of the fifth axis appears to be low but modifications suggested by VanGoor-Lambo (1987) have been shown to improve it.

DSM-III-R

DSM-III has been widely used on the North American continent and it is likely that DSM-III-R will be employed as widely. Unlike ICD-9, DSM-III and DSM-III-R are designed as multiaxial schemes. The five axes of DSM-III-R are:

- Axis I: Clinical syndromes and V codes.
- Axis II: Developmental disorders and personality disorders.
- Axis III: Physical disorders and conditions.
- Axis IV: Severity of psychosocial stressors.
- Axis V: Global assessment of functioning.

Axis I: Clinical syndromes and V codes
The first axis starts with a list of 'disorders usually first evident in infancy, childhood or adolescence'. These are subdivided as follows:

I.   Disruptive behaviour disorders
        Attention-deficit hyperactivity disorder (ADHD)
        Conduct disorder
        Oppositional defiant disorder
II. Anxiety disorders of childhood or adolescence
        Separation anxiety disorder
        Avoidant disorder of childhood or adolescence
        Overanxious disorder
IV. Eating disorders
        Anorexia nervosa
        Bulimia nervosa
        Pica
        Rumination disorder of infancy
V.   Gender identity disorders
VI. Tic disorders
VII. Elimination disorders
        Functional encopresis
        Functional enuresis
VII. Various other disorders: Cluttering, stuttering, elective mutism, identity disorder, reactive attachment disorder of early childhood, stereotypy/habit disorder.

The other Axis I categories may also be used for children's and adolescents' disorders. The principal categories are:

Organic mental syndromes and disorders
Psychoactive substance use disorders
Schizophrenia
Delusional (paranoid) disorders
Psychotic disorders not elsewhere classified
Mood disorders
Anxiety disorders (or anxiety and phobic neuroses)
Somatoform disorders
Dissociative disorders (or hysterical neuroses, dissociative type)
Sexual disorders
Sleep disorders
Factitious disorders
Impulse control disorders not elsewhere classified
Adjustment disorders
Psychological factors affecting physical condition
'V' Codes for conditions not attributable to a mental disorder that are a focus of attention or treatment

Axis II: Developmental disorders and personality disorders
This axis comprises 'developmental' and personality disorders. The developmental disorders catagories are:

Mental retardation
Pervasive developmental disorders
Specific developmental disorders
Other developmental disorders

The various categories of personality disorder are discussed in Chapter 12.

Axis III: Physical disorders and conditions
These are to be classified according to a modification of the ICD-9, developed in the USA and known as the ICD-9-CM.

Axis IV: Severity of psychosocial stressors
Stressors are assessed on a 6-point scale, ranging from 1 (none) to 6 (catastrophic), with a code (0) for 'inadequate information or no change in condition'.

Axis V: Global assessment of functioning scale (GAF scale)
In using this scale 'psychological, social, and occupational functioning on a hypothetical continuum of mental health-illness' are to be

considered. A numerical score in the range 1 to 90 is awarded, 1 indicating severely impaired functioning and 90 absent or minimal symptoms.

DSM-III-R provides precise operational definitions of the disorders it recognizes. Its forerunner (DSM-III) was criticized because 'many of the supposedly unambiguous criteria are actually quite vague and value-laden' (Rutter and Gould, 1985, page 316), as when it used such phrases as 'often doesn't seem to listen' or 'needs a lot of supervision'. How far DSM-III-R has overcome these difficulties is not yet clear.

The relative merits of the two classification schemes

It is important to classify psychiatric disorders, so that meaningful communication can occur between those who work in the field. This is necessary in day-to-day clinical work, but especially so in research. If different workers do not have a common, agreed language with which to describe and discuss the conditions they are treating or studying, our subject cannot advance. Unfortunately, as we have seen, most child psychiatric disorders are not discrete, well-defined entities, though some come near to being so, for example infantile autism and syndromes with very specific symptoms, like Gilles de la Tourette's syndrome.

Devising a classification scheme involves difficult choices. On the one hand is the Scylla of defining disorders in broad, clinical terms which may lack precision; on the other is the Charybdis of attempting to define in precise, scientifically objective terms conditions which in reality are not distinct, clear-cut entities, even though they have properties in common. ICD-9 tends towards the first of these alternatives, DSM-III-R towards the second.

A valuable aspect of DSM-III-R is the inclusion of the 'V' codes. Some of these refer to interactional processes, such as parent-child problems or marital problems, for which people are increasingly seeking professional help. Others refer to problems for which the help of mental health professionals may be sought but which may not be manifestations of mental disorders. Included are antisocial behaviour in the absence of mental disorder, academic problems, occupational problems, uncomplicated bereavement, malingering, and 'phase of life or other life circumstance problems'. Some of these issues are addressed in the fifth axis of the scheme of Rutter *et al.* (1985), but ICD-9 itself does not cover them.

The prevalence of child psychiatric disorders

A major epidemiological study of children's disorders was carried out in the Isle of Wight in 1965. All the 10- and 11-year-old children in the island were surveyed. The prevalence of psychiatric disorders, as the researchers defined them, was found to be 6.8 per cent. Psychiatric disorder was considered to be present if 'abnormalities of behaviour, emotions or relationships were sufficiently marked and sufficiently prolonged to be causing persistent suffering or handicap in the child himself, or distress or disturbance in the family or community' (Rutter, Tizard and Whitmore, 1970). There were nearly twice as many boys with psychiatric disorder as there were girls.

The Isle of Wight is an area of small towns and rural areas and, as we have seen, the prevalence of psychiatric disorders is higher in urban areas. A subsequent survey, using similar methods, in an inner London borough showed a rate of disturbance about double that in the Isle of Wight (Rutter *et al.*, 1975). Prevalence rates also vary according to the age range studied.

Leslie (1974) studied 13- and 14-year-olds in Blackburn, a British industrial town. The prevalence rates she found for psychiatric disorder, expressed in percentages, were:

	Boys	Girls
Moderate disorder	6.2	2.6
Severe disorder	14.6	11.0
Total	20.8	13.6

A study in an Australian town of about 2000 inhabitants suggested prevalence rates of 10 per cent in children and 16 per cent in adolescents (Krupinski *et al.*, 1967).

The Ontario Child Health Study has recently yielded data on the prevalence of psychiatric disorders in children aged 4 to 16 in the Canadian province of Ontario (Boyle *et al.*, 1987; Offord *et al.*, 1987). In this study a representative sample of households from various parts of the province was selected. Of the eligible households (principally those containing children in the age range being studied), 91.1 per cent agreed to participate in the survey. These contained a total of 3294 children aged 4 to 16. The households of native North Americans living on Indian Reserves were not included; nor were children living in institutions. The percentage prevalence rates that were found are shown in Table 2.1. 'Somatization' refers to the presence of somatic symptoms without evident physical cause.

The Ontario prevalence rates are considerably higher than those found in the Isle of Wight, but the latter study was confined to children aged 10 and 11 and the Isle of Wight comprises only rural areas and

Table 2.1: Prevalence of disorders by age and sex (percentages): Ontario Child Health Study (Offord *et al.*, 1987).

Age	Sex	One or more disorders	Conduct disorder	Hyperactivity	Emotional disorder	Somatization
4–11	Boys	19.5	6.5	10.1	10.2	–
4–11	Girls	13.5	1.8	3.3	10.7	–
12–16	Boys	18.8	10.4	7.3	4.9	4.5
12–16	Girls	21.8	4.1	3.4	13.6	10.7
4–16	Boys	19.2	8.1	8.9	7.9	–
4–16	Girls	16.9	2.7	3.3	11.9	–

small towns; on the other hand the rates are lower than those found in urban areas in some other studies. The Ontario data confirm that there are marked sex differences in the prevalence of many child psychiatric disorders; they also highlight the differential changes in prevalence rates with age. In the younger age group emotional disorders are about equally prevalent in the two sexes but in the older group they are nearly 3 times more common in girls; on the other hand conduct disorders are in both age groups much commoner in boys than girls.

Chapter 3

Assessing Children and their Families

A flexible approach is necessary when assessing children and their families. Some psychiatrists like to interview child and parents separately, while others start by seeing the whole family. If the parents are seen first, the child may feel, perhaps with justification, that the parents have been reporting unfavourably on him or her. This may make it hard to gain the child's confidence. But if the child is seen first, the interviewer will probably know less of the problems for which help is being sought, and so may be unable to steer the interview accordingly. With children the merits of the two approaches are generally quite evenly balanced. Adolescents are usually best seen first if they are to be seen apart from their parents.

I prefer to start by seeing the whole family as a group, making it clear, when an appointment is first made, that all family members in the household should attend. Seeing the family members together, and observing how they interact, provides information of great value in the assessment of a child. While some facts concerning the child's and the family's history may not emerge in an interview designed to explore the current functioning of a family, this information can always be obtained in later interviews with child, parents or others.

The option of seeing the whole family together may not be available in some situations, for example when children are brought to emergency departments of hospitals, or in residential institutions. In such circumstances one must work with whoever is available.

Family interviews

Chapter 5 of the companion volume *Basic Family Therapy* (Barker, 1986) describes several of the models available for the assessment of families, and provides a practical scheme for the diagnostic interviewing of families. What follows is a shortened version of that scheme. The reader who plans to interview whole families and lacks experience in this area of clinical work, should read the fuller account or consult another source of information on family interviewing. In developing family interviewing skills, supervised practice is also essential.

The assessment of a family should proceed through the following stages, which may overlap:

(1) the initial contact;
(2) joining the family and establishing rapport;
(3) defining the desired outcome;
(4) reviewing the family's history, determining its present developmental stage and constructing a genogram;
(5) assessing the current functioning of the family.

The initial contact

If you decide to interview the whole family as part of your initial assessment, the family should be told, when the appointment is made, that all family members in the household should attend. (You may not at this stage want to see non-members of the family who may be living in the household.) If the family question the necessity of this, they should be told that it is easier to gain a proper understanding of a child's problems if you know the family of which the child is a part; that the behaviour of any one family member inevitably affects the other members; and that the other family members can often be part of the solution of the problem. It is not usually a good idea to suggest that they are a part of the problem.

It is usually easy to persuade parents that *they* are important to their children, but they may be reluctant to bring siblings whom they consider to be well adjusted and problem-free. In that case the point can be made that the well-functioning children may have much to offer the problem child, in that they have acquired the skills to function well in the family – skills the identified patient needs.

Joining the family and establishing rapport

Rapport may be defined as a state of understanding, harmony and accord. People who are in rapport with one another have a sympathetic relationship and feel warmly towards each other. The establishment of rapport starts with the initial contact, and should be a primary objective in your first interviews, whether with individuals or families.

Establishing rapport has been given other names, such as 'joining' the family (Minuchin, 1974), or 'building working alliances' (Karpel and Strauss, 1983). As it develops the participants become increasingly involved with each other. Hypnotherapists have long recognized the importance of rapport, and know that failure to induce an hypnotic trance is usually due primarily to the lack of sufficient rapport. Rapport has been described as:

> '... that peculiar relationship, existing between subject and operator, wherein, since it [hypnosis] is a cooperative endeavour, the subject's attention is directed to the operator, and the operator's attention is directed to the subject. Hence, the subject tends to pay no attention to externals or the environmental situation.' (Erickson *et al.*, 1961, page 66.)

When rapport is well developed the therapist can say almost anything, even quite outrageous things, without the client becoming upset; even remarks which could be construed as insulting will be taken as being meant jokingly, or at least not seriously.

Rapport may be fostered by both verbal and non-verbal means. The non-verbal ones are probably the more important.

The non-verbal communications start at the first contact, even if it is a telephone conversation, since one's tone of voice and manner of speaking convey powerful messages. A warm, friendly tone of voice, and a respectful, interested and accepting approach are important. When the family arrives it is best to greet them personally in the waiting room and to make the acquaintance briefly of each family member. I like to address them by name, if I know their names, and shake hands with each (except for very small children); if I do not know their names I ask for them as I greet them. I tell the family who I am and express my pleasure at their arrival.

Comfortable physical surroundings assist in promoting rapport. A pleasantly furnished room is desirable. It should be well ventilated and unobtrusively lit, with comfortable chairs, paper tissues (in case of tears, which are not too uncommon in family therapy sessions) and ashtrays (since there are smokers in many families, and it does not usually help to ban smoking). Your dress should conform to cultural norms; dress which is too formal can lead some children to feel ill at ease, as can the white coats which doctors tend to wear in hospitals.

Most important of all is the therapist's behaviour, and excellent rapport can be established in prison cells, classrooms, public parks or on the beach. Rapport is promoted by matching or 'pacing' the behaviour of those with whom you wish to establish rapport. You can do this by matching their body postures and movements, respiratory rhythm, speed of talking, and voice tone and volume. You can also 'mirror' or 'cross-match' their movements; mirroring is the moving of, say, your left arm or leg in response to similar movements of the client's right arm or leg. 'Cross-matching' occurs, for example, when the therapist's hand or finger is moved in rhythm with movements of the client's foot. Movements which may be matched include such things as crossing and uncrossing the legs, the tilting of the head to one side or the other, and leaning forward or settling back.

Pacing should be done sensitively and unobtrusively and it is only necessary to match some of the client's behaviours. When these guidelines are followed the subjects do not become consciously aware that you are matching their behaviours. While it is not possible to pace simultaneously the behaviours of all members of a family, you may observe common things about their behaviour which you can use. With families it is usually sufficient to match the behaviours of the different family members in turn, perhaps as you speak to each one.

The developers of 'neuro-linguistic programming' (NLP) have paid much attention to rapport-building processes. They point out that:

> 'When you pace someone – by communicating from the context of their model of the world – you become synchronized with their own internal processes. It is, in one sense, an explicit means to 'second guess' people or to 'read their minds', because you know how they will respond to your communications. This kind of synchrony can serve to reduce resistance between you and the people with whom you are communicating. The strongest form of synchrony is the continuous presentation of your communication in sequences which perfectly parallel the unconscious processes of the person you are communicating with – such communication approaches the much desired goal of irresistibility.' (Dilts *et al.*, 1980 pages 116–117.)

Verbal communications are also important. Rapport is helped when you match your predicates with those used by your clients (Bandler *et al.*, 1976; Bandler and Grinder, 1979). A predicate is a word that says something descriptive about the subject of a sentence; predicates include verbs, adjectives and adverbs. Some people use mainly visual, rather than auditory or feeling, predicates – as in the phrases, 'I see what you mean', or 'things are looking brighter'.

Examples of the use of auditory predicates are, 'I hear what you're saying', 'that sounds terrible', or 'it was like music to my ears'. Sentences such as 'I have a lot of heavy problems,' 'that feels like a good idea', or 'that's a big weight off my shoulders', illustrate the use of 'kinesthetic' or feeling-type predicates. Although we all use predicates of all three types – as well as some olfactory ('this business smells fishy to me') and gustatory ('it leaves a bad taste in my mouth') ones, and many that are non-specific, most of us have a preferred way of processing information. This uses one of the three main sensory channels. Noting this, and using the information to 'join' others in processing information as they do, is a powerful rapport-building technique.

In addition to matching predicates, you should listen carefully to the vocabularies of those you are interviewing, noting the words and expressions they use. Few things impede the establishment of rapport as much as repeatedly using words and expressions with which those to whom you are speaking are unfamiliar. This is especially important when dealing with children, but it applies also to adults. Thus the vocabulary of a university professor will be different from that of a person who left school at the age of 15.

Other rapport-building devices are:

- Accepting people's views of things without initially challenging them.
- Adopting a 'one-down' position.
- Talking of experiences and interests you have in common with whoever you are interviewing.

The 'one-down' position can help, for example, with parents who are convinced their views about the nature of their child's problems are correct. Rather than confronting them with a conflicting opinion which may lead to an unproductive argument, you might say that you do not understand the situation as yet and thank them for coming up with this suggested explanation. Some people, especially children, are overawed or intimidated by the therapist. For them a one-down approach might consist of asking them, from a position of ignorance, about something in which they have expertise and you have not – their job perhaps, or skate-boarding, or how to spell their names.

Common experiences might be having lived in the same city, country, province or state as the family has in the past. Hobbies, sports and pastimes you have in common with family members may be used in similar ways.

Defining the desired outcome

Almost invariably children are brought for psychiatric consultation because someone wants some change to occur – in their behaviour, emotions, school performance, relationships with others, mental or physical development, or whatever. Defining, and if necessary clarifying, the changes sought is important for several reasons:

- It formally acknowledges the family's concerns.
- It defines your involvement as therapeutic and oriented towards promoting change.
- It helps avoid misunderstandings about the purpose of the child's or the family's attendance.
- It provides an opportunity for the family to clarify their thoughts, and if necessary to consider the situation they *do* want, rather than

complaining about how they do not like the present one.

- It can inspire hope by having the family look forward to a better future, rather than dwelling upon the past.
- If all, or even several, family members are present it offers an opportunity for them to discover whether they all have the same objectives.
- There is no way to define success if no desired outcome has been established.

The goals of a consultation should be defined in positive, rather than negative terms. It is not sufficient for parents to say they want their child's tantrums to cease; they should be asked how they would like the child to react in situations in which tantrums have been occurring. Other points to consider are:

- What consequences will follow once the goals have been achieved?
- Are there any drawbacks which may be associated with these consequences?
- Under what circumstances are the changes desired? Most behaviours have value in some situations.
- What has prevented the changes occurring in response to whatever has been tried so far?
- How quickly should the changes occur? Change that is too rapid can itself be stressful and adjusting to new situations takes time. There is also embedded in this question the idea that change *will* occur.

The establishment of treatment goals is discussed in more detail in *Basic Family Therapy*, Chapter 6 (Barker, 1986).

Reviewing the family's history, determining its developmental stage and constructing a genogram

These tasks can conveniently be tackled together in a session with the whole family. A good way to approach the family's history is to start with the parents' births and childhoods. The parents can be asked where they were born and brought up, what kinds of families they were raised in, how they got along at school and what they did when they left school. As they answer these questions they will probably speak of their parents and siblings. They can next be asked how they met and courted, and invited to outline the course of their married life so far.

Enquiry may next be made about the births of the children and their development to date. It will be clear by now what stage in its life cycle the family has reached; there may also have emerged evidence of any difficulty the family is having in passing from one stage to the next.

The construction of a *genogram* (sometimes called a geneogram), or family map, is often helpful and much of the above information may be obtained during this process. A genogram gives a concise, graphic summary of a family's current composition. It should also show the extended family network, the ages of the family members, the dates of the parents' marriage, and of any previous marriages, divorces or separations; and it indicates how the family members are related. It can also show who is the identified patient, although I prefer to omit this information when I am working on a genogram with family members. The geographical locations of the family members can be indicated. Brief summaries of the salient points concerning each family member – for example occupation, school grade, health, and past illnesses, accidents, losses, incarcerations and so forth may also be noted.

While some therapists prepare the genogram later using the information they have obtained from the family during sessions with them, I prefer to have the family members participate. An example of a genogram, reproduced from *Basic Family Therapy* (Barker, 1986), is shown in Figure 3.1.

In this family the parents of the identified patient, Brad (distinguished by a double boundary), cohabited in a 'common law' relationship from 1965 to 1969, after which they got married. They separated in 1973 and were legally divorced in 1980. Carmen, Brad's mother, lived with Eric from 1973 to 1976 and they had two daughters, Jane and Audrey. Eric subsequently married Fay and they now have a daughter, Holly. Carmen commenced living with Ken in 1978 and they were married in 1982. Her two children by Eric, and one by Ken make up their present family unit. Brad and his father, Dave, live with Katrina and her 10-year-old daughter by her former husband, Len. Katrina also had a previous pregnancy which ended in a miscarriage in 1974. Carmen is an only child and both her parents are dead; Dave is the fourth in a family of one girl and four boys.

There is a fuller discussion of genograms in *Basic Family Therapy* (Barker, 1986). *Genograms in Family Assessment* (McGoldrick and Gerson, 1985) provides comprehensive information on the construction, interpretation and clinical uses of genograms, with many illustrations.

Assessing the current functioning of the family

You will usually learn more about how a family functions from the experience of interacting with it, than by asking the members how they think they function. Information about family relationships may be obtained during interviews in three ways:

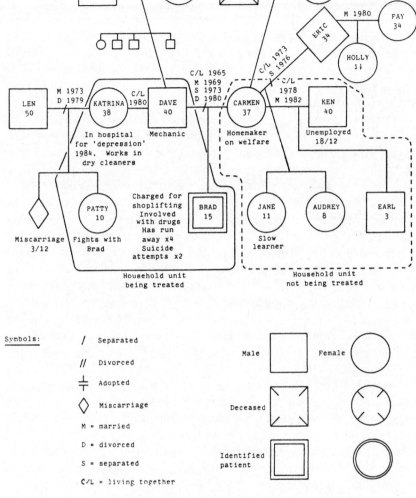

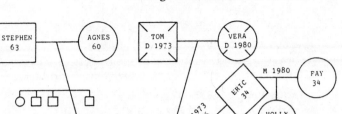

Figure 3.1 The Green family genogram, 1985

- by the experience of interacting with the family;
- by observing the interactions between family members;
- by asking questions which bear on the relationships between the members, and studying carefully the family's responses, both verbal and non-verbal.

A family cannot adequately describe how it functions. The formal organizational structure may be described, but this says little about how the different parts habitually interact and about the functioning of the system as a whole. The questions asked of family members are not, therefore, usually about *how* the family functions as a group or organization; instead they are designed to reveal this indirectly.

There are many ways of interviewing families. An important contribution was made by the Milan group of therapists in their paper, 'Hypothesizing – circularity – neutrality: three guidelines for the conductor of the session' (Palazzoli *et al.*, 1980). As the paper's title suggests, these authors recommend that the interviewer should first develop some hypotheses about the family system; one always knows something of a family, even before the first interview – for example, its composition and the fact that it contains a rebellious child, an anorexic adolescent or a depressed adult. Whatever information *is* available is the basis of the hypotheses with which the therapist starts.

An hypothesis is 'an unproved supposition tentatively accepted to provide a basis for further investigation, from which a verification or refutation can be obtained' (Palazzoli *et al.*, 1980, page 5). The interview is designed to test the hypotheses, and often leads to the formulation of new ones. This is an active process in which the therapist asks questions to explore the patterns of the family's relationships. The Milan authors believe that if the therapist were to behave in a passive fashion, that is as an observer rather than a mover, the family, 'conforming to its own linear hypothesis, would impose its own script, dedicated exclusively to the designation of who is "crazy" and who is "guilty", resulting in zero information for the therapist' (Palazzoli, *et al.*, 1980, page 5).

Hypotheses should be systemic, that is they should concern the family system as a whole. The objective of the family interview is to understand the relationships between the family members, rather than to explore the mental states of the individual members.

Circularity is a way of thinking which led the Milan group to develop their process of 'circular interviewing'. The therapist responds to information the family gives about relationships by formulating more questions, to which the family then responds again, and so on. The questions are framed in a circular way too; their method is to ask one member of the family to describe the interactions or relationships between two others. This 'triadic interviewing' is an example of triadic thinking.

Triadic theory – which is the idea that two people (or groups or even agencies) in conflict tend to involve a third person or group in the conflict – has been described as 'one of the cornerstones of many models of family therapy' (Coppersmith, 1985). The process of bringing in a third person is sometimes referred to as 'triangulation', and the ability to think in terms of triads (or triangles, which are essentially the same thing) is an important skill for the family therapist. The questions asked of family members, or group of members, are often about differences between the behaviours or responses of two other members or groups of members; and the emphasis is on relationships between people rather than on the behaviour of individuals.

Other practical points about using the ideas of Palazzoli *et al.* (1980) are:

- It is better to ask questions about specific behaviours than about how people feel about the situation, or how they interpret or understand it. For example, the therapist might ask one of the children in a family questions such as the following:

  'What does your father do when Billy loses his temper and swears at his mother?' Then, when the father's reaction has been described: 'And what does your mother do then? And if your big sister is around, what would she be doing?'

- Differences may be revealed by asking people to rank the family members in terms of specific behaviours. Thus the members of a family in which one child is physically aggressive to a younger one, might be asked:

  'When Chad hits Dorothy, who is most likely to step in and try and stop him? And who is the next most likely to do this? And then?' ... (And so on, until it is determined who is least likely to intervene.)

- Questions concerning changes in the patterns of relationships are often revealing. These may concern differences before and after certain specific events. Thus members of a family which has recently moved, or in which there has been a marital separation, a remarriage, an illness or accident affecting a family member, or a child's entry into school or departure to university, might be asked about differences in the behaviours of members relative to one another before and after the event.

- Questions can be asked about how behaviours or relationships vary in different circumstances, real or hypothetical. For example:

  'Who would be most upset if Eric was seriously ill?'

  'Do Frances and Gillian fight more when Dad is at home than when he is not?'

  'What does Mummy do when Harry misbehaves? Does she react differently when Dad is at home?'

Neutrality means taking care not to become allied with any family member or members. Nor should the therapist accept a particular family member's view of the situation. Some of the above questions might seem to ally the therapist with the person being questioned, but the alliance shifts when the questioning moves to another family member. So the therapist will be allied in turn with all the family members, and 'the end result of the successive alliances is that the therapist is allied with everyone and no one at the same time' (Palazzoli *et al.*, 1980). The interviewer should also declare no judgments, whether implicit or explicit, while interviewing the family.

Other sources of information on interviewing families are *Basic Family Therapy* (Barker, 1986) and *Family Evaluation* (Karpel and Strauss, 1983).

Taking the history

At some stage during the assessment a history of the child's problems and development should be obtained. If possible both parents should be interviewed. It is important that both are concerned with the study and treatment of the child from the outset and it should be made clear, when the appointment is made, that both should attend. If only one comes, I arrange to see the other later. This applies equally if one is a step-parent, or the parents are unmarried. When the parents are permanently separated or divorced, involvement of the non-custodial parent at some stage is usually helpful, but not at the initial interview.

It is best to let the parents start by talking freely about the child's problems. They should be allowed to explain the situation as they see it, in their own way and with a minimum of prompting. When they have finished speaking of one issue or problem they can be asked if there are any others and, if so, again allowed to explain them in their own words. During this process information is often obtained about the nature of the relationship between the parents.

I prefer to discuss symptoms in terms of the changes the parents seek. If they complain of the child's behaviour at mealtimes, I ask how they would like the child to behave. If they want a certain behaviour to stop, for example hitting a sibling, I ask them how they would like the child to respond in circumstances in which the hitting currently occurs.

The development of symptoms, their duration and frequency, whether they are getting better or worse or have remained much the same for a while, and how the parents have attempted to deal with them – and with what success – all need to be explored.

The next step is to enquire about any of the following areas not yet covered:

(1) *The digestive system:* Eating habits, nausea, vomiting, abdominal pain, constipation, diarrhoea, faecal soiling, pica.

(2)   *The urinary system:* Bedwetting, wetting by day, over-frequent or painful micturition.

(3)   *Sleep:* Problems of going to bed, problems in sleeping, nightmares, sleepwalking, night terrors, excessive sleepiness.

(4)   *The circulatory and respiratory systems:* Breathlessness, cough, palpitations.

(5)   *The motor system:* Restlessness, overactivity, underactivity, clumsiness, tics, abnormal gait, motor weakness, whether right- or left-handed.

(6)   *Habitual manipulations of the body:* Nail biting, thumb sucking, nose picking, head banging, rocking and other repetitive habits.

(7)   *Speech:* Over-talkativeness, mutism, faulty speech of any type, including late development of speech and stuttering, comprehension of what is said.

(8)   *Thought processes:* Poor concentration, distractibility, disordered thinking, day dreaming. Delusional ideas.

(9)   *Vision and hearing:* Any defects, evidence suggesting hallucinations.

(10) *Temperamental traits:* See Chapter 2.

(11) *Behaviour:* Follower or leader, relationships with siblings, parents, teachers, friends. Fearfulness, sensitiveness, tearfulness, sulking, irritability, temper tantrums. Obedience/ disobedience, co-operativeness/negativism, constructiveness/ destructiveness, truthfulness/untruthfulness, stealing, wandering from home, staying out late, group or gang membership, smoking, drinking, drug-taking. History of involvement with police, court appearance, probation, or placement away from home. Involvement of social agencies.

(12) *Mood:* Whether mood is appropriate or the child is depressed, elated, angry, anxious, fearful, or showing evidence of other mood disturbance. Does the mood vary a lot? If so, is this related to environmental circumstances, or does it appear to be independent of them?

(13) *Fantasy life and play:* The types of games the child plays. Content of play. Does he/she have a lot of imagination? Fantasy friends, transitional objects. Content of fantasy as expressed in play, drawing, painting, conversation or dreams.

(14) *Sexual issues:* Sex instruction given, child's reaction to it, sexual attitudes, masturbation, heterosexual or homosexual experiences, onset of menstruation, dysmenorrhoea, any history of sexual abuse.

(15) *Attack disorders:* Epilepsy, fainting, other alterations of consciousness, breath-holding attacks.

(16) *School:* Attitude to school, behaviour at school, school class or

grade, progress in school, social adjustment at school.
(17)   *Physical abuse:* Has the child ever been physically abused?

Although the above list consists mainly of possible problems, it is important to ask about and note strengths and areas of healthy functioning. Thus information that a child does well at school, has much musical talent, gets on well with siblings and friends or has an easy temperament, is as important as that concerning problem areas.

As you obtain the history you should ask about the duration, frequency and degree of both problem behaviours and strengths. Observe also how parents describe symptoms: do they make light of the child's problem behaviour, or do they describe it in over-dramatic or rejecting terms?

A series of studies of interviewing techniques was undertaken at the Maudsley Hospital, London, to assess the effectiveness of different approaches in eliciting facts and feelings from the parents of children referred for psychiatric assessment (Rutter and Cox, 1981; Cox, Hopkinson and Rutter, 1981; Rutter, Cox *et al.*, 1981; Hopkinson *et al.*, 1981; Cox, Rutter and Holbrook, 1981; Cox, Holbrook and Rutter, 1981). Left to themselves, mothers raised most key issues, but suitable specific questioning was necessary to obtain 'good quality factual data'. An active, structured approach, used sensitively and with the inter-viewer alert for clues to the presence of unusual symptoms, is best for eliciting facts. It is often important to establish the absence of certain symptoms as well as discovering which ones are present – hence the merits of going through the above list.

In eliciting feelings, the use of 'open' questions, a low level of talk by the interviewer, and direct requests for the expression of feelings combined with interpretations and expressions of sympathy, were found to be most helpful.

Some non-verbal behaviour was studied during this research, but the results were not clear-cut. Nevertheless clinical experience suggests that it is important.

The developmental history

An account of the child's development from conception to the date of the interview should be obtained, as follows:

- The course of the pregnancy, any complications, whether the mother used alcohol or drugs, and if so, how heavily.
- The child's birth and neonatal condition.
- The subsequent progress of the child's development (motor, speech, feeding, toilet training, social behaviour and adjustment, progress in school and so on).

- Any previous illnesses, injuries or emotional problems.

It is useful to have a description of the child's behaviour as a baby, a toddler, over the period of starting school and up to the present time.

Examining the child

There can be no set routine for the psychiatric examination of children. Much depends on the child's age, language skills, willingness to talk and personality. With children below the age of five, contact usually has to be largely through the medium of play, though even pre-school children can sometimes reveal a lot about themselves in conversation. Older children, and especially adolescents, can often be approached much as adult patients are. In the intermediate age range a mixture of play and conversation is usually appropriate.

It is seldom the presenting child who is complaining of symptoms. Usually an adult, often a parent or teacher, is either complaining on the child's behalf or is objecting to some aspect of the child's behaviour. So it is usually unwise to start the interview by discussing the presenting complaints. Indeed to do so can be a serious error; it can lead the child to identify the person carrying out the assessment with other disapproving adults, and so develop a guarded or suspicious attitude. A trusting relationship with the child will thus be more difficult to establish.

The first step is to establish rapport and gain the child's confidence, rather than to ascertain facts. Rapport-building techniques were described in the foregoing section on interviewing families. The same principles apply to individuals, whether children or adults, as to families. Nevertheless there are some particular points which are important in dealing with children.

Children being interviewed should feel that they and their points of view and opinions are respected and valued. The atmosphere in the consulting room should be relaxed and friendly, but not condescending. Toys, play materials, and painting and drawing materials, appropriate to the child's age, should be available and in view. Younger children are best seen in a playroom. It is best not to have a desk between child and interviewer; to do so tends to distance child and interviewer emotionally as well as physically, making it harder to establish rapport.

It should be made clear to young children that the toys and materials are there for their use. If they do not wish to talk this should be accepted, and they should be allowed to play for a while. A conversation may then be started while the child plays.

It is best to start talking with children about topics well away from the symptom areas, such as how they travelled to the clinic or office, their interests and hobbies, games they like to play, toys they have at home, any recent birthday, school (unless this is an area of difficulty), friends, siblings, and their ambitions for the future. If Christmas, Easter, Thanksgiving, a holiday or other such events have occurred recently, these can be brought up.

The symptoms or presenting problems may come up as the interview proceeds; if not, they can be dealt with later. This is especially so with children who have been engaging in antisocial acts, such as stealing. There is little point in asking, 'Did you steal such-and-such?' If the question is answered at all, the child must say yes or no. If yes, the interviewer is usually none the wiser; if no, the child has been forced into the position of witholding information, which may damage the developing relationship with the interviewer and erect a barrier to communication. Still less should one say, 'Why did you steal?' Such a question is futile. It tends to put the interviewer in the same category as other authority figures who may have been questioning, lecturing and perhaps punishing the child for whatever the problems may have been. While one wishes to understand why the child has been stealing, it is naive to suppose that this can be achieved simply by asking the child. The child may in due course bring the subject up, but this is a different matter.

The early part of the first interview, sometimes the whole of it, is thus spent gaining the child's confidence. Once this has been achieved, at least to a reasonable extent, it is justifiable to ask, in a general way, what has brought the child to the clinic, office or hospital. An accurate reply is often given, but if not the subject should not be pressed.

Once rapport has been established, particular areas of the child's life may be explored. This should be done gently, using words and in a manner appropriate to the child's age and personality. It is not a matter of asking a series of direct questions. Such an approach seldom gives the desired result. It is more a matter of saying, 'Lots of people have dreams when they are asleep at night ... I wonder if you do?' The child who admits to having dreams can then be invited to recount one, and perhaps asked whether the dreams are mostly nice ones or nasty ones. The child who denies having or remembering dreams may be told, 'Often when people who don't have dreams come to see us, they like to make up a dream ... to pretend they've had one ... perhaps you'd like to do that?' This is one way of exploring children's fantasy lives. Another is to ask them to imagine they can have three magic wishes and that whatever they wish will come true; what would they then most like to happen? Children often take their wishes very seriously. The interviewer can go on to say something like, 'Now I'd like you to pretend you were all alone on a desert island (or in a boat) and you could choose one person to be with you ... anyone you like but just one person ... I wonder who you would have?' The child may then be asked to choose a second person, then a third.

The interviewer should enquire in a similar way for fears, worries, and somatic and other symptoms. Conversation about family, friends (whom the child can be asked to name and describe), and school should also be encouraged. Throughout all of this the interviewer must respond appropriately to what the child is saying, trying to share the child's sorrow at the loss of a pet, or pleasure at being a member of a winning sports team. Above all it is important to convey interest in the child's point of view. This does not necessarily imply approval of what the child does or thinks.

Children who have not reached adolescence should be invited to draw, paint and/or play with some of the toys. This enables their concentration, attention-span, distractibility and motor dexterity to be observed. The content of their play, and their artistic productions, frequently give helpful information. I usually ask any child I see to draw her or his family. The appearance of the different family members, their relative sizes and positions, and even who is included and who is left out can be revealing. It can also be useful to invite the child to draw a 'person' and then discuss the person (let us assume it is a boy) the child has drawn, asking questions like, 'What makes him happy?' 'What makes him sad?' 'What makes him angry?' 'What makes him laugh?' 'How many friends does he have?' 'Does he make friends easily?' 'Do people like him?' ... and so on. The answers can reveal much about children's views of the world and their relationships to it.

Much can be learned about children from what they draw or paint. For example, some pictures bristle with aggression; guns are firing, people are being hurled over cliffs or otherwise killed, and violence of all sorts is occuring. Others equally obviously portray sadness with people looking unhappy or crying, or being represented as feeling ill or even being about to die. Yet others show happy scenes, or illustrate the fulfilment of the artist's ambitions. Children's artistic productions should be kept with their clinical records. What they say as they draw, paint or make models should also be recorded; otherwise it is not always obvious what their productions represent. Moreover these can change with time; even in the course of a few minutes a picture may be redefined as something quite different.

What children draw, paint or model must always be interpreted in the light of the whole clinical picture, taking into account all other available information about them. There is much more to the understanding of children's artistic productions than can be covered here. The book *Interpreting Children's Drawings* (DiLeo, 1983) is a valuable source of further information, and refers also to earlier work on the subject.

Adolescents may or may not wish to paint, play or draw, but it is usually possible to judge whether it is appropriate to suggest such activities.

By means of interviews such as have been described it should be possible to make an assessment of the child as follows:

(1) *General appearance:* Are there any abnormalities of facial appearance, head, body build or limbs? Are there any bruises, cuts or grazes? What is the mode of dress and is it appropriate for the climate and time of year? Does the child look happy or unhappy, tearful or worried? Attitude to the examiner and the consultation?

(2) *Motor function:* Is the child overactive, normal or underactive? What motor activities are carried out? Are they performed normally, or clumsily, quickly or slowly? Abnormal movements such as tics? Right- or left-handed? Can the child distinguish right from left? Is the gait normal, and if not in what way is it abnormal? Can the child write, draw and paint, and if so, how well?

(3) *Speech:* Articulation, vocabulary and use of language should be noted. Does the child speak freely, little or not at all? Any stuttering? Receptive and expressive language? Ability to read and write?

(4) *Content of talk and thought:* What does the child talk about? How easy is it to steer the conversation towards particular topics? Are any subjects avoided? Does the stream of thought flow logically from one thing to another? Is there any abnormal use of words or expressions? Is there evidence of hallucinations or delusions?

(5) *Intellectual function:* A rough estimate of the child's level of intelligence should be made, based on general knowledge, conversation, level of play, and knowledge of time, day, date, year, place and people's identity, taking into account what is normal for the child's age.

(6) *Mood and emotional state:* Happy, elated, unhappy, frankly depressed, anxious, hostile, resentful, suspicious, upset by separation from parents and so on? Level of rapport which has been established. Has the child ever wanted to run away, or to hide, wished to be dead or contemplated suicide? Does the child cry, and if so, in what circumstances? Specific fears and if present how are they dealt with? Appropriateness of emotional state to subject being discussed?

(7)   *Attitudes to family:* Indications during conversation about family members or during play.

(8)   *Attitudes to school:* Does the child like school? Attitudes towards school work, play, staff, other pupils? Child's estimate of own abilities and progress in school?

(9)   *Fantasy life:* The child's three magic wishes. The three most desired companions on a desert island. What kind of dreams are reported or made up? What is the worst thing – and the best thing – that could happen to the child? What are the child's ambitions in life? Material expressed in play, drawing, painting, modelling and so on.

(10)   *Sleep:* Does the child report any difficulty in sleeping? Fear of going to bed or to sleep? Nightmares, night terrors (not usually reported by children unless they have been told they have them by others), pleasant dreams?

(11)   *Behaviour problems:* Does the child reveal anything about behaviour problems, delinquent activities, illicit drug use, running away, sexual problems or appearance in court?

(12)   *Placement away from home:* Has the child been placed, or lived, away from home? If so where, when, for how long, and what is the child's understanding of this? What is the child's reaction to this experience?

(13)   *Attitude to referral:* How does the child see the referral, and the reasons for it? Is he or she aware of a problem, and if so what?

(14)   *Indications of social adjustment:* Number of reported friends, hobbies, interests, games played, youth organizations belonged to, how leisure time is spent. Does the child feel a follower or a leader, or bullied, teased or picked on? If so, by whom?

(15)   *Other problems:* Do any other problems come to light during the interview, for example, worries, pains, headaches, other somatic problems or relationship difficulties?

(16)   *Play:* A general description of the child's play is required. What is played with and how? To what extent is play symbolic? Content of play? Concentration, distractibility and constructiveness?

(17)   *The child's self-image:* This cannot usually be assessed directly, but must be inferred from the sum total of what the child does and says, the ambitions and fantasy ideas expressed, and the child's estimate of what others think of him or her. There is evidence that disturbed children may overrate their self-esteem, as compared to ratings by adults, whether these are parents, therapists or teachers (Zimet and Farley, 1986).

Children's behaviour should always be described as objectively as possible. A good account of how to do this is provided by Savicki and

Brown (1981, Chapter 15).

It may not be possible to obtain all the above information at the first interview. Assessment should be regarded as an ongoing process, continuing as long as the child or family are being seen. With non-speaking children, it is possible to assess their condition by making all the observations that do not require spoken replies from the child, and by obtaining information from others. The fact that a child who can talk declines to do so is itself an important clinical observation.

Further information on interviewing and examining children is available in books by Goodman and Sours (1967) and Simmons (1987). *Anxiety in Children* (Varma, 1984) contains a chapter on the recognition of anxiety in children by means of psychiatric interview (Barker, 1984). Rutter and Graham (1968) reported an investigation of the reliability and validity of a procedure, which they described, for interviewing children.

The physical examination

Unless the child's physical state has already been assessed or is being investigated by a colleague, a physical examination should be carried out as part of the assessment. This may be done by a colleague, and if the interviewer is not medically trained it has to be. Some psychiatrists prefer to arrange for the physical examination to be done by another physician, believing that the procedure may impede the development of a psychotherapeutic relationship.

A convenient time for the physical examination may be at the end of the first diagnostic interview. With younger children it is usually best to ask the mother to come into the room during the examination, and if necessary help undress and dress the child. Doing this provides a further opportunity to observe the interaction between child and parent.

Other sources of information

Useful information can often be obtained from other sources, notably the child's school. When a child is seen who is or has been at school the parents should be asked to consent to a report being obtained from the school. This applies whether or not the reported problems are manifest at school. The fact that a child is symptom-free and making good academic progress at school, while perhaps showing signs of serious problems in other situations, is itself of significance.

While written reports from schools are helpful, talking with the child's teacher(s) is often better, especially when problems in school are reported. This may be done on the telephone, but a personal visit to the school may be more informative. A joint meeting with the parents, the relevant school staff including the head teacher or principal, and the school psychologist or counsellor if they are involved is often productive. It can be therapeutic as well as providing information of diagnostic significance. Sometimes the referred child can usefully be included in this meeting.

Aponte (1976), a family therapist, recommended that when the main problems are at school the first face-to-face contact should be a family – school interview. This may be hard to arrange and is probably not the practice of most child psychiatrists. Yet the idea has merit, especially when the initiative for referral comes from the school.

The following may also supply useful information:

- schools the child has attended in the past;
- physicians or other professionals who have assessed or treated the child or family in the past;
- any professionals who are currently involved with child or family;
- any social agencies which have been involved with the child or the family, especially child protection and child welfare agencies and probation services;
- hospitals or institutions in which the child has been treated or has received care;
- foster-parents and others who have cared for the child.

Permission to contact any of the above must be obtained from the family. It is usually wise to get the written consent of both parents.

Psychological tests

Psychological tests can add to the information obtained in clinical interviews. Such tests should be administered and the results interpreted by psychologists trained in their use. They should especially be considered when it remains unclear how a case should be formulated when the assessment procedures described above have been completed; when the patient has been uncooperative or has given inconsistent or confusing information; and when decisions with very serious consequences have to be made. Examples of the latter are criminal prosecution and the discharge from hospital of patients who may be suicidal or homicidal.

The main groups of tests available for use with children are:

- intelligence tests;
- tests of academic attainment;

- personality tests;
- tests of specific psychological functions.

Intelligence tests

Intelligence tests are designed to assess children's cognitive abilities. They yield scores which show how a child's abilities to perform various tasks compare with those of other children of similar age. They give an indication of the general intellectual ability of a child in relation to the whole population of the same age; they also provide information about how the child performs on the different tasks of which the test consists. The 'intelligence quotient' (IQ) was originally conceived as the child's 'mental age' divided by the chronological age, multiplied by 100:

$$IQ = \frac{\text{mental age}}{\text{chronological age}} \times 100$$

The concept of 'mental age' is used less nowadays than it was in the past. It is another way of describing a child's level of functioning on the test concerned. For example, if a boy has an IQ of 100, this means that he performs on the test at the level of an average child of that age in the same population. Thus an eight-year-old boy with an IQ of 100 would have a mental age of 8. If he performed on the test like a seven-year-old, that is he had a mental age of 7, this would correspond to an IQ of $\frac{7}{8} \times 100$, or about 88. A mental age of $9\frac{1}{2}$, in an eight-year-old, corresponds to an IQ of $\frac{9.5}{8} \times 100$, or 119.

The intelligence tests most used with children are:

- the Wechsler Intelligence Scale for Children, revised (WISC-R);
- the Wechsler Pre-School and Primary School Intelligence Scale (for children aged 4 to $6\frac{1}{2}$);
- the Stanford-Binet Intelligence Scale;
- the Merrill-Palmer Scale (for children from 18 months to 6 years of age);
- the Kaufman Assessment Battery for Children.

Intelligence tests are standardized on large populations, to determine how the average child functions in performing the test's tasks, and what variance there is within the population. The WISC-R, one of the most-used tests, has two sets of subtests. One consists of verbal tasks and the other of non-verbal ones, the 'performance' subtests. It is designed so that the mean verbal, performance and full-scale IQs at any age are 100. Each of the twelve subtests (only ten of which are normally used) has a mean (scaled) score of 10. The standard IQ deviation is 15, which means that about 66 per cent of the population will have IQs between 85 and 115. Two standard deviations (IQ 70-

130) will cover about 95 per cent of the population and three (55-145) over 99 per cent.

The other tests listed above, although constructed differently, have similar objectives. Many other tests are available, designed to measure abilities of various sorts. Raven's Progressive Matrices are a series of patterns, from each of which a part is missing; the child has to decide which shape will complete each matrix. This test provides an estimate of non-verbal skills. The Peabody Picture Vocabulary Test is an easily administered test of verbal skills.

Tests are also available for infants and young children. They include the Griffiths Scale of Mental Development, the Bayley Infant Scales of Mental and Motor Development and the Gesell Developmental Schedule.

Intelligence tests were originally designed to detect the mentally retarded, and to determine which children required special educational placement, or perhaps were not suitable for any existing school programmes. They subsequently came to be overvalued, however, and sometimes an IQ figure became attached to a child as a sort of permanent label, an abuse of the intended purpose of intellectual assessment. One is entitled only to say that on a particular date the child achieved a certain score on a named test. The psychologist's comments should also be taken into account. These should state how cooperative or disturbed the child was during testing and how reliable the results are thought to be. To reduce the misuse of IQ figures, it is accepted practice nowadays to quote a range, or a verbal description of intelligence (e.g. 'the upper end of the average range'). The child's approach to the cognitive tasks of the test is generally considered to be at least as important as the test scores.

Despite these reservations, intelligence tests still have their uses. They may assist in detecting children who are underfunctioning, that is not making full use of their intellectual potential; and those of whom more is being demanded than is appropriate in light of their current cognitive functioning. Often of more importance, though, is the pattern of the child's performance, and the detection of areas of weakness with which special help may be needed, and of areas of strength upon which the child's teachers and parents may capitalize.

Tests of educational attainment

Tests are also available to assess a child's current level of educational attainment. Tests of reading, arithmetic and spelling have been devised and standardized on large populations. These can be used to discover whether children are performing at the expected level for their age. Reading, arithmetic and spelling ages can be derived in the same way as the mental age. Children's assessed intelligence levels (or mental ages) should also be taken into account, since a higher level of academic attainment can be expected from an intellectually higher functioning child. There is a well-established association between behaviour problems and poor reading skills. In assessing and treating children with behaviour problems the detection and remediation of reading difficulties can be important.

Group tests

Both intelligence and academic attainments can be assessed by means of group tests. These are often used in schools. A group of children, large or small, writes answers to a series of questions and/or instructions on a form which is often constructed using a multiple choice format. These tests can be of practical value in assessing the progress of large numbers of children, but the results are less reliable than those of individual tests and it is harder to detect the child who is not cooperating, perhaps because of illness, fatigue or hostility. These tests are also predominantly verbal. Their results may differ from those of individual tests and reassessment by individual testing is indicated when abnormal or unexpected results are encountered.

Personality tests

The assessment of personality is more difficult than the estimation of intelligence or educational attainment. It is easier to define average reading attainment or average intelligence than to define average personality. Nevertheless , the administration of personality tests can contribute to clinical diagnosis.

Projective personality tests are those in which the subject is presented with vague or ambiguous material, with the aim of eliciting responses which may reflect the person's personality or mental state. The oldest and best known projective test is the Rorschach Test. The subject is presented with a series of printed shapes, originally derived from ink blots, and asked to say what they resemble. The blots themselves have no designed meaning, so any response must be a projection. Interpretation is difficult and special training and experience with the test are needed.

The Children's Apperception Test (CAT) is probably more commonly used than the Rorschach. It consists of a number of somewhat ambiguous pictures about which the child is asked to tell a story. The Thematic Apperception Test (TAT), although designed for adults, is sometimes used instead of, or as well as, the CAT. It has more realistic pictures than the CAT, and also offers a wider variety of pictures and situations. Two other widely used tests are the Draw-a-Person Test and the House-Tree-Person Test. In each case the child is asked to draw the items mentioned. The results can be analysed qualitatively and quantitively to give information about the child's personality and emotional state.

The above tests do not give results as valid and reliable as, for example, tests of educational attainment. They are especially useful with children who do not talk or play freely at interview and for those presenting particularly puzzling clinical pictures. Even if not scored they may reveal valuable information about a child's inner life, information which may not emerge during a routine clinical interview. Some of these tests resemble techniques used by psychiatrists who ask children to make up stories, draw or comment on pictures, or make up dreams.

The Children's Personality Questionnaire of Catell is an example of the many questionnaire-type tests that are available. The parent or other adult familiar with the child answers a series of questions. From the responses an estimate of the child's personality and emotional state is made.

Various tests of 'social adjustment' are available. The Vineland Social Maturity Scale is a series of questions put to the child's parent(s) or to someone else with a good knowledge of the child. It covers such things as dressing, feeding oneself, walking and talking, and is a quick way of assessing the social development of infants and young children. The Bristol Social Adjustment Guides are questionnaires designed to examine the adjustment of children in school, in residential care and in the family. There are questionnaires for use by parents, teachers, residential child care staff and social workers, and there are boy and girl versions.

Tests of specific psychological functions

Countless other tests are available to assess language development, self-esteem and self-perception, motor development, the presence of emotional disturbance, perceptual skills, temperament, the presence of organic brain damage, and many other aspects of children's functioning.

How to use psychological tests

Psychological tests are not items to be 'ordered', as blood counts or X-rays sometimes are. Rather than asking for a particular test to be administered, it is better to explain to your psychological colleague the clinical problem and how you hope testing will help solve it. This may lead to a discussion of the tests available for the clinical situation and the kind of information each is likely to give. Whether testing may be expected to help, and if so which tests should be used, can then be decided. The psychologist is a professional colleague with expertise in, among other things, the use of these tests, not a technician carrying out set routines. Moreover, the range of tests is so large that it is hard for those without training as psychologists to keep up to date and be aware of what is available.

Psychological tests also have important uses in research. Because they use standardized procedures, and normative data derived from large populations are often available, they lend themselves to the measurement of psychological functioning and the statistical treatment of the resulting data.

Information on available tests is to be found in the many reference books on the subject (for example Anastasi, 1982; Reynolds and Gutkin, 1982).

EEGs, X-rays and laboratory tests

It is not usually necessary to arrange any additional investigations of the child's physical state, if there are no symptoms suggesting organic disease and physical examination reveals no relevant abnormality.

Although children with psychiatric disorders show a higher rate of abnormalities in the electroencephalogram (EEG) than is found in the general population, these abnormalities are mainly non-specific, and for the most part do not help in planning treatment. The EEG is, however, a valuable aid in the diagnosis and management of epilepsy. Apart from this, its main roles at present are in the diagnosis of suspected physical disease of the brain and in research. The EEG has been said to provide information useful in planning the treatment of autistic children. A recent study, however, showed no significant correlation between EEG changes and language patterns in autistic children, contrary to previous assertions (Dorenbaum *et al.*, 1987).

The main value of X-ray studies of the skull, and special radiological investigations, is also in the diagnosis of physical conditions affecting the brain. In such cases X-ray studies are usually part of the neurological assessment.

Computerized axial tomography (the CAT scan), and the more recently introduced procedure of nuclear magnetic resonance (NMR) promise to be of value in the investigation of possible neurological correlates or causes of child psychiatric disorders, for example infantile autism. Their use is still in the research stage but there are indications that CAT scan results correlate with the results of tests of neuropsy-chological functions, which themselves often show evidence of impairment in disturbed children (Tramontana and Sherrets, 1985).

Other laboratory investigations, such as blood counts and biochem-ical tests, have little role to play in the routine investigation of child psychiatric patients, unless there is reason to suspect an associated physical disorder. A study of laboratory tests carried out on a population of 100 adolescent inpatients by Gabel and Hsu (1986) showed that the results contributed little or nothing to the manage-ment of these young people.

The formulation

When the assessment of child and family is complete, a formulation of the case should be developed. Where staff function as teams, the formulation is usually worked out at a meeting attended by the team members. The practitioner working alone should carry out the same procedure.

The formulation is a concise summary of the case in the light of all the information available. It should start with a brief statement of the presenting problem(s). This is followed by a description of how the clinician understands the case. The construction of the formulation is a vital part of the assessment, for it is the basis of the management and treatment plan. A good way of developing a formulation is to consider possible causative factors as follows:

(a) *Predisposing:* What pre-existing factors contributed to the development of the disorder? Constitutional, temperamental, physical and environmental factors should all be considered.
(b) *Precipitating:* Has evidence emerged of anything that helped precipitate the disorder? Why did the problem appear at the particular time reported? Again, constitutional, temperamental, physical and environmental factors must be considered.
(c) *Perpetuating:* What is maintaining the condition? The four sets of factors should again be considered.
(d) *Protective:* What are the child's and the family's strengths? What factors are limiting the severity of the disorder and promoting healthy functioning?

The grid in Figure 3.2 may be used to get the process of developing the formulation started. It is essential to remember, though, that a formulation is not just a list of causative, contributing or associated factors but a description of their interplay and relative importance.

Figure 3.2   Formulation grid of contributing factors.

	Constitutional	Temperamental	Physical	Environmental
Predisposing				
Precipitating				
Perpetuating				
Protective				

Based on the information in the grid, if one is used, the formulation should be a clearly written, logical, dynamic explanation of the case, leading to a plan of treatment, management or further assessment. Strengths as well as weaknesses should be included. The expected outcome should be stated. If a 'problem-oriented' or 'goal-oriented' system of clinical recording is used, the formulation should be the basis of the problem and strength lists.

Formulations should be updated from time to time during treatment, since new information usually comes to light as treatment or further investigation of the case proceeds, and as circumstances in the family, school or elsewhere change. The following is an example of a formulation.

Angela B. presents as a reserved, anxious twelve-year-old girl with a three-year history of failure to attend school despite three changes of school arranged by her mother at Angela's insistence. She is a physically fit girl who has just reached puberty. She is said always to have been a quiet child, slow to adapt to change and overdependent on her mother. The latter has long been unable to resist Angela's demands, and behaves similarly towards Angela's nine-year-old sister who seems, however, to have a more assertive personality than Angela and is developing more independence than her sister.

Before the onset of school refusal Angela did well at school and she appears to be of above average intelligence. Non-attendance was precipitated by a change to a stricter, male teacher and a period of illness in mother. Now attempts to get Angela to go to school result in panic and an acute exacerbation of anxiety symptoms. Angela has, however, a keen interest in horses and attends riding school on her own with no difficulty. In this area of her life her self-esteem appears good, but in others it is poor and she feels unable to cope with many situations without the support of others, especially her mother.

Mrs B. and the two daughters have a close, enmeshed relationship; there is a clear boundary between their family subsystem and Mr B., who makes only a small contribution to the upbringing of the children and volunteered little during the family interview. He spent part of his childhood in a group home and seems uninvolved in family life. He has an adequately paid job working in a bank.

The whole family appears to need support over sending Angela to school. At the same time the relationship between the parents requires to be strengthened; boundaries must be established between the parents on the one hand and the two daughters on the other.

Although the problem is a longstanding one, the parents are strongly motivated to receive help and are concerned about the amount of schooling Angela has missed. Mr B. seems willing, even keen, to get more involved in the parenting process but at present lacks the necessary skills or confidence. Other strengths are Angela's good physical health, her above average intelligence and her interests outside the home, notably in horses. With treatment, which will have to address the family system problems as well as being concerned simply with getting Angela back in school, the outlook for improvement is good. Angela may require some individual therapy as well as the family work. If early return to school is not achieved a short period of inpatient treatment may be indicated.

This formulation is written using many concepts derived from structural family therapy but any theoretical orientation may be employed in a formulation.

Using the first of the two multiaxial classifications described in Chapter 2, the diagnosis made in this case was:

Axis I: Neurotic disorder: anxiety state.
Axis II: No specific delay in development.
Axis III: Normal intelligence.
Axis IV: No associated medical condition.
Axis V: Familial over-involvement (referring to the over-involvement of Angela and her mother).
            Inadequate or distorted intrafamilial communications (referring to the lack of communication between the parents).

The DSM-III-R diagnosis in this case was:

Axis I: 309.21 Separation Anxiety Disorder.
Axis II: V71.09 No Diagnosis on Axis II.
Axis III: No Physical Disorder.

Axis IV: Psychosocial stressors: change of teacher; illness in mother; enmeshment of Angela and mother, lack of involvement by father):
Severity: 3 – Moderate (acute events and enduring circumstances).
Axis V: Global assessment of functioning:
Current: 51
Highest past year: 62.

It is clear that the formulation gives considerably more information about the case than either of the five-axis schemes. But being free-flowing literary vignettes, formulations are not suitable for statistical analysis, nor for grouping disorders together for research or clinical purposes.

Recording clinical information

In child psychiatry, as in all branches of medicine, it is essential to keep good clinical records. The information obtained when children and their families are assessed should be summarized, preferably system-atically in a format developed for the purpose. If this is done important points are less likely to be omitted. The headings in this chapter may be used as a basis for such a format. A typed summary, which may be prepared in the form of a letter to the referring physician, is much to be desired. Children's drawing and paintings should be preserved as part of the clinical record.

Records should be stored in a secure place, access to them being limited to those who have legitimate reasons to examine them. Issues concerning the confidentiality of clinical information are discussed further in Chapter 17.

Chapter 4

Conduct Disorders

Definition and classification

Conduct disorders are characterized by antisocial behaviour. ICD-9 defines 'disturbances of conduct not elswhere classified' as disorders 'involving aggressive and destructive behaviour and involving delinquency'. The behaviour should not be part of some other psychiatric disorder, such as a neurotic disorder (see Chapter 5) or a psychosis (Chapter 6), but 'minor emotional disturbance' may be present.

DSM-III-R states that the 'essential feature' of a conduct disorder is a persistent pattern of conduct in which the basic rights of others or 'major age-appropriate societal norms or rules' are violated. The problems are more serious than those seen in 'oppositional defiant' disorders. The problems must have existed for 6 months or longer and at least three out of a list of 13 behaviours must be present. Three types of conduct disorder are distinguished:

(1) *The group type.* In this category the conduct problems occur 'mainly as a group activity with peers'. Physical aggression may or may not be a feature.
(2) *The solitary aggressive type.* The predominant feature of this category is physically aggressive behaviour, usually towards both adults and peers. This is initiated by the person, rather than being a group activity.
(3) *The undifferentiated type.* In this category there is a 'mixture of clinical features that cannot be classified' as either of the above two types.

This is a simpler system of classifying conduct disorders than was offered in DSM-III. There is research data supporting a distinction between 'socialized' and 'undersocialized' disorders (Hewitt and Jenkins, 1946; Field, 1967; Jenkins, 1973), though in practice the distinction is not always easy to make. DSM-III-R's distinction of a 'group' type and a 'solitary' type is in keeping with this data, but whether it is valid or clinically useful to restrict the 'solitary' category to disorders in which there is physical aggression is less clear.

DSM-III-R also distinguishes 'oppositional defiant disorders', in which there is 'a pattern of negativistic, hostile, and defiant behaviour without the more serious violations of the basic rights of others that are seen in conduct disorder'.

'Juvenile delinquency' is usually defined as behaviour leading to the conviction of the young person of a criminal offence, or an offence which would be criminal in an adult. The definition is thus a legal, rather than a psychiatric one, but delinquent behaviour often develops in children who have been displaying conduct disorder symptoms. Most delinquents have conduct disorders, often severe and longstanding ones.

Shamsie (1981), writing of adolescents, suggests that antisocial behaviour may be best regarded as 'a problem arising from lack of socialization'. For whatever reason – and we will consider possible reasons shortly – the young person has failed to learn, or has not effectively been taught, society's norms.

Prevalence

Conduct disorders are the commonest psychiatric disorders in older children and adolescents. In the Isle of Wight study (Rutter, Tizard and Whitmore, 1970) nearly two-thirds of the 10- and 11-year-olds with psychiatric disorders were found to have conduct disorders. Including the children with mixed neurotic and conduct disorder, the prevalence of conduct problems was 4 per cent. In a London borough studied later it was 12 per cent (Rutter, Cox *et al.*, 1975). Leslie's (1974) survey of adolescents in Blackburn, England, showed prevalence rates of 13 per cent for boys and 6 per cent for girls, on the basis of the sample seen by the psychiatrist. Conduct disorders have repeatedly been shown to be commoner in boys than in girls.

The Ontario Child Health Study (Offord *et al.*, 1987) revealed the following percentage prevalence rates for conduct disorders:

Boys aged 4-11:	6.5	Girls aged 4-11:	1.8
12-16:	10.4	12-16:	4.1
4-16:	8.1	4-16:	2.8

In the Ontario study the urban and rural prevalence rates for conduct disorders were quite similar at 5.6 per cent and 5.2 per cent respectively.

Causes

Antisocial behaviour illustrates well the complexity of the causation of child psychiatric disorders and their multifactorial aetiology. Seldom is it possible to pinpoint one specific cause for a conduct disorder.

The essential problem in these disorders is a failure to learn society's norms for behaviour, a failure to observe these even though aware of them, or a combination of the two. Factors in any or all of the categories discussed in Chapter 2 may contribute to this.

(1) Constitutional factors

(a) Genetic factors
Polygenic factors may play some part in predisposing to these disorders. Both twin and adoption studies suggest a genetic predisposition to adult criminality (Vandenberg *et al.*, 1986, Chapter 10), though the evidence is less strong in the case of children.

(b) Chromosome abnormalities
The possession of an extra Y chromosome or of a long arm on the Y chromosome may slightly increase the risk of antisocial behaviour or other emotional problems (Nielson and Christensen, 1974; Ratcliffe and Field, 1982), but the great majority of those with these anomalies are free of such problems.

(c) Intrauterine disease or damage
We have discussed in Chapter 2 the various intrauterine hazards a fetus may face. These may contribute to antisocial behaviour indirectly by causing brain damage. This is known to predispose to psychiatric disorders in general (Rutter, Graham and Yule, 1970).

(d) Birth injury and prematurity
These may predispose to antisocial behaviour in the same way as intrauterine damage. Babies who require intensive medical care in the neonatal period may also be separated from their parents in special care units for weeks or even months. This can adversely affect the bonding process, which may contribute to later difficulties.

(2) Physical disease and injury ·

Physical damage to the brain after birth is associated with an increased likelihood that a child will develop antisocial behaviour. Various explanations of this association are possible. Because of brain damage the child may be more difficult to train, the neurological pathways or mechanisms involved having been damaged. We know also that behavioural problems are more frequent in children of lower intelligence (Rutter, Tizard and Whitmore, 1970) and brain damage can lower intelligence. Occasionally oppositional behaviour or conduct disorder symptoms are associated with epilepsy, especially when this arises from a temporal lobe focus.

Non-neurological mechanisms may also operate. The presence of handicap, whether neurological or not, in the child may provoke rejecting, fatalistic or other unhelpful attitudes in parents and others. These may affect the child's self-esteem and may be associated with adverse rearing practices.

(3) Temperamental factors

Temperament, and the importance of the various possible constellations of temperamental factors, have been discussed in Chapter 2. A temperamentally 'difficult' child has more chance of developing behavioural problems than one with an 'easy' temperament. As we have seen, however, much depends on the goodness of fit between the child's temperament and the temperaments and responses of the parents. A clash of temperaments is sometimes the basis of difficulties that may become serious and longlasting. On the other hand, some families are able to rear children with difficult temperaments quite successfully.

(4) Environmental factors

(a) The family
There is no satisfactory substitute for a stable, loving and united parental couple in the rearing and socialization of a child, at least in western cultures. (This may not necessarily be true for cultures in which extended family systems are the units in which children are reared, as for instance in many traditional African societies.) This does not mean that children cannot do well in single-parent families or other settings, but the task a single parent faces is greater than that confronting a stable parental couple.

Children who lack a permanent family group in which to grow up suffer grave disadvantages. Those who move repeatedly from one home to another, or live in large, impersonal orphanages, are often deprived of the consistent learning experiences needed for the process of socialization. They also lack consistent, permanent and stable figures with whom to identify. Children who have been 'in care' earlier in childhood have been found to show significantly more deviant behaviour later, and this most often takes the form of antisocial behaviour (Wolkind and Rutter, 1973).

Living in a permanent family group, however, even one containing both the natural parents, does not guarantee a childhood free of antisocial behaviour. So what are the factors in a family that affect the socialization process, and help determine whether antisocial behaviour becomes a problem in the children? Many have been suggested, including disharmonious relationships between the parents, broken homes in both the parents' and the grandparents' generations (Wardle, 1961), working mothers (Bowlby, 1951), day care for young children (Blehar, 1974), brief separations or admissions to hospital, bereavement, father absence (Biller, 1970), a poor fit between the personalities of parents and child (Chess and Thomas, 1984), large family size, socioeconomic disadvantage, and various other disorders of family systems. While any or all of these may be associated with problems, they are also compatible with healthy child development. Thus even very young children placed in day care usually develop normally if the quality of the day care is good. Similarly, many children of working mothers are well adjusted. The crucial question is: *What actually happens to the child?* The various circumstances listed above may increase the chances that the child's social training will go awry, but they need not do so.

What do children require in order to give them the best chance of learning to behave in socially acceptable ways? The generally agreed requirements are a stable and consistent environment, acceptance, affirmation of their worth as individuals and proper social training. The latter is provided partly by parental precept and example, and partly through the setting of rules and expectations, rewards and consequences being used as needed. In the setting of a happy home characterized by warm, loving relationships between the family members, the rewards and punishment may need be no more than a smile or word of encouragement, or a frown or minor reproof. This sort of family environment helps promote children's emotional security and self-esteem and facilitates the process of socialization.

What exactly does 'proper social training' mean in practice? According to Patterson (1982) antisocial behaviour is associated with:

- lack of 'house rules' – that is, no set routine for meals and other activities, and a lack of clarity about what the children may do or how they are expected to behave;
- failure by the parents to monitor children's behaviour, and to know what they have been doing or how they feel;
- lack of effective contingencies – that is, inconsistent responses to

undesired behaviour, with failure to follow through with threatened consequences or with rewards for desired behaviour;
- lack of techniques with which to deal with crises or problems in the family, so that tensions and disputes arise but are not satisfactorily resolved.

Wilson (1980), in a study of delinquents, found weak parental supervision to be the factor most strongly associated with delinquency, among those she investigated. Poorly supervised children roam the streets without their parents knowing where they are; they do not know when they are supposed to be home; and they engage in many activities independently of their families. The conclusions of these two investigators are thus quite similar.

The following is an example of a severely dysfunctional family.

Robin, aged 11, had been treated in two child psychiatric units because of his aggressive, disobedient, restless and generally difficult behaviour. When he, his two brothers, his sister and his parents were interviewed as a group, chaos was evident. Everyone spoke, or more usually shouted, at once and no-one seemed to listen to what anyone else was saying. Instructions by the parents were ignored by the children; the mother was more active in issuing orders than the father, who seemed in semi-retirement from the fray, but neither parent apparently expected to be obeyed. All family members seemed to compete on equal terms. No differentiated parental system was evident, nor any clear boundary between parents and children. Robin had become the identified patient perhaps because, as a big, strong, active and out-going boy for his age, his antisocial behaviour was more threatening than that of the others. But the behaviour of the other children was little different. Only if the whole family system was restructured could the antisocial behaviour of Robin and his siblings be eliminated, unless they were removed to live long-term elsewhere, that is in a different family or other social system.

It is easy to see how the criteria for the development of antisocial behaviour set out by both Patterson (1982) and Wilson (1980) would be met in a family such as Robin's. But not all dysfunctional families are as grossly disorganized as that one; indeed it is fortunate for therapists that most are not! Family dysfunction may take many other forms, not all of which are incompatible with successful child rearing. But some involve children adopting roles, such as that of 'scapegoat' (see Chapter 2), which require them to be the 'bad' child. Families which fail to provide satisfactory social training for their children often prove also to have many of the problem-solving, communication, role behaviour, affective involvement, control and other difficulties described by family therapists. These are discussed in *Basic Family Therapy* (Barker, 1986, especially Chapters 5 and 9)

(b) Extrafamilial factors

These comprise the school, the wider social setting in which family and school are situated and the child's peer group. We have seen, in Chapter 2, how important a child's school can be in influencing both academic progress and behaviour. The features of family functioning which Patterson (1982) found to be associated with antisocial behaviour probably have similar effects when they occur in schools. Clinical experience also suggests that dramatic changes in the course of children's development sometimes occur when they change schools.

Several studies have found a higher prevalence of conduct problems in urban than in rural areas. It is especially high in the more run-down and deprived areas of big cities. This cannot be entirely explained by the migration to cities of poorly functioning families or the mentally ill (Rutter, 1981). It seems that cities are less healthy places in which to rear children, though the prevalence of problems can vary a lot in different areas of the same city. The effects of city life may operate more at the family level than on the individual child, but at present they are far from being fully understood. Close supervision of children is, however, more difficult in large urban areas than in villages and rural areas; in the country everyone tends to know everyone else's business and children can perhaps get away with less without being caught!

We have seen that adolescents are often greatly influenced by their peer groups. How far group pressures and dynamics lead to antisocial behaviour is however unclear, though it does seem that most serious delinquent activities are carried out in the company of others, rather than alone. This has been found to apply to girls even more than it does to boys (Emler *et al.*, 1987). Possible explanations for these findings are discussed by Emler and his colleagues. Involvement with the group could be a causal factor; another possibility is that delinquent youths choose to associate together but do not become any more delinquent as a result; or the explanation might be that young people tend to do things together and that this applies no more to delinquent than to other activities. A causal connection seems most probable.

(5) The interaction of factors

The different categories of causative factors we have considered are not independent. Thus temperament is in part genetically determined. Physical disease in a child may lead to adverse parental attitudes such as overprotection of the child. The 'goodness of fit' between child and environment may be a crucial issue ... and so on. The causes of antisocial behaviour are complex and multiple, and the result we see is the outcome of the interplay of many forces. Some of these may be difficult or impossible to modify but there are usually some that are open to intervention.

Description

Conduct disorders usually first become evident within the family group. Early signs of trouble may be persistent or repeated stealing, lying, disobedience or aggressive behaviour. As the disorder progresses similar problem behaviours may be manifest outside the home, either in the school, the neighbourhood or both. The child may play truant from school, stay out late, run away from home or commit acts of vandalism. Some children go on to engage in criminal activities such as breaking into houses and stealing from them, shoplifting or stealing from cars.

Sometimes the problem behaviours first appear in school. They may be accompanied by a deterioration in the quality of school work, as the child's hostile attitude to the world in general, or to the adult world, is expressed as defiance of the teachers' instructions.

In some cases, particularly when conduct disorders develop in adolescence, the problems are first manifest in the wider community. Careful enquiry may, however, provide evidence of co-existing problems at home and/or in school.

Symptoms of 'unsocialized' (ICD-9) conduct disorders include disobedience, quarrelsomeness, aggression, destructive behaviour, temper tantrums, solitary stealing, lying, teasing, bullying, disturbed relationships with others and sexual misconduct. These children are less likely to have lasting peer group friendships, to extend themselves or show concern for others, to show feelings of guilt and to avoid blaming or informing on others. Using DSM-III-R the disorders of many of these children would be classified as of the 'solitary aggressive' type.

Children with 'socialized' conduct disorders are more inclined to engage in antisocial activities as members of groups to whom they show some loyalty, though the behaviours themselves may be quite similar to those seen in the unsocialized types. They may have established peer group friendships and be prepared to help other group members out even when there is nothing in it for them; they avoid blaming or informing on their companions, and may show evidence of guilt or remorse when these emotions are appropriate. Some of these children are members of established delinquent gangs.

Specific symptoms

Stealing is common in conduct disorders. It only becomes abnormal when it is severe and persistent and fails to respond to commonsense measures instituted by parents or others. Virtually every child takes another's property without permission from time to time, but persistent failure to respect the possessions of others is a sign of deviant development. It is often associated with rejecting, inconsistent or indifferent parental attitudes.

Aggressive behaviour is another common cause of referral. It may present as temper tantrums, verbal threats or physical attacks on others. These may occur with minimal or no apparent provocation. Other conduct disorder symptoms are frequently reported along with aggressive behaviour.

Truancy is the wilful and unjustifiable avoidance of attendance at school by a child who is supposed to be there. It differs from school refusal (or 'school phobia', see Chapter 5), in which it is neurotic anxiety that keeps the child from school. The truant stays away from school not because of overwhelming anxiety associated with the idea of going, but because of a stronger desire to do something else, like play in the park, attend the video arcade or sit at home watching television. Children may leave home and return there at the appropriate times, but without having attended school. The parents may think they are at school, while the school staff assume there is a legitimate reason for their absence, such as illness. It is surprising how long this situation sometimes continues. If both parents work outside the home, or there is a single working parent, the child may sit at home all day, failing to answer the doorbell or telephone and destroying letters from the school.

Truancy is seldom purely the child's problem. Some parents take little interest in their children's schooling and do not bother to take steps to ensure attendance. They may not regard school and its benefits as important. Some actively encourage their children's non-attendance; they may even tell them to stay at home to help with housework or shopping or to babysit for younger children. Most truants have poor academic records; their consequent failure to get satisfaction from doing school work is an additional factor discouraging attendance. They often come from materially and culturally impoverished homes, though some are rebellious teenagers from affluent homes.

Factors in school may also contribute to truancy. Other things being equal, a child is more likely to attend a school if it provides an enjoyable, rewarding and affirming experience, and if its staff are willing and able to help the child with any personal or family problems that may exist.

As with most child psychiatric problems, the causes of truancy are complex and a multitude of factors combine to bring it about. Current knowledge is reviewed in a magnificently concise way by Reid (1986), who has also written about it at greater length in *Truancy and School Absenteeism* (Reid, 1985). Berg's (1985) review is another source of information.

Vandalism, the wanton damage to or destruction of property, is often a group activity of adolescents. Whether carried out by a group or an individual, however, it is usually a means of expressing hostile, aggressive feelings towards the adult world. Such feelings often arise from similarly disturbed relationships with parents. In the child whose development is following a healthy course, aggressive drives are channelled into constructive activities (or 'sublimated'). Failure of sublimation may be due to faulty relationships and identifications. Social factors may operate too; in some places there are few outlets available for the energies of young people. The influence of antisocially inclined groups may also pressurise their members to commit destructive acts.

Closely related to vandalism is the raising of false alarms, for example summoning an ambulance or the fire brigade to a non-existent emergency. These behaviours may occur as part of either socialized or unsocialized conduct disorders.

Firesetting is a relatively uncommon but serious symptom. Many children go through a phase of playing with matches and lighting fires, but this usually responds to parental training and precept. Children who instead develop a pattern of deliberately setting fires, are often expressing severe, deep-seated feelings of aggression, arising from profoundly disturbed family relationships.

Some 2 per cent to 3 per cent of child psychiatric outpatients have set fires (Vandersall and Wiener, 1970; Jacobson, 1985a). Many are referred with other conduct disorder symptoms, along with the firesetting, but a small group are referred specifically because they have set fires (Yarnell, 1940; Jacobson, 1985b).

Jacobson (1985a) reviewed the cases of 104 'definite firesetters' seen in an inner London clinic, and compared them with 'age-, sex- and class-matched non-firesetters with equivalent diagnoses'. The majority were diagnosed as having conduct disorders. Specific reading retardation was more common in the firesetters than in the non-firesetters. When the firesetters were compared with conduct-disordered controls, they were found to show 'marked antisocial and aggressive behaviour, rather than a broad range of syndromes'. Family discord was 50 per cent more frequent in the firesetters, who comprised 5.5 per cent of the children with conduct disorders.

Jacobson (1985b) also reports that the overall boy:girl ratio was 5.1, much higher than the overall clinic ratio (1.58) or that for all conduct disorders (1.82); in firesetters under 11 it was 14.25, there being only 4 girls in a total of 61. Over the age of 11 the ratio was 2.3. There were age peaks at 8 and 13.

Bradford and Dimock (1986) studied 46 adolescent arsonists 39 (85 per cent) boys and 7 (15 per cent) girls, referred for a forensic psychiatric examination and compared them with a group of 57 adult arsonists similarly referred. The backgrounds of the juveniles were characterized by parental alcoholism and major psychiatric illness, physical abuse, and father absence (the latter in 40 per cent of cases). Seven (15 per cent) were mentally retarded. There was a history of significantly more violent behaviour in the juvenile group. Half of both groups set their own homes alight, most commonly in acts of revenge.

The Psychology of Child Firesetting (Gaynor and Hatcher, 1987) provides a comprehensive overview of this subject. It emphasizes the scale of the problem, pointing out for example that 48 per cent of all those arrested for arson in the USA in 1984 were under 18 years of age; and that children under 13 constituted 17.1 per cent of arson arrests in 1977. The authors believe that it is important how the 'natural curiosity about fire' that most children display is handled. This can lead to 'fire-safe' or 'fire-risk' behaviour. The various individual, social and environmental factors which may lead to serious firesetting behaviour are examined. Gaynor and Hatcher (1987) proceed to summarize factors which tend to be associated with pathological firesetting. Firesetters are mainly boys 10 years or older; they are usually of normal intelligence but may have learning disabilities; they experience overwhelming anger and express aggression inappropriately; they may have previously been diagnosed as having conduct or personality disorders; their relationships with peers are unsatisfactory; their behaviour and achievements in school are poor; and previous firesetting behaviour and other behavioural problems have not been well handled. They often belong to single-parent families and have parents who are distant and uninvolved. In these families there is much aggressive behaviour and there have often been stressful events such as repeated geographical moves. One or both parents may have a psychiatric history.

Drug abuse is a frequent feature of conduct disorders, especially in adolescents, though younger children are not immune. The latter may sniff glue, solvents, benzine or petrol (gasoline), often in the context of severe social and emotional deprivation (O'Connor, 1979). In the black townships of South Africa it is said to be common in middle childhood; many of the children who use inhalants have been abandoned by or have left their families. In Soweto an interesting pilot project to treat such children has been set up. Children addicted to inhalants are to be

found among the deprived urban populations of Third-World countries, and in deprived subgroups of more developed countries.

The abuse of other drugs more often commences in adolescence,
and is discussed in Chapter 15; it is by no means unknown in
prepubertal children, however.

Disapproved sexual behaviour is a feature of some conduct disorders. It
may take the form of engaging in intercourse at a socially unacceptably
early age, or at an age before the law permits it (which varies in
different jurisdictions, but is usually between 16 and 18).

Rape and other sexual offences may be part of a general pattern of
antisocial behaviour, especially in teenagers with severe conduct
disorders; but sometimes those who commit sexual offences have not
displayed other conduct disorder symptoms, their psychopathology
being mainly in the area of their psychosexual development.

Juvenile delinquency

Whether a young person is legally defined as a delinquent may depend
on circumstances, including luck (whether the police are nearby at the
time of an offence); the effectiveness of the police in tracking down
offenders; local policy concerning the prosecution of juveniles (many
are initially let off with warnings); whether the accused has a lawyer,
and if so the skill of the lawyer in court; and the witnesses the police
produce. In most jurisdictions there is also a minimum age of legal
responsibility for one's acts. This is commonly in the range 10-12
years. Below this age it is impossible to become a delinquent, in the
legal sense, however grave the offences. Although it is partly
fortuitous whether a youth becomes a legal delinquent, those who do
tend to be more seriously disturbed than the non-delinquent
population.

An example of a conduct disorder

Paul R. was referred at age 10. He was reported to be one of a group of boys who
had been staying out late, damaging public telephones, stealing from cars and
breaking into shops and a school. His school attendance had been poor for two
years, and his teacher reported that his performance was the worst in his class. He
was usually badly dressed and dirty, and the school staff described him as hostile
and uncooperative. A few weeks earlier he had been placed in the care of the local
authority by the juvenile court, as being beyond his parents' control and because of
his failure to attend school.

At interview Paul answered questions guardedly and made no spontaneous
conversation. He spoke in a matter-of-fact way and showed little emotion. He said
he did not like either of the schools he had attended. He referred quite freely to his
truancy and to having stayed out for periods of up to two days and nights, during

which, he said, he and his friends slept rough. He showed little evidence of any affection for his parents, though he looked a little unhappy when speaking of how they argued. His 'three wishes' were to go to London, to have a bicycle, and to go to a seaside town. His only ambition seemed to be membership of a pop group. Psychological testing showed him to be of low average intelligence, with marked retardation in reading and arithmetic.

The parents' marriage had been far from happy. They had been separated for several short periods and Mr R. had served a prison sentence a few years previously. During this Mrs R. lived with another man and became pregnant by him, though this boy (aged 4 when Paul was referred) was accepted into the household by Mr R. An older brother had been educated in a residential school for disturbed children since the age of 8; he had been placed there because of repeated stealing and truancy.

Throughout Paul's childhood his parents' marriage had been precarious; he had no secure and consistent background for his emotional development, and his parents had failed to set for him, or to demonstrate in their own lives, any clear and consistent pattern of socially acceptable behaviour. Little interest was taken in his schooling. Indeed, the parents, who themselves both grew up in chaotic homes in which there was much abuse of alcohol, were so preoccupied with their own problems that they had little time for their children. So Paul grew up insecure and without any strong relationships in his family. He came to get most satisfaction from relationships with a delinquent gang of older children, but mainly he lived for the moment.

After careful investigation it was recommended that Paul be placed in residential school, as his brother had been, returning to live at home during the school holidays. Simultaneously a social worker undertook to give help and support to the family, though the difficulty of doing so was recognized.

Comment

Throughout his childhood Paul had been deprived of a stable, dependable background. He had lacked the relationships needed for normal emotional development. Although it is impossible to know what part polygenic heredity may have played in his problems, there was no evidence of any physical or constitutional abnormality to account for his deviant development, apart from his slightly dull intelligence, to which his deprived background probably contributed. Questioning his parents about his behaviour when younger did not suggest that he was a temperamentally 'difficult' child, but the parents' recollection of his early behaviour was poor. In a more stable family he would probably have progressed better, and indeed his response to the treatment measures described was good. At follow-up six years later he had left school and was well settled working in a factory.

The DSM-III-R diagnosis was:

Axis I: Conduct Disorder, Group Type.
Axis II: Developmental Arithmetic Disorder.
           Developmental Reading Disorder.
Axis III: No Physical Disorder.

Axis IV: Psychosocial Stressors: parental indifference and
                              inconsistency.
                              unstable parental marriage.
                              inadequate family communication.
          Severity: 4-Severe (enduring circumstances).
Axis V: Current Global Assessment of Functioning: 44.
           Highest GAF in past year: 38.

   Using the ICD-9-derived multiaxial system (Rutter, Shaffer and
Sturge, 1975) the diagnosis was:

Axis I: Unsocialized Conduct Disorder.
Axis II: Mixed Specific Developmental Disorder.
Axis III: Normal Intelligence.
Axis IV: No Associated Physical Disorder.
Axis V: Discordant intra-familial relationships.
            Lack of warmth in intra-familial relationships.
            Inadequate or inconsistent parental control.
            Inadequate or distorted intra-familial communication.

Associated disorders

Conduct disorders often occur along with other psychiatric disorders,
notably attention deficit/hyperkinetic syndromes (see Chapter 8),
specific reading disability (Chapter 10), and depression (Chapter 6).

Attention-deficit hyperactivity disorder (ADHD) and the hyperkinetic syndrome

The distinction between these disorders and conduct disorders is not
as clear in clinical practice as reading the DSM-III-R manual, for
example, might suggest. Shapiro and Garfinkel (1986), studying a
population of 315 elementary school children, found 'inattentive-
overactive symptoms suggestive of attention deficit disorder (ADD)
(the DSM-III predecessor of ADHD) in 2.3 per cent and 'aggressive/
oppositional symptoms suggestive of conduct disorder' in 3.6 per cent;
but another 3.0 per cent had both ADD and conduct disorder
symptoms. The symptoms of the two disorders could not be clearly
differentiated. The two types of behavioural reaction may lie on a
continuum with overlap in the middle.

Reading disability

The association between conduct disorders and reading retardation emerged clearly in the Isle of Wight study (Rutter, Tizard and Whitmore, 1970). One-third of the children with conduct disorders were retarded in reading, and one-third of those with reading retardation had conduct disorders. The same association was found in a later study in a London borough (Rutter *et al.*, 1975). Research has not yet determined whether the behaviour problems are a consequence, in part, of the reading problems, or *vice versa*; or whether there are common factors contributing to both sets of problems. Follow-up studies suggest, however, that the combination of reading retardation and behavioural problems often leads to serious difficulties later (Maughan *et al.*, 1985).

Depression

Puig-Antich (1982) reported that 37 per cent of 47 pre-pubertal boys with 'major depression' also met the DSM-III criteria for conduct disorder. Moreover the boys' behaviour improved when the depression responded to treatment with the antidepressant imipramine, and worsened again in cases in which the depression later recurred.

Marriage *et al.* (1986) report that of 33 children and adolescents with affective disorders, 11 (33 per cent) also met the DSM-III criteria for conduct disorder. Ten of these had dysthymic disorders (see Chapter 9) and one suffered from major depression. These two studies, and that of Chiles *et al.* (1980), suggest that it is advisable to look for associated depression or dysthymia in children with conduct disorders.

Oppositional defiant disorders

DSM-III-R distinguishes 'oppositional defiant disorders' from conduct disorders, as being characterized by generally milder antisocial behaviour which does not violate 'the basic rights of others'. Minor rules may be violated, and there may be temper tantrums, argumentativeness, provocative behaviour and stubborness.

Oppositional defiant disorders probably represent problems in the socialization process similar to those responsible for conduct disorders but of a lesser degree. The difference between the two syndromes appears more quantitative than qualitative. Some oppositional disorders progress to become conduct disorders, while others resolve, with or without professional help.

Treatment of conduct and oppositional disorders

In both these groups of children there has been a failure of the process whereby children learn social rules and customs. Treatment should therefore correct or promote this process. A' basic prerequisite is a careful assessment of child, family and the wider environment, especially the school. This assessment, and the formulation arising from it, should point to the factors that have led to failure in the socialization process, so that treatment can address these.

Some causative factors are more susceptible to therapeutic intervention than others but we will consider in turn each of the categories we have defined. In the early stages of the development of antisocial behaviour, attention to the following issues may prevent the emergence of a serious conduct disorder later.

Constitutional factors

Chromosome abnormalities or a child's *genetic make-up* cannot, in the present state of our knowledge, be altered. Yet their consequences sometimes can be, as in the dietary treatment of children with phenylketonuria. We know also that genetic factors, and the results of intrauterine and birth hazards, play their parts in determining a child's intelligence and temperamental characteristics, and this knowledge can be useful in treatment. Thus explaining to parents, and sometimes teachers, what a child's intellectual and temperamental attributes are, may help them provide a suitable environment for that child's development. Many parents blame themselves when their child proves to have a 'difficult' constellation of temperamental traits, or below average intelligence. Being reassured that their upbringing of the child is not the cause may relieve the guilt they feel; also being told how they can promote their child's healthy development may encourage them and enhance their self-esteem as parents.

Physical disease and injury

Similar considerations apply to physical handicaps and disorders, problems with reading and other specific learning difficulties. When these can be rectified they should be; in other cases the nature of the child's handicap(s) or difficulties should be explained to all concerned, and the necessary modifications made to school and other programmes.

Temperamental factors and 'goodness of fit'

Although there is little systematic knowledge of how to improve the goodness of fit between children's temperaments and those of their parents, efforts to do this are indicated when the fit is poor. Counselling the parents, especially of young children whose behaviour is developing along antisocial lines, is probably the best approach. Once a child's temperamental style has been determined, a programme to deal with those features of it which are causing difficulty can usually be worked out. The principles of learning theory, discussed in Chapter 19, are useful here. Simply clarifying the nature of the temperamental clash may help, especially when dealing with the more perceptive and motivated families.

Environmental factors

Changes in the family environment are needed in many cases. Based upon Patterson's (1982) criteria for the development of antisocial behaviour, the parents may require to learn:

- to develop and apply well defined house rules, with clearly set expectations concerning routines for meals and other activities;
- to monitor consistently the behaviour of their children, so that they know what their children are doing and how they are feeling;
- to apply effective contingencies, that is consistent responses to the children's behaviour, following through with appropriate rewards and consequences when these are needed;
- effective techniques for dealing with crises or problems in the family, so that tensions and disputes are resolved before they get out of hand.

The following are possible means of achieving the above:

(a) Parental counselling
This may be done individually with parental couples (or with single parents when only one is available), or in group settings. The use of behaviour therapy principles and techniques (see below and Chapter 19) is a good basis for this work. Many centres offer group counselling for the parents of disturbed children and there are also many 'self-help' groups with similar aims.

(b) Family therapy
The range of family therapy approaches and techniques now available offers many possible ways of improving family functioning. They are discussed below and in Chapter 19.

Changes in the school environment may also be required. How these may be achieved is also discussed below and in Chapter 19.

Treating severe, established conduct disorders

Many gloomy statements have been made about the response of conduct disorders to treatment, and most conventional treatment approaches yield poor results (Shamsie, 1981). Anna Freud (1970) believed that children with seriously defective conscience formation, a characteristic of many of those with severe conduct disorders, needed not psychotherapy, but specially skilled substitute parents. Nowadays things look more hopeful, mainly because we have developed effective methods of behaviour therapy, and techniques for improving the functioning of families.

Family Therapy
When children present with severe conduct disorders, there are often found to be major problems in their family systems, as in the cases of both Robin and Paul, mentioned earlier in the chapter. Radical changes in such families may be needed before the children's behavioural problems can be resolved. It is often not enough to tell parents they should provide the 'house rules' and make the other changes advocated above; these families are too disturbed for straightforward instructions of this sort to be effective. Changes in the family system are necessary first. Treatment of the whole family is usually needed to achieve this. In a sense the child's behaviour problems are reframed as features of the way the family as a whole functions; the latter then becomes the focus of treatment.

Family therapy is discussed further in Chapter 19, and more fully in *Basic Family Therapy* (Barker, 1986). Some of the concepts and techniques of *Comprehensive Family Therapy* (Kirschner and Kirschner, 1986) are valuable in these cases. Metaphorical approaches (Barker, 1985, Chapter 6) can also be useful.

Behaviour therapy
Well planned behaviour therapy programmes, instituted with attention to detail, seem to be the most effective direct means of treating severe conduct disorders. The active participation of parents and other involved adults is essential, and some preliminary work to stabilize the family system may be needed. Patterson (1976) has been a pioneer in the development of such programmes. His books *Living with Families* (Patterson and Gullion, 1968) and *Families* (Patterson, 1971), both of which are designed for use by parents, are excellent adjuncts to such

programmes. Behaviour therapy is also discussed further in Chapter 19.

Other therapeutic options

The school environment often requires attention too. Sometimes changes in the way children are dealt with in school, including the use of behaviour therapy techniques, can contribute to the treatment plan. We cannot usually bring about radical changes in the social structures of schools but contacts with teachers, school counsellors and school psychologists can be invaluable. They may provide school staff with a better understanding of the needs of the child and the family. Also important are good relationships and close co-operation between family and school. In cases of truancy it is essential that the parents have an arrangement with the school staff to ensure that any failure to attend on their child's part is immediately detected.

Berg (1985) provides an excellent summary of how truancy is managed in Britain. A wide variety of services and professionals may be involved, including the legal system. A remarkably successful device for the 'less disturbed' truants seems to be the 'adjournment procedure'; the court simply adjourns the case for a few weeks to give time for school attendance to be re-established. A few adjournments 2 to 4 weeks apart may be enough to restore satisfactory attendance and 'possibly to reduce delinquent behaviour' (Berg, 1985).

In some cases a change of school or teacher can be helpful. The question of 'goodness of fit' between teachers and pupils has not, as far as I know, been investigated scientifically. But clinical experience suggests that some teachers find children with certain kinds of temperament particularly exasperating. Moving a child to another teacher's class may then be of salutory benefit. We know also that the social climates of schools vary (Rutter *et al.*, 1979). This is probably why a change of school can be helpful, occasionally marking a turning point in the school career of a child who seemed headed for behavioural disaster.

Individual psychotherapy has long been the mainstay of much child psychiatric treatment, but it generally yields poor results in the treatment of children with conduct disorders. These children usually have little or no motivation to engage in psychotherapy. It is rarely they who are complaining about the presenting problems, and they may get some vicarious satisfaction from their behaviour. But in the minority of children in whom there is a high level of consciously felt anxiety, or who have a strong conscious desire to alter their way of life, individual therapy may be of benefit. In such cases, an emphasis on enhancing self-esteem, combined with Ericksonian techniques designed to enable the subject to gain access to psychological resources which hitherto have not been used (see Chapter 19), seem most helpful.

Group psychotherapy suffers from some of the same disadvantages as individual therapy. Nevertheless, groups which enhance the young person's self-esteem, or provide these children with opportunities to learn new social or vocational skills – for example drama, dance, martial arts, ceramics, gymnastics, carpentry or metalworking – can help.

Residential treatment has often been advocated for children with severe conduct disorders but its results have been generally disappointing (Romig, 1978; Shamsie, 1981). The best results seem to be those of centres using well planned and intensive behaviour therapy methods. These should be combined with family work, designed especially to teach the parents the behaviour therapy principles and practices used in the residential setting. It is relatively easy, by providing a highly structured residential environment and strict behavioural controls, to achieve improvement in the behaviour of most conduct disordered children, but such changes are of little value if they do not persist after return to the community. Intimate involvement of the parents seems to help achieve this.

Some programmes use the 'therapeutic community' concept. This may be applied in both residential and day treatment, especially of adolescents. The treatment is structured so that the main therapeutic agent is the community, and the considerable pressure it can exert on individuals. Related to such programmes is 'positive peer culture', a treatment approach in which group process and the influence of the young person's peers are used as the main change-promoting agents (Vorrath and Brendthro, 1985).

Day treatment offers an alternative to residential treatment, and has the advantage that the young person is not separated from the rest of the family full-time. When the child is at home in the evenings and during weekends, the family members are together and can practise what they are learning in treatment. Progress must be monitored, and input offered as necessary, by the treatment staff.

Other environmental change. The influence of the neighbourhood environment is even harder to modify than that of the school, unless the family can move to another neighbourhood. When you consider suggesting such a move it is well to bear in mind that neighbourhood influences are not usually the central problem, but merely contributory. The family system is more important, though some families function better after a move to a different environment.

Medication. Pharmacological treatment has little if any role to play in the treatment of conduct disorders, unless there is associated epilepsy, in which case anticonvulsant medication is indicated. In some treatment centres tranquillisers such as chlorpromazine or haloperidol are occasionally used to control acutely and violently aggressive young people, but in adequately staffed units this should not be necessary. Drugs are not an effective treatment for conduct disorders. Their use also runs the risk of giving the young person and the family the message that there is a 'magical' pharmacological solution to the problems. In reality what is usually needed is the learning of new social skills, the incorporation into the subject's personality of new values and beliefs, the acquisition of improved relationship skills and, usually, changes in the family system. The danger of drug dependence, or at least espousing the idea that there is a chemical solution to these problems, is real.

Treatment of associated conditions

Reading retardation, when present, should be tackled energetically by means of intensive remedial education. Although the reading problem may not be the cause of the behaviour problems, its persistence makes it harder to achieve improvement in the child's self-esteem, as well as making school a difficult environment for the child. By the time they present for treatment, many of these children are so retarded in their reading that much of what their peers are doing is beyond them; they may even be unable to read the instructions relating to other subjects such as mathematics or science.

Depression should also receive appropriate treatment (see Chapter 9). Puig-Antich (1982) reported behavioural improvement in depressed children with conduct disorder symptoms when the depression resolved, the symptoms returning with recurrence of depression.

Associated attention deficit disorders should be treated as set out in Chapters 9 and 19. This may involve the use of methylphenidate or one of the other available drugs.

Severe emotional deprivation, when it accompanies conduct disorders, presents a special therapeutic challenge. Children who have suffered such deprivation from early in life, or through a long period of their childhood, often seem lacking in the capacity to form deep and satisfying emotional relationships. Neither psychotherapy nor a simple change of environment is likely to be a sufficient treatment. Sometimes a long period of treatment in a specialized residential setting offers the best hope of effecting improvement, but highly skilled care and continuity of staffing are essential. Theoretically a good foster home might be better, but few foster parents have the resources to cope with such children, from whom they may get little response over a long period, while at the same time being subject to constant, and often very distressing 'testing out' behaviour. Furthermore, failure and rejection from the home would be yet another adverse experience for the child. Some schemes have, however, been specially devised to select, train and support suitable alternative families (Hazel, 1977; Rubinstein, 1977; Barker *et al.*, 1978).

Outcome

Most minor and some major conduct disorders clear up without treatment. Some are related to difficulties the child or the family may be having in surmounting developmental hurdles; when these are overcome the behavioural symptoms may subside. In other cases psychosocial stress, in the family or outside it, contributes and the resolution of the stress results in improvement in the child's behaviour. Much depends on the basic stability of the family, parental attitudes, the child's personality and temperament, and whether there are continuing stresses facing the child or the family as a whole.

Children with severe conduct disorders, especially those who have appeared in court, tend in adult life to have a high incidence of psychiatric illness and often show antisocial and criminal behaviour (Rutter, 1980b). Robins' (1966) study of a large child guidance clinic population, almost all of whom were traced in adult life, suggested a poor outlook for the later social adjustment of children who had had conduct disorders. The group she followed up, however, had little treatment when they were children. It may be that modern treatment has altered this, though hard data are lacking.

The combination of conduct disorder symptoms with reading retardation seems often to lead to a particularly poor outcome, at least in boys with severe reading problems, of average ability or below, from mainly working class backgrounds, such as were followed up by Maughan *et al.* (1985). They had high rates of early school leaving, unstable work records and seriously depressed skill levels.

Chapter 5

Neurotic, Anxiety and Emotional Disorders

Definition and classification

Each of the three terms in the chapter title has been used to describe disorders in which the basic feature is an abnormally high level of anxiety. The anxiety may not be expressed directly, however. These disorders sometimes present as unduly severe reactions to environmental stress, which may be quite minor; in other cases there is no obvious stress to which they can be attributed.

Psychiatrists are not agreed on how these disorders should be labelled and classified. ICD-9 has categories for 'neurotic disorders' and for 'disturbance of emotions specific to childhood and adolescence'. The latter are defined as 'less well differentiated emotional disorders characteristic of the childhood period', and the following subcategories are listed:

- with anxiety and fearfulness;
- with misery and unhappiness;
- with sensitivity, shyness and social withdrawal;
- relationship problems;
- other or mixed.

DSM-III-R, in its section on 'disorders usually first evident in infancy, childhood, or adolescence', has a category for 'anxiety disorders of childhood and adolescence'. These are divided into:

- separation anxiety disorder;
- avoidant disorder of childhood and adolescence;
- over-anxious disorder;

In the general sections of DSM-III-R, which apply to adults and children, there are also listed many categories, all of which may be regarded as being expressions of or reactions to anxiety. They are listed in three groups:

(1) Anxiety Disorders:

- Panic disorders, with or without agoraphobia.

- Agoraphobia without a history of panic disorder.
- Social phobia.
- Simple phobia
- Obsessive compulsive disorder (or neurosis).
- Post-traumatic stress disorder.
- Generalized anxiety disorder.
- Anxiety disorder not otherwise specified.

(2) Somatoform disorders:

- Body dysmorphic disorder (dysmorphophobia).
- Conversion disorder (or hysterical neurosis, conversion type).
- Hypochondriasis (or hypochondriacal neurosis).
- Somatization disorder.
- Somatoform pain disorder.
- Undifferentiated somatoform disorder.
- Somatoform disorder not otherwise specified.

(3) Dissociative disorders (hysterical neuroses, dissociative type).

- Multiple personality disorder.
- Psychogenic fugue.
- Psychogenic amnesia.
- Depersonalization disorder.
- Dissociative disorder not otherwise specified.

As a group these conditions are distinct from conduct disorders, in which the primary symptom is antisocial behaviour rather than anxiety. Hersov (1985a) prefers the term 'emotional disorders' to cover the broad spectrum of conditions in which emotional distress, rather than antisocial behaviour, is the essential feature. He points out that there is good evidence, from research studies, of the many distinctions between these two major groups of child psychiatric disorders (Hewitt and Jenkins, 1946; Quay, 1979; Achenbach and Edelbrock, 1983). He also includes depressive disorders with this group, though we shall consider them separately in Chapter 6.

Prevalence

'Emotional' disorders were detected in 2.5 per cent of the 10- and 11-year-olds in the Isle of Wight (Rutter, Tizard and Whitmore, 1970). In the London borough studied later, the prevalence rate was found to be about twice that in the Isle of Wight (Rutter, Cox *et al.*, 1973). In the Ontario Child Health Study (Offord *et al.*, 1987), the following percentage prevalence rates for emotional disorder and 'somatization' were found:

Age	Emotional disorder	Somatization	Age	Emotional disorder	Somatization
Boys 4–11	10.2	–	Girls 4–11	10.7	–
12–16	4.9	4.5	12–16	13.6	10.7
4–16	7.9	–	4–16	11.9	–

'Somatization' was defined as the presence of recurrent, multiple and vague physical symptoms without evident physical cause in children who perceived themselves as sickly. Many of these symptoms may have been somatic expressions of anxiety.

These results are rather different from those of the Isle of Wight study. The discrepancies are probably due to a combination of factors including the wider age range studied in Ontario, real differences between the two populations, and the use of different research methods and definitions. A striking feature of the Ontario study is the high overall prevalence of emotional disorder (11.9 per cent) as compared with conduct disorders (2.7 per cent) in girls. In boys the prevalence rates for emotional disorders (7.9 per cent) and conduct disorders (8.1 per cent) are similar, but these figures conceal the fact that neuroses were more common in younger boys and conduct disorders in adolescent boys.

Causes

As usual we have to consider constitutional, temperamental and environmental factors, and the effects of physical disease and injury. The role of genetic factors is not well established except that in some family trees there has been shown to be a genetic relationship between obsessive-compulsive disorders, Gilles de la Tourette's syndrome and chronic tics (see Chapter 12). It seems that autosomal dominant transmission is involved, and that the inherited disorder may be expressed either as chronic tics, Tourette's syndrome or obsessive-compulsive disorder (Pauls and Leckman, 1986). It is probable, however, that only some obsessive-compulsive disorders are inherited in this way.

The threshold for the development of neurotic anxiety (that is anxiety that is excessive in relation to the realities of the individual's situation) varies from person to person. We know very little, however, about the precise roles of constitutional and temperamental factors in contributing to this variation. In practice we are limited to making clinical judgments. These are based on the history of the child's past anxiety-proneness, and consideration of how far other factors, such as parental handling of the child or family systems problems, can explain current anxiety levels and ways of reacting to stress. It is clear, though, that some children are relatively anxiety-prone, while others are relatively invulnerable.

Physical diseases and disorders may contribute to the development of anxiety in either of two ways. They may lead to the child becoming anxious, for example as a result of having severe attacks of asthma which may realistically arouse fear of dying; or they may provoke anxious and overprotective attitudes in parents and others concerned with the care of the child. Sometimes both processes operate, and it can be difficult to distinguish the two.

Environmental contributory factors are often prominent. Sometimes the appearance of anxiety symptoms marks the culmination of a long series of stresses. The adverse or unhelpful attitudes of parents and others over the years may have had cumulative effects. Relevant questions are: How much has the child been allowed to mix with other children, and to make his or her own decisions? Has too much been done or decided for the child? How secure is the relationship of the child to the parents and the rest of the family? These and related issues all affect a child's capacity to cope with particular situations, especially stressful ones. Children brought up by worrying, anxious parents, perhaps themselves suffering from neurotic conditions, tend to become that way themselves. It is impossible in clinical practice to know how far this is due to the operation of genetic factors and how much the anxious atmosphere in the home is responsible; but children of parents who see the world as an anxious, threatening place in which they feel insecure, tend to view it that way too.

The concept of emotional maturity is helpful. At any particular age, the normal child has learned to cope with a range of emotionally stressful situations, and the extent to which a child can deal with stress without becoming excessively anxious is one measure of emotional maturity. Childhood should be a process of progressively decreasing dependence on parents, as the child learns to cope with more and more challenges without outside support. When this process has been slowed, halted or even reversed, the likelihood of neurotic symptoms appearing is greater. Children who are faced with more anxiety and stress than they can cope with may regress to an earlier stage of development. The symptoms often express the child's conflicts in a symbolic way. Anna Freud (1966) defined 'fixation points' as points at which psychosexual development is held up, as a result of excessive frustration, excessive gratification or a traumatic experience. The point at which fixation occurs depends on development to date; fixation will normally occur where a developmental phase has not been negotiated successfully, nor the relevant conflicts resolved.

How do the family and other environmental factors work to cause, or contribute to, the disorders we are discussing? According to psychodynamic theory, consciously felt anxiety is always due in part, and often almost entirely, to causes of which the subject is unaware at the conscious level. The repressed conflicts are considered to be concerned with difficulties over the handling of sexual, aggressive and other impulses. Such difficulties are likely to arise in children who have experienced unsatisfactory and insecure relationships with their parents, especially during their early years. The processes of development outlined in Chapter 1 have been distorted. The anxiety and guilt aroused by the Oedipal conflict, for example, are more easily, quickly and satisfactorily overcome in the context of secure relationships with the parents. If these relationships are tainted by anxiety and unpredictable, gross changes of parental mood, the child may have difficulty dealing with the stresses associated with the various demands of growing up. Children who do not feel able to depend on and trust their parents may come to see the world generally as threatening and hostile. Yet because of children's different strengths, temperaments and personalities, there is much variation in how they respond to situations of this sort.

Behaviourists, such as Eysenck (1959), view the genesis of neurotic symptoms rather differently. They regard neurotic symptoms as learned behaviour. The symptoms themselves are the neurosis and, behaviourists in their purest culture would say, there is no need to postulate unconscious or other underlying causes. Indeed they believe that behaviours generally, whether considered normal or abnormal, are due to the effects on the individuals concerned of environmental contingencies.

Rossi (1986a; 1986b) draws attention to the concept of 'state-dependent' learning and its relevance to the development of psychiatric symptoms. Information learned and experiences undergone can often be recalled only in situations similar to those in which they were first learned or experienced – that is, they are 'state-bound' or 'state-dependent'. Rossi goes on to suggest that:

'So-called "psychological conflict" is a metaphor for competing patterns of state-dependent memory and learning. Reframing therapeutic concepts in terms of state-bound patterns of information and behaviour renders them immediately (1) more amenable to operational definition for experimental study in the laboratory, and (2) more available for active, therapeutic utilization than the traditional process of "analysis" and "understanding".' (Rossi, 1986b, page 233.)

The idea that neurotic and other psychiatric symptoms may be understood in terms of state-dependent learning has not yet been widely accepted by psychiatrists. There is nevertheless much evidence to support it. Both the Isle of Wight study (Rutter, Tizard and Whitmore, 1970) and the Ontario Child Health Study (Offord *et al.*, 1987) found that children were rarely identified as disturbed both by their teachers and by their parents. Of the children with neuroses identified in the Ontario study, 50 per cent of the boys and 23.9 per cent of the girls were identified by their parents only; 43 per cent of the boys and 64.6 per cent of the girls either by the teacher or the youth concerned; and only 6.9 per cent of the boys and 11.5 per cent of the girls by both sources. These findings suggest that children's emotional disorders are highly context-dependent, and support the idea that they are manifestations of state-dependent learning.

Another way to understand how environmental factors may lead to the development of anxiety in a child (or in any family member) is by means of family systems theory (see Chapter 2). This takes the family group as the basic unit to be considered. Pathological degrees of anxiety in children are often associated with dysfunctional family situations. In such families children may find themselves playing idiosyncratic and stressful roles. These can lead to high levels of anxiety. The relationship of anxiety to family functioning is discussed more fully in Chapter 6 of the book *Anxiety in Children* (Barker, 1984).

Yet another way of looking at the environmental causes of childhood anxiety is to use the concepts of attachment theory (Bowlby 1969; 1979). Heard (1982) discusses the roles of 'care-giving' and 'care-seeking' behaviours, which she considers in-built, interpersonal and complementary; also of exploratory behaviour which may be contrasted with attachment behaviour. The caregiver normally assists the child in dealing with anxiety-provoking situations; these stimulate attachment behaviour (see Chapter 1), and lead the child to go to the caregiver for help. Heard (1982) describes two forms of ineffective caregiving. In the first, this is experienced as underactive, fear-evoking and unresponsive; in the second it is experienced as overactive, fear-evoking and impinging. The child may react to ineffective caregiving in various ways:

● continuous unassuaged attachment behaviour;
● frustrated, inhibited and anxious exploratory behaviour;
● anxious exploration;
● frustrated and inhibited exploration.

In all of the above there is a failure of the caregiver to respond in such a way as to terminate the attachment behaviour, and relieve the anxiety which led to it.

This approach is but another way of looking at processes that may occur in dysfunctional families; no doubt the problems some parents have in acting as effective caregivers are related to some of their own personal problems, and to the properties of the family system.

Finally we must not overlook the importance of the wider social environment, especially the school. Academic or social problems in school may contribute to neurotic disorders, especially in anxiety-prone children.

In summary, there are several ways the development of anxiety disorders in children can be understood. The individual psychotherapist will examine the child's intrapsychic processes for factors there; the behaviourist will investigate the child's learning experiences in terms of environmental contingencies; the family therapist will look at the total family system to try to understand the child's symptoms in light of the functioning and structure of the system; and the therapist with a special interest in attachment theory will look closely at attachment processes for difficulties there. In addition, the concepts of the 'goodness of fit' between the parents' and the child's temperaments (see Chapter 2), and of state-dependent learning and behaviour, offer yet other ways of looking at these situations. These approaches are not mutually exclusive and all may be of practical value to the clinician seeking to understand the genesis of anxiety and neurotic disorders.

Description

Anxiety disorders are rarely diagnosed in infancy. While infants can certainly appear upset, as evidenced by crying, sleeplessness and irritability, it is uncertain whether such reactions are of the same nature as the anxiety states of older children. There are many things that may cause such behaviour, for example hunger, cold, physical diseases, tension in the family and disruption of routine.

According to DSM-III-R, 'avoidant disorder of childhood' may develop as early as two-and-a-half, and 'separation anxiety disorder' at 'pre-school age'. In practice these disorders can rarely be defined and diagnosed with any confidence before about four or five years of age, that is the period when the child's use of mental defence mechanisms is emerging. At this age, many children who are developing quite normally display irrational fears of such things as flies, birds, dogs, earthworms, wind, the dark and other items they have not yet become familiar with and do not understand. In older children such fear would be abnormal and might be a symptom of an anxiety disorder, so in diagnosis the patient's age, and the normal stress tolerance for that age, must be taken into account.

Neurotic/anxiety disorders in children tend to be less fixed and chronic than the equivalent disorders occurring in adults, so that response to treatment and prognosis are generally better. They often disturb the family and people in the child's environment as much as, or more than, they do the child; in this respect neurotic children differ from neurotic adults, who often live their lives without causing distress to others.

We will now review the various categories of neurotic/anxiety disorders, though some of the sub-groups, especially those distinguished in DSM-III-R, will be grouped together for discussion.

Anxiety states (or anxiety neuroses)

We will consider here a broad group of syndromes, covering ICD-9's 'disturbance of emotions specific to childhood and adolescence, with anxiety and fearfulness'; DSM-III-R's 'separation anxiety disorder', 'avoidant disorder' and 'over-anxious disorder'; ICD-9's 'anxiety states'; and DSM-III-R's 'anxiety disorders', with its subcategories listed above. The subcategory of 'obsessive-compulsive disorder' is considered separately later.

In anxiety states and related disorders, the subject's anxiety is directly expressed. These children may be shy, timid and clinging, emotionally immature, overdependent on their parents and poor at mixing with other children. They may fear loss of family, or death or other disaster. They may have difficulty in getting to sleep, and their sleep may be disturbed by dreams, nightmares or frequent waking. There may be 'free-floating anxiety', that is anxiety which comes to be associated with any situation the child may be experiencing. Such anxiety is often perceived as arising from within, rather than from the environment. Distractibility and impaired concentration may accompany feelings of general apprehension.

Common somatic manifestations of anxiety in these children are loss of appetite, feelings of nausea, abdominal pain, diarrhoea, vomiting, headaches, dry mouth, rapid heart beat, cold and clammy hands, dizziness, sweating, increased frequency of micturition and palpitations. Restlessness and feelings of tension are also often present. Symptoms of this type characterize the 'generalized anxiety disorders' of DSM-III-R.

Panic attacks may occur in the course of an anxiety state. They are characterized by the sudden onset of extreme fear, sometimes with a sense of impending doom and often with such physical symptoms as shortness of breath, palpitations, sweating, faintness and trembling or shaking. Subjects who suffer panic attacks may or may not also have agoraphobia (see below).

Separation anxiety is manifest on separation, or the threat or fear of separation, from attachment figures, usually the parents and more often the mother than the father. DSM-III-R's 'separation anxiety disorder' is defined as a disturbance lasting at least two weeks, characterized by unrealistic fears or worries about separation from a 'major attachment figure'; reluctance or refusal to be separated from, or go to sleep without being near to, such a person; and excessive distress, perhaps with physical symptoms such as headaches, abdominal pain or vomiting, on separation, or the threat of separation from an attachment figure. There may be nightmares involving separation themes. The symptoms of school refusal, discussed in a later section, are often present.

DSM-III-R's 'avoidant disorder' and 'overanxious disorder' are variants of anxiety states. In the former there is persistent and excessive shrinking from strangers. At the same time the child seeks social involvement with family members and other familiar figures. DSM-III-R's 'overanxious disorders' are anxiety states of milder severity than generalized anxiety states. These children worry excessively about future events such as examinations, the possibility of injury, meeting deadlines, inclusion in peer activities, performing chores and the like. Physical concomitants of anxiety and sleep problems may also be present.

Most of these disorders would be classified as 'disturbances of emotions specific to childhood and adolescence – with anxiety and fearfulness', on the ICD-9 scheme. Whether there is any real advantage in dividing them into the more numerous categories of DSM-III-R is uncertain. The DSM-III-R descriptions do however provide an overview of the range of symptoms these children may experience.

Phobic states or disorders

In phobic disorders there is persistent and irrational fear of specific objects, activities or situations. This leads to avoidance of the objects or situations. The fear may be due to the defence mechanism of displacement, that is it is transferred from its true, but unconscious, source to the phobic object. Thus the agarophobic person who is afraid of going out of the house is effectively prevented from having to deal with many situations which might be met with away from the security of home.

The phobic object or objects may change during the course of the illness. While they may dominate the clinical picture, phobias are sometimes but one feature, even a minor and transient one, of a neurotic disorder with predominantly, for example, anxiety symptoms as described in the previous section. There is an almost infinite variety of phobic objects, for example buses, dogs, cats, doctors, dentists, heights, enclosed spaces, open spaces, shops, crowds, snakes, insects and so on.

Monosymptomatic phobias, called 'simple phobias' in DSM-III-R, are sometimes encountered in children. The child has a severe and perhaps handicapping fear of a particular object or situation. Such isolated phobias may differ in their etiology from other neurotic disorders, in that they are not usually accompanied by general emotional immaturity and their development is more easily under-. stood on the basis of learning theory. Their development may be understood in terms of state-dependent learning; fear and avoidance of a particular situation sometimes seems to be learned in the course of experiencing a single frightening experience. These phobias respond better to behaviour therapy than the more complex phobic disorders.

Agarophobia is uncommon in childhood and early adolescence, though it sometimes starts in late adolescence. Its main feature is severe and handicapping fear of being alone or in public places from which escape is difficult. Panic attacks are sometimes a feature of the condition.

Social phobia, which may occur in late childhood or adolescence, is defined in DSM-III-R as a persistent, irrational fear of situations in which the subject is exposed to possible scrutiny by others. It may be manifest, for example, when the person is asked to speak or perform in public, or when using public lavatories, eating in public, or writing in the presence of others. As in the other phobic conditions we have discussed, the subject recognizes that the fear is excessive or unreasonable, and is consequently distressed by it.

Although the term 'school phobia' has long been used to describe a certain form of reluctance to go to school, it is a complex condition and better termed 'school refusal'. It is discussed below.

Fears and phobias of childhood are discussed by Berecz (1968), Miller *et al.* (1974) and Ferrari (1986).

Obsessive-compulsive disorders

These disorders are characterized by obsessional thoughts – that is, intrusive thoughts and ideas which persist despite conscious awareness of their unreasonableness and resistance to them. Compulsions are actions arising from such thoughts.

Prevalence

The prevalence of obsessive-compulsive disorders in children and adolescents may be about 0.3 per cent (Rapoport, 1986). Adams (1973) reported that they comprised about 1 per cent of referrals to a child psychiatric clinic.

Description

Although minor forms of obsessive-compulsive behaviour, like avoiding the cracks in concrete paths, touching lamp standards as they are passed, and feeding and bedtime rituals, are quite common, in obsessive-compulsive disorders the symptoms are more severe and persistent, and interfere with the child's life. There is a 'discontinuity from normal development' (Rapoport, 1986). There are often repetitive, ritualistic activities which may seem purposeful, such as hand washing. Yet they are carried out needlessly because of an irrational, 'magical' belief that they will prevent some undesired event from happening or otherwise influence the course of events. Complex rituals are sometimes observed. One boy had to shut the dining room door three times and then touch each corner of the table before he could start his meal. Obsessions and compulsions are unwelcome, unpleasant and disturbing to the individual. Psychodynamic theory regards them as the results of a mental defence mechanism against unconscious anxiety, a sort of magical means of coping with an underlying problem.

Adams (1973) reviewed the cases of 49 obsessive-compulsive children, 29 boys and 20 girls. The symptoms usually started about age 6, with referral coming on average about 4 years later. More than half the children also had phobias.

> Barry was referred at age nine. He was said always to have been fussy about cleaning his hands, which he washed unduly frequently. For six months he had been avoiding imaginary lumps in the carpet. He would take a long time saying his prayers at night in case 'something' went wrong or because he thought he might have made a mistake and so had to start over again; and he had other obsessive-compulsive symptoms. Barry acknowledged that these ideas and actions were irrational and tried to resist them, but without success.

After outpatient treatment had failed and because Barry was becoming increasingly depressed and withdrawn and was expressing a fear of dying, he was admitted for inpatient treatment. On admission he was tearful and communicated little with the other children. He was always clean and well dressed, but quiet and unassertive. It soon became clear that his whole life was ruled by rituals. For example, he had to get his clothes out of his locker without touching the locker; he had to cut his food into very small pieces before he would eat it; when getting his books out of his 'tidy box' in school he had to bring them backwards and forwards, four times, across the side of the box; and he would only walk across the dining room by a particular route. He also had complicated rituals for going to bed.

Eventually Barry told us that the reason for most of his habits, as he called them, was that he was afraid something would happen to his parents if he did not carry them out. He was an intellectually bright boy but reluctant to say much about his feelings or to talk about family relationships.

Psychotherapy with Barry proved difficult. He was passive and uncommunicative at interview. Instead, a behaviour modification approach (see Chapter 19), to be applied both in the treatment centre and at home during weekends was developed. This had considerable success, reducing his symptoms almost to none. His parents were cooperative professional people, and the family seemed a stable one, though his mother presented as unduly anxious about Barry. This seemed to antedate the onset of the obsessive-compulsive symptoms and Barry's mother had probably tended to 'infantilize' him long after he had ceased to be an infant.

Comment

This is an example of quite a severe obsessive-compulsive disorder in a prepubertal child. Treatment was difficult and extended, with outpatient treatment following Barry's inpatient stay, over more than two years.

Obsessional symptoms are sometimes seen in children who have other anxiety symptoms or neurotic disorders. For example, Tracie, whose case history appears later in this chapter, showed compulsive hand washing before admission. This continued for a few days after admission but disappeared as her anxiety lessened. Obsessive-compulsive symptoms frequently accompany Tourette's syndrome (see Chapter 12), though Tourette's syndrome less often occurs along with obsessive-compulsive disorders (Rapoport, 1986). As we have seen, there is a genetic connection between obsessive-compulsive disorders and Tourette's syndrome in some families (Pauls and Leckman, 1986).

Treatment of obsessive-compulsive disorders

Psychodynamic treatments are generally ineffective (Rapoport, 1986). Behaviour therapy may yield better results. The technique of 'response prevention' comprises a programme of consistently preventing the compulsive behaviours, if necessary by physically restraining the patient from carrying them out (Stanley, 1980). In many instances, by the time the child is referred for treatment the family and others concerned with the child have fallen into the habit of 'giving in' to the rituals; that is they modify the environment so that the child is allowed extra time to dress, prepare for bed and so on. This usually makes things worse rather than better.

I report elsewhere (Barker, 1985, pages 120-122) the case of an 11-year-old girl with a severe obsessive-compulsive disorder,who was successfully treated by prescribing alternative rituals. These were specific forms of exercise which she did not much enjoy, to be carried out whenever any ritualistic activity was observed. Devising such therapeutic rituals may hold promise as an approach to these disorders, since it uses the subject's obsessive characteristics to therapeutic advantage.

The results of a controlled trial of the antidepressant drug clomipramine suggest that this may be a useful adjunct in the treatment of these children, as it appears to be in adults (Flament *et al.*, 1985).

Outcome in obsessive-compulsive disorders

Adams (1973) reported that the outcome is usually good for a first attack of mild obsessional symptoms, but that chronic, long-established cases can be very difficult to treat. However, he relied on dynamic psychotherapy, which nowadays is not thought to be effective. Behaviour therapy, perhaps combined with medication, yields better results and the substitution of other symptoms when the obsessive ones disappear does not seem to happen.

Impulsions

Obsessive-compulsive symptoms should be distinguished from 'impulsions', as described by Bender and Shilder (1940). Impulsions include behaviour such as constantly looking at or handling an object, drawing the object, being preoccupied with an object in fantasy or thought, hoarding things, counting repeatedly and being preoccupied with numbers. The behaviour resembles compulsive behaviour, but there is a lack of conscious resistance to it. Impulsions are commoner in younger children (aged four to ten), while obsessive-compulsive phenomena occur more often in prepubertal children, adolescents and adults. Some older children and adolescents who present with obsessive-compulsive disorders have had impulsions when younger. Impulsions and compulsions sometimes occur together around puberty.

Hysteria, conversion disorders and dissociative states

These disorders fall into two main groups:

(1) Those characterized by physical symptoms which may suggest organic disease, although such disease cannot be demonstrated. DSM-III-R calls these 'somatoform disorders'.
(2) Dissociative disorders, in which there are psychogenic changes in the subject's consciousness, identity or motor behaviour. In all these conditions, the symptoms are usually understood as expressions of anxiety. The subject is consciously unaware of the underlying problem and is not malingering – that is, consciously elaborating symptoms which are not present. The symptoms are real to the patient, who is imperfectly aware or unaware of their psychogenic cause.

(1) Disorders with Physical Symptoms, or Somatoform Disorders

(a) *Somatization disorders*
These are also known as hysteria or Briquet's syndrome. The main feature is the presence of recurrent and multiple physical complaints, often described in dramatic, vague or exaggerated terms. The complaints may include visual problems, paralyses, seizures, pain in various parts of the body, especially the back and abdomen, dizziness, shortness of breath and headache. In older patients there may be complaints of psychosexual problems, painful menstruation and excessive menstrual bleeding. DSM-III-R arbitrarily requires there to be 13 symptoms, out of the list it provides, for the diagnosis to be valid.

Although the DSM-III-R manual states that the onset is usually in the teen years, disorders of this type occur also in younger children. They may not meet all the DSM-III-R diagnostic criteria, either because there are as yet too few symptoms or because they have not been present for 'several years'.

(b) *Conversion disorders or conversion hysteria*
Traditionally many of those who meet the DSM-III-R criteria for somatization disorder would have been regarded as having conversion disorders. In this condition the physical disorders are believed to represent the 'conversion' of anxiety into physical form. DSM-III-R, however, makes more restrictive use of this term, confining it to cases where there is evidence of 'primary' or 'secondary' gain, and in which there is usually only a single symptom, suggesting physical disease, during each episode. The symptom may be blindness, paralysis, aphonia (the inability to speak except in a whisper), anaesthesia of a part of the body, seizures, disturbance of coordination or some other

symptom that bears a relation to the patient's understanding of neurological disorders.

'Primary gain' is a term used when the symptom serves to keep 'an internal conflict or need out of awareness'. Thus aphonia, or paralysis of an arm, may be a reaction to an argument in a person who has an inner conflict about the expression of rage; the symptom thus has symbolic significance in relation to the conflict.

'Secondary gain' is the term used when the symptom enables the subject to avoid situations that are unpleasant or anxiety-provoking to the person. The following is an example.

Joan, aged 13, was anxious about leaving home to go to school. Despite superior intelligence and a place at the top of her class, her relationships with other children in the school were poor. One Monday morning she complained of pain and weakness in her legs. The doctor was consulted and advised aspirin and a few days' rest in bed. The symptoms subsided and Joan returned to school. The same problems recurred on the first day of school after the half-term break. This time Joan was taken to a paediatrician who could find no evidence of physical illness. After two weeks off school, Joan again appeared well and she returned to school and completed the term.

On the first day of the next term Joan was again unable to go to school because she could not walk and had painful legs. A psychiatric cause was now considered by the parents and the family doctor. Joan had to be carried into the psychiatric consultation but despite her inability to walk she showed a bland indifference to her symptoms. Her social difficulties at school and a considerable fear of leaving her mother soon emerged in discussion; after three sessions she understood her physical symptoms as a means of avoiding going to school and the attendant anxieties. It appeared that she had unconsciously seen them as the only way available to her of avoiding school, which was acceptable to her ambitious parents. Her problems were tackled in the course of a series of psychotherapeutic interviews, while another therapist worked with the parents to help them recognize their part in the situation.

Joan's physical symptoms did not recur but she remained anxious about school and it was ten weeks before she was able to return. She then did so, without recurrence of pain or paralysis, and subsequently made good progress.

Comment

In this case the 'conversion' symptoms were partly a way of expressing anxiety, but also a means of avoiding an anxiety-provoking situation. Joan had some conscious awareness of her desire to remain at home rather than cope with the other children at school. Initially, however, she did not recognize that her physical symptoms were unconsciously motivated in the way in which they turned out to be. Her 'choice' of symptoms was probably related to her father's longstanding limp and pain, the result of a war wound.

While abdominal pain, sickness and other physical symptoms may arise in similar ways, the term 'conversion disorder' is usually reserved for conditions in which there is at least one major physical symptom and in which the anxiety has been repressed and replaced by the physical symptom(s). Because the symptoms serve the unconscious purpose of reducing consciously felt anxiety, the patient may show little or no concern about them, despite what appears to be a crippling disability. This is the oft-described *belle indifférence*, well displayed by Joan who, when first seen, expressed little concern about her inability to walk and smiled when describing the severity of her pain.

(c) Somatoform pain disorder
This DSM-III-R term simply describes conditions in which there is severe and prolonged pain, arising in much the same way as the symptoms in the two previous categories. It is really another form of conversion disorder.

(d) Hypochondriasis
In this disorder there is unrealistic interpretation of physical symptoms as indicating serious disease. The symptoms complained of may be quite minor ones such as awareness of the heart beat, sweating, supposed constipation, or intestinal peristalsis. The physically healthy person thus becomes convinced that he or she has a serious disease. This can become a major preoccupation seriously affecting the subject's life. Such conditions also have financial implications, since they can lead to large expenditures by the individuals concerned, or by health insurance agencies or state-run health services.

(e) Undifferentiated somatoform disorders and somatoform disorders not otherwise specified
These are DSM-III-R terms for disorders in which there are physical symptoms or complaints not due to demonstrable physical disorder, or grossly out of proportion to the severity of any organic condition present, and which do not fit into any of the above categories.

2. Dissociative disorders

These are uncommon in childhood and will therefore be considered only briefly. Dissociative disorders should only be diagnosed in the absence of evidence of physical disease which could explain the symptoms.

(a) Psychogenic amnesia
This is characterized by loss of memory for some past period or for particular events or people during some period of time.

(b) Psychogenic fugue
These patients suddenly leave their current lives, often to travel elsewhere to start new lives with new identities. They have no memories of their previous lives or identities.

(c) Multiple personality
In this condition the subject displays two or more distinct personalities and identities at different times. The transition from one to the other is usually sudden.

(d) Depersonalization disorder
In this disorder there are feelings of altered perception or experience of the self, with lost or altered experience of one's own reality. Derealization, a similar alteration in the perception of one's surroundings, often accompanies the depersonalization.

The relative frequency of different anxiety disorders in children

Reliable data on the frequency with which the various neurotic expressions of anxiety occur in childhood are scarce. Moreover, cultural factors play their part, so that any statement on the subject must take cultural factors into account. Turgay (1980), in an extensive review of conversion disorders in childhood, points out that the incidence of such disorders varies greatly in different cultures; in Turkey, where Turgay has studied conversion disorders, they are apparently commoner than in western countries.

Another example of a culture-dependent neurotic condition is the 'brain fag syndrome', perhaps better called 'school anxiety'. This was first described by Prince (1962) in Nigerian school children but it occurs also in many other parts of Africa. Mbanefo (1966) and German (1972) described it in East Africa; Minde (1974) described a controlled evaluation of a group of Ugandan high school children suffering from the syndrome and a programme of treatment by group therapy. Its often strikingly florid presentation is unlike anything commonly seen in western psychiatric practice. The following is a mild example.

> Lindiwe presented at a Swaziland clinic at age 16, complaining of severe, incapacitating headaches, blurring of vision, dizziness and buzzing in the ears. She was in 'Form 3' (that is the third year of a high school course). The sixth of seven children in her family, she was the only one to have reached Form 3. She and her impoverished family lived in a semi-rural part of the country, and paying the school fees and supporting Lindiwe through high school was a considerable financial burden to the family. In Africa formal education is widely seen as the passport to a

good job and a better life, and the hopes and aspirations of Lindiwe's family were pinned on her. The pressure on her to succeed was therefore great.

Lindiwe's history revealed that she was an average student who had always passed her exams but had to work hard to do so. As the high school years passed the work became harder, and many of the concepts she was supposed to learn about were difficult for her to comprehend.[1]

It was not possible for Lindiwe to admit defeat or indeed to face the possibility of failure, and as the year-end examinations loomed near her anxiety level rose. There is in Swaziland a deep-rooted cultural belief in bewitchment and the operation of supernatural forces. Lindiwe's symptoms were compatible with her having been bewitched by some ill-intentioned person. Many Swazis would regard this as the most likely explanation of symptoms such as Lindiwe's and indeed Lindiwe and her family were inclined to think she had been bewitched. But careful history taking revealed a close relationship between school attendance and the symptoms, which had been absent during a recent two-week school holiday. The headaches also came on as Lindiwe entered the classroom at the start of the school day and remitted at the end of the day.

Comment

There is widespread agreement that 'school anxiety' is a culturally determined reaction. It occurs in African children who are subject to intense and often unrealistic pressures to perform in school at a level they believe to be beyond them. Guinness (1986) describes it as not 'associated so much with personality or intelligence factors as with sociocultural stresses and ... the historical development of education in Africa'. The extended family system with its attendant obligations, the high regard in which education is held, the perceived economic advantages of a good education and the immense difficulty which achieving success presents in an educational system based upon European practices of times gone by, combine to put the child in an intensely anxiety-provoking situation. Prevalent beliefs about bewitchment add to the anxiety of all concerned. All these factors appeared to be operating in Lindiwe's case. It is unlikely she would have developed the symptoms she presented with if circumstances had not placed her in the particular predicament she faced.

Anxiety states are seen quite commonly in children and panic may be a feature of them. Phobic symptoms are well recognized but severe, chronic, phobic disorders are quite rare. Somatization/conversion disorders are quite common and are more likely to be seen in paediatric than psychiatric units, since children with physical symptoms are

[1] In Swaziland, as in much of Africa, schooling is neither free nor compulsory, fees being payable at all schools. The children sit the Cambridge external 'O' level examinations, which often involve the study of subjects far removed from Swazi culture and experience, such as Shakespeare's plays or the rise and fall of the Weimar republic. Moreover, the teaching and examinations are in English, their second language.

usually first referred for paediatric attention. As we have seen, established obsessive-compulsive disorders are quite uncommon in childhood and more often have their onset in adolescence. Hypochondriasis also starts more often in adolescence than in childhood, though neurotic antecedents may have been present earlier. Dissociative disorders are rare in childhood, except for those associated with disturbed sleep (sleepwalking and night terrors), which are in a different category. They are rare, too, in adult life, but when they occur their onset may be during adolescence.

A word of warning

Caution is in order in diagnosing conversion disorders or any of the disorders in which physical symptoms are attributed to emotional causes. There is a real danger of misdiagnosing organic disease. In one study of neurological disease presenting as child psychiatric disorder (Rivinus *et al.*, 1975), it was found that falling-off of school performance, loss of vision, disturbance of balance and variability of symptoms were common features. As well as trying to establish that organic disease is *not* present, it is desirable to establish also that there *are* adequate psychological causes for the symptoms. If the symptoms can be understood on neither basis, it is better to leave the diagnosis open until further information is available and the progress of the condition has been observed for a longer period.

School refusal (school phobia)

The main feature of school refusal is reluctance to attend school associated with anxiety and, often, depressed mood. It is sometimes called school phobia, because the child appears frightened to go to school.

Prevalence

The prevalence of school refusal varies with age and socioeconomic and cultural circumstances. In the Isle of Wight study of 10- and 11-year-olds (Rutter, Tizard and Whitmore, 1970), it was present in fewer than 3 per cent of the children identified as having psychiatric disorders. It appears to be commoner in early adolescence, at which age it is more often accompanied by symptoms of depression (Rutter *et al.*, 1976).

Weiner (1982), reviewing a number of studies, suggested a prevalence of 1 per cent to 2 per cent in school-age children. The condition is most frequently seen on entry to school (about age 5 or 6); around the age of 11, often in association with a change to a new school containing older children; and in early adolescence. When the onset is in the teen years there are more often associated depression and difficulties in the school situation. The disorder affects boys and girls equally.

Clinical picture

While fear of school, implied by the term 'school phobia,' can certainly be a feature of the condition, it is not usually the primary one, even though at first sight it may seem to be. Separation anxiety, and the fear of leaving home are generally more important. Many children with this condition meet the DSM-III-R criteria for separation anxiety disorder.

Hersov (1985b) has reviewed the development of the concept of school refusal, and its distinction from truancy, which he himself did much to clarify (Hersov, 1960a; 1960b). As we saw in Chapter 4, truancy is the wilful avoidance of school, whereas in school refusal it is an excessively high level of anxiety, sometimes combined with depression, that makes it hard for the child to attend. If attempts are made to force the child to go to school, increased distress usually results, though in some cases this is the best treatment. Physical symptoms such as poor appetite, nausea, vomiting, pains and diarrhoea are common, especially at breakfast time. They may disappear once the time for going to school has passed. This may lead parents and school staff to the erroneous conclusion that the child is malingering. In more severe cases symptoms persist and may be present throughout the day; there may also be sleep disturbance. There is usually an exacerbation of the symptoms when the child is faced with pressure to attend school.

These children are often emotionally immature and so have difficulty in coping with the everyday social stresses of life at school. They may find relationships with other children difficult and they become acutely anxious away from what they feel is the safety and protection of home and family. School attendance may finally cease in response to a minor additional stress, like a change of teacher, bullying by other children or transfer from one school to another. The emotional immaturity of these children is often manifest also in their covert aggressiveness. Having grown up in anxious and often indulgent atmospheres, they have not learned to accept frustration and to channel their aggressive drives into socially useful and constructive activities. Their anger may seldom have been aroused, since they have always been given their way. When this situation is challenged they may become both panic-stricken and very angry. The anger is often expressed verbally but some of these children become physically violent with their parents, for example if the latter try to force them, by physical means, to go to school. Anger may also be expressed silently through refusal to speak or cooperate, both with the parents and with therapists and others trying to help.

In practice either anxiety, depression or anger may dominate the clinical picture. These children may also feel resentful because they are aware, perhaps at an unconscious rather than a conscious level, of their inability to fulfil age-appropriate roles. Some authors, for example Davidson (1960) and Tisher (1983) have emphasized the role of depression in school refusal, the former reporting it in 77 per cent of a series of 30 cases. Hersov (1960a; 1960b) reported it in 20 per cent of 50 cases. More recently, Bernstein and Garfinkel (1986) reported that 69 per cent of a sample of 26 early adolescent, chronic school refusers met DSM-III criteria for depressive disorders (either major depression (see Chapter 6) or adjustment disorder with depression (see Chapter 12)). In that study there were more subjects with depressive disorders than anxiety disorders, though the number with both was greater still.

How often depression is diagnosed in children with school refusal depends on age, the diagnostic criteria used for both depression and school refusal, and the severity and chronicity of the condition. In the following case anxiety dominated the clinical picture but there was also an element of depression.

> Tracie, aged 10, was referred because of school refusal. Her symptoms dated back two months to the start of the new term. At first she became very anxious about her school books, worrying unduly about small mistakes in her work. Then, after being persuaded by other children in the playground to eat a horse chestnut, she became acutely fearful that she was being poisoned. Afterwards she would eat only if her mother ate the same food with her. At this time she was also washing herself needlessly often, despite acknowledging that it was unnecessary when her mother spoke to her about it.
>
> During the month before she was first seen, Tracie became overdependent on her mother, to whom she confided that she had frightening fantasies and dreams. Her mother responded to this by reassuring and comforting her. Tracie frequently wept for her father and any attempt to get her to go school led to an acute state of panic. At night she would not go to sleep until she knew her mother was in bed. She sucked two of her fingers almost all day.
>
> Four years previously Tracie's father had died of a subarachnoid haemorrhage after a short illness. Tracie, the sixth of eight siblings, was said always to have been her father's favourite child. After his death she cried bitterly for days and she continued over the next four years to cry for him whenever upset. Her mother also was depressed after the father's death but did her best to comfort Tracie. This seemed to have led to a mutually overdependent relationship between them. It

appeared that Tracie had made little progress in becoming independent of her mother during the previous four years.

Tracie was admitted to an inpatient unit for treatment. On separation from her mother she was very upset, crying constantly and insistently demanding to go home. For a few days she required constant attention but it was not difficult to get her to go to the unit school, where she worked well and made steady progress. At first she was reluctant to mix with the other children but her relations with them gradually became more normal. After eight weeks in the unit she was able to spend weekends at home without becoming upset on return to the unit. Towards the end of her three-month stay she was able to attend an outside school daily.

During the early part of her stay Tracie declined to see the doctor who was looking after her in the inpatient unit, as she was invited to do each day. Instead she hung around the building sucking her fingers. This was at first accepted but later she was persuaded to come to individual interviews. She then began to talk about the obsessive thoughts which previously had distressed her so much, but she seemed to feel guilty about them and would give not details of their content. She spoke also of her relationships with her mother, her siblings and various friends, including another girl in the unit with whom she developed a rather ambivalent relationship. She also played out scenes in the dolls' house; in these the figure of father was always left out.

While Tracie was in hospital her mother was seen weekly by another therapist. She responded well to discussion of Tracie's difficulties and her part in them. She became less protective towards Tracie and learned to handle her firmly when this was required, despite her own strongly felt desire to 'baby' her.

Tracie went home after three months and was seen for a time as an outpatient. At follow-up $3\frac{1}{2}$ years after admission she was attending school regularly and making good progress there, without showing signs of undue anxiety or any other symptoms. The whole family also seemed to be functioning at a better level than when Tracie was first seen.

Comment

This case is a little unusual in that the father was dead and the anxious overprotection of Tracie by her mother developed in the context of the reactions of each to the father's death. Nevertheless the combination of an anxious and overprotective mother with a weak, passive, ineffectual or absent father is common (Skynner, 1975). In such a situation the child may become increasingly emotionally immature. This can lead to the development of overt neurotic symptoms. In Tracie's case these consisted of school refusal coming on following a minor stress, namely the start of a new school term with a new teacher. Little fantasy material emerged during Tracie's treatment; this is often the case in children with school refusal. A period of specialized treatment in an inpatient setting nevertheless enabled her to overcome her problems.

In Tracie's case, as in many others, there was a strong element of separation anxiety. Berney et al. (1981) found separation anxiety to be 'moderate to marked' in 87 per cent of 51 school refusers aged 9 to 15.

In older school refusers, especially those presenting in adolescence, it tends to be less marked. In that age group stress at school often seems more important.

Other neurotic syndromes

Some cases of anorexia nervosa present as neurotic disorders. Neurotic processes also operate in many cases of elective mutism. These disorders are considered separately, in Chapter 12 and 13 respectively. Anxiety is also a prominent feature of some adjustment disorders; these are considered in Chapter 12.

Treatment

(a) Psychotherapy

Psychotherapy, in one form or another, plays a major role in the treatment of the disorders discussed in this chapter. It usually needs to involve child and parents and is often best focused on the family group as a whole. The diagnostic assessment and the formulation emerging from it should give a clear indication of where the main therapeutic efforts are required.

Individual therapy with the child may or not involve the working through of unconscious conflicts. Whether it need do so will depend on the severity and chronicity of the disorder, and the child's response to changes in the environment, especially the family environment.

Therapy for the parents is likely to be required when there is evidence of overanxious, overprotective or otherwise unhelpful attitudes to or handling of the child. In many such cases one or both parents have their own psychiatric problems which need to be addressed in therapy.

Family therapy is often indicated. When the child's disorder can be understood as a feature of the way the family system functions, therapy is best addressed to promoting systems change in the family. In school refusal, especially in adolescence when the family psychopathology is often complex and chronic, family therapy can be particularly valuable.

When family systems problems are prominent, as is often the case, I prefer to address these problems first. This frequently leads to amelioration of the child's symptoms, or their resolution. If it does not, individual work with the child may be needed, perhaps combined with help also for the parents.

(b) Behaviour therapy

We have seen that behavioural approaches may be effective in the treatment of phobias and obsessive-compulsive disorders. Behavioural analysis may also reveal that environmental contingencies are reinforcing or promoting other neurotic symptoms. Thus the response of family, teachers and others to the symptoms of children with conversion disorders, somatization disorders and hypochondriasis may serve to reinforce those symptoms too.

(c) Daypatient and inpatient treatment

Children living in particularly insecure and anxiety-provoking home environments may benefit from a period of daypatient or inpatient treatment. This can be an effective, if drastic, way of countering anxious parental overprotection, such as may be encountered in severe school refusal.

(d) Pharmacotherapy

Drugs have but a small part to play in the treatment of childhood neuroses, unless there is associated depression. If depression is present antidepressant medication may help. Small doses of anxiolytics such as diazepam or chlordiazepoxide may occasionally be indicated to bring about a temporary reduction in the anxiety level of an acutely disturbed child, particularly when this is a reaction to severe, current environmental stress which cannot immediately be alleviated. These drugs should not be prescribed for more than a few days; a week is usually too long.

The disadvantages of anxiety-relieving drugs generally outweigh any merits their use may have. Prescribing them tends to imply that the problem is the child's, whereas it is usually at least as much that of the family or wider environment; it may also cause the real problems to be ignored, especially if it leads to a short-term reduction of symptoms. The prescription of drugs also carries the message that there is an easy pharmacological cure for these problems, which in reality are concerned with such issues as relationships, emotional maturity and family functioning. The model of a 'magical' chemical cure for human problems is not one we should offer to our young people.

(e) Special points about the treatment of school refusal

Since family systems problems often exist in the families of children with school refusal, family therapy is often useful in this condition. The fathers are often uninvolved (Skynner, 1975) and one of the objectives of treatment may be to increase the father's participation in the affairs of the family.

Whatever treatment is employed with family or child we have to consider when to make efforts to get the school refuser back to school. For children who are still attending, even with difficulty and with symptoms, efforts to make the school environment temporarily less stressful and to provide emotional support to the child at school are well worthwhile. In mild cases and those of recent onset, an early return to school is advisable and usually leads to good results (Kennedy, 1965).

The return to school needs to be well planned and carefully orchestrated. All concerned should first be agreed on a plan. This includes the parents; the school principal and child's teacher(s); the family doctor and any other physicians who have been involved; and any other people who are actively involved in the treatment of child or family. The child should be aware of the plan and if possible should be in agreement with it. A meeting of the above people to work out and agree on a plan is often useful. By the end of the meeting everyone should know precisely what is to happen on the day appointed for the child's return to school; it must also be agreed what is to be done if the child refuses to get up, leave the house or enter the classroom or whatever.

Firm, calm handling of the return to school is desirable. It is sometimes necessary physically to take the child to school, even if not properly dressed, in order to break the cycle of events that has seemed to make attendance impossible. Usually, however, once these children know that all concerned with their care are agreed about the timing and other details of their return, they go back with little difficulty. The plan should provide for what is to happen if the child becomes acutely anxious at any point; whatever this is it should seldom be that the child returns to or stays at home.

In more severe and chronic cases a period of psychotherapy may be required before plans are set up for the child's return to school. Attempts to force severely anxious and depressed children and those who have had repeated severe panic attacks, to attend school can aggravate the problems. In some such cases a period of treatment in a daypatient or an inpatient unit, combined with psychotherapy for the family or for child and parents, can lead to more rapid resolution of the problems (Barker, 1968; Hersov, 1980).

Blagg and Yule (1984) describe a 'flexible, behavioural approach'. This involves:

- a detailed clarification of the child's problem;
- a realistic discussion of child, parental and teacher worries;
- contingency plans to ensure maintenance once the child has returned to school;
- *in vivo* flooding, that is an enforced return to school, under escort if necessary;
- follow-up, consisting of frequent contacts until the child has been attending full-time for at least six weeks, then careful steps to ensure return after 'genuine illness', holidays and long weekends, and at the start of a new academic year and after any reorganization of the child's timetable.

The authors reported that 28 out of 30 children treated using the above approach returned rapidly to school. A comparison group treated in a hospital inpatient unit did less well, and another group treated by home teaching and outpatient psychotherapy did very poorly indeed.

Although the antidepressant drug imipramine has been advocated as a treatment for school refusal, there is little evidence that it has any specific effect. When there is an associated major depressive disorder, however, it may be useful. A controlled trial of clomipramine, a related drug, used along with psychotherapy, failed to demonstrate any short-term effect of the drug in the doses used (Berney *et al.*, 1981).

Sometimes the parents and/or the child ask for a change of school. This can on occasion be helpful, especially if there are real-life stresses at school or the child has gained the reputation of being a 'cry baby' or 'crazy' in the school. In itself, however, it is seldom an adequate treatment. It may represent an attempt by child or parents to deal with anxiety or guilt by projecting it on to an outside source, namely the school or a member of the school staff.

The treatment approaches mentioned above are all discussed further in Chapter 19.

Outcome

The disorders we have discussed in this chapter generally have a good outcome. Neurotic and anxiety symptoms often clear up completely and are not followed by any observable psychiatric abnormality. Many milder ones and some more severe ones resolve without any specific treatment. Such an outcome is more likely in children whose emotional development has been satisfactory and in cases in which the symptoms developed in response to severe, but temporary, environmental stress.

In other instances the symptoms of these disorders are more persistent, especially in the absence of suitable treatment. Emotionally immature children, who are often overdependent on their parents, tend to do less well. Much depends, however, on the family's response to treatment. Constitutional predisposition, suggested by a positive family history and the appearance of symptoms with little apparent environmental cause, may be associated with a poorer outlook.

If psychiatric disorder persists, the type of disorder diagnosed in adult life is likely to be a neurosis or an affective psychosis (Robins, 1966). This stands in contrast with conduct disorders which, if disturbed behaviour persists into adult life, are more likely to be followed by antisocial or criminal behaviour.

Many aspects of the anxiety disorders of children and the findings of research in this and related areas are discussed by the contributors to *Anxiety Disorders of Childhood* (Gittelman, 1986).

Chapter 6

Major Affective Disorders and Suicide

In major affective disorders the main feature is a major disorder of mood. The term 'affective psychosis' may be used when there are psychotic symptoms such as delusions or hallucinations. The mood disorder is most often in the direction of depression. Mania, in which there is undue elation, is rare before puberty but less uncommon in adolescence.

Classification

Apart from those characterized by anxiety, DSM-III-R does not recognize any category of affective disorder occurring specifically in childhood. The following categories appear under 'mood disorders' in the general section and may be used with individuals of any age:

- Major depression. This term may be used for a single episode of depression or it may be applied when the depressive attack is one of a series of such episodes, with periods of normal mood in between.
- Bipolar disorders. These have in the past been called manic-depressive disorders. They are characterized by one or more manic or hypomanic episodes (see below) with periods of normality and/or depression between these. DSM-III-R does not require that there be depressive episodes between the manic ones, though it states that there usually are.
- Cyclothymia. These are milder forms of recurrent mood disturbance involving depression and elation.
- Dysthymia (or depressive neurosis). This is a chronic condition of depression, but less severe and not meeting the DSM-III-R criteria for major depression.
- Adjustment disorder with depressed mood. The patient has symptoms such as depressed mood, tearfulness and hopelessness, but these follow an identifiable psychosocial stress. The reaction is greater than the normal and expectable one, and impairs social

functioning. This category appears in a different section of DSM-III-R to that dealing with mood disorders. Adjustment disorders are discussed in Chapter 12.

ICD-9 has a rather different scheme:

- Affective psychoses. These correspond roughly to the major mood disorders of DSM-III-R, but ICD-9 uses the time-honoured term, 'manic-depressive psychosis', rather than 'bipolar disorder'. As in DSM-III-R there are various subcategories.
- Neurotic depression. In neurotic depressions the degree of depression is milder, there are other neurotic symptoms and there is no evidence of psychosis – that is, no delusions, hallucinations or other signs of loss of contact with reality. This category covers roughly the same disorders as the dysthymia of DSM-III-R.
- Depressive disorders not elsewhere classified. This is a residual category. (Similar categories appear in DSM-III-R.)
- Adjustment reaction with depression, which may be either brief or prolonged.
- Disturbance of emotions specific to childhood and adolescence – with misery and unhappiness.
- Other non-organic psychosis. This is for conditions 'largely or entirely attributable to a recent life experience'. 'Depressive' and 'excitative' types are described.

The validity of the quite complex subdivision of affective disorders in both schemes, but especially in ICD-9, is unclear.

The current practice in many centres is to use criteria derived from the study of adult patients in the study and diagnosis of affective disorders in children. Whether there are distinct affective disorders that occur specifically in children, as ICD-9 implies by having a special category for such disorders, is uncertain.

Depression and depressive disorders

It has long been recognized that children can experience moods of depression, but the occurrence in childhood of major depressive illnesses of the type encountered in adult patients has, until recently, been less generally accepted. It is now clear, however, that children can suffer from major depressive conditions, though whether these are essentially the same as those occurring in adults is less certain. Puig-Antich (1986, page 345) believes they are and asserts that the basic phenomenology of major depression, and also of dysthymia and manic disorder, is 'quite similar from age 6 to senescence'. He asserts that the developmental variations which do occur are 'minor compared to the steadiness of the symptomatology'.

The above quotations are from a discussion of psychobiological markers of depression (such as the sleep EEG, and the pattern of secretion of hormones such as cortisol and growth hormone). Despite the above statements, Puig-Antich's review indicates that the markers found in adult patients with depressive disorders are by no means generally found in depressed children. These differences may, though, be 'secondary to maturational factors, which modify the expression of depressive illness' (Puig-Antich, 1986, page 350).

Depression, like other children's problems, must be considered in the light of the developmental processes that occur during childhood, a factor that complicates comparisons with adult disorders. Much of what is known about childhood depression and its developmental aspects is discussed by the 31 contributors to the book *Depression in Young People: Clinical and Developmental Perspectives* (Rutter, Izard and Read, 1986).

Prevalence

While depressive feelings are relatively common in prepubertal children, major depressive conditions are considerably less so. Of the 2000 10-year-olds studied in the Isle of Wight (Rutter, Tizard and Whitmore, 1970), 13 per cent showed depressed mood at interview, 9 per cent seemed preoccupied with depressive ideas, 17 per cent failed to smile, and 15 per cent showed poor emotional responsiveness. But according to the criteria used, which required there to be persisting social impairment or handicap, only 3 (0.15 per cent) had a depressive disorder. If DSM-III-R criteria had been used the prevalence might have been higher. A study of 9-year-olds in New Zealand did yield a higher prevalence rate, namely 1.7 per cent for 'major depression' and 3.6 per cent for 'minor depression'; this study used the Research Diagnostic Criteria which are similar to those of DSM-III-R (Kashani *et al.*, 1983).

Both depressive feelings and depressive disorders become commoner after puberty. When the Isle of Wight children were studied at age 14-15, over 40 per cent reported feelings of misery and depression, 20 per cent described feelings of self-depreciation, 7 per cent reported suicidal feelings and 25 per cent ideas of reference. Moreover there were 9 cases of depressive disorder and another 26 with 'mixed affective disorder' (of which depression was a feature), an elevenfold increase.

In reviewing these findings, Rutter (1986) points out that, at least for boys (data are lacking for girls), the increase is due to the appearance of depressive phenomena in postpubertal subjects. The sex ratio also changes at puberty. Before puberty there are about twice as many boys as girls with depressive symptoms, whereas after puberty the situation is reversed. Not only does depression with onset before puberty affect boys more than girls, but such cases are frequently 'secondary' ones, with accompanying serious academic problems. A family history of alcoholism and/or antisocial behaviour is present in about half these prepubertal cases but one of major affective disorder is uncommon.

Children with onset after puberty are more often girls; the disorder is usually of the 'primary' type; and there is much more often a family history of major affective disorder, most often depression, rather than of alcoholism or antisocial behaviour.

Causes

Affective disorders may be primary or secondary as indicated in Figure 6.1.

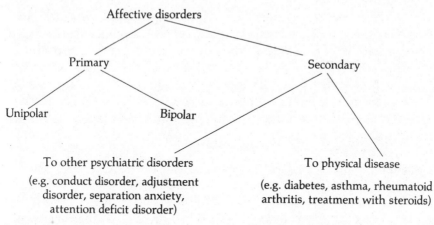

Figure 6.1. The types of affective disorder.

Genetic factors probably play a significant role in predisposing to primary depressive states in children, as they are known to do in adults. Children of parents with affective disorders, especially depression, have a high rate of psychiatric problems (Weissman *et al.*, 1984; Cytryn *et al.*, 1986). Cytryn and his colleagues (1986, page 179) state that:

'Already at the age of 12 months the infants of manic-depressive parents show disturbances in attachment behaviour and dysregulation of affect...similar to the central characteristics of adults with affective illness.'

The presence of such disturbances, even so early in life, is not proof that genetic processes are operating. The children's behaviour could also be due to the effects of living with manic-depressive parents; or both genetic and environmental processes could be contributing. From a clinical point of view, however, the important thing is to be aware that such children are more at risk of developing psychiatric, including depressive, problems.

Environmental stress often seems to contribute to depression. Precisely what stresses are most likely to do so is less clear. Separation from an attachment figure (see the discussion of attachment theory in Chapter 1) has been blamed. Bowlby (1969) has described the sequence of protest, despair and detachment seen in toddlers separated from their parents, for example on admission to hospital. He believes that separation experiences contribute to the later development of depression (Bowlby, 1980). But whether children undergoing separation experiences are depressed in the same way as those presenting for psychiatric treatment, or identified in research surveys, is uncertain (Rutter, 1986a).

Clinical experience and research data suggest that bereavement, especially the loss of a parent, can lead to depression but that the grief reactions are briefer in young children than in adolescents and adults (Rutter, 1986). But this is a complex issue, since bereavement frequently involves other things besides the loss of the loved one; these may include break-up of the home, geographical moves, the arrival in the family of a step-parent, and emotional problems in other family members, especially the surviving parent (see the case history of Tracie in Chapter 5).

Other possible causative factors are the break-up of the child's family by divorce or separation of the parents and 'learned helplessness'. As with bereavement, it is difficult to separate out the effects of parental separation or divorce from those of related circumstances, such as the marital dysharmony and general family disruption which often precede such events.

'Learned helplessness' is a term originally used to describe the state of dogs that had been subjected to a series of electric shocks over which they had no control. The dogs subsequently showed motivational, cognitive and emotional deficits (Maier et al., 1969; Seligman and Peterson, 1986). Their state bore some resemblance to human depression. It is possible that the development of self-esteem in children might be impaired by similar experiences of being in painful or unpleasant situations over which they have no control. An important aspect of self-esteem is a sense of mastery of the environment. Children brought up in predictable environments might be expected to learn more easily what to expect from them and thus gain a sense of mastery and control of their lives. It is possible that those brought up in environments in which events occur in random fashion and cannot be predicted or anticipated, might lack a sense of mastery and so be predisposed to depression. This is far from being proved but Seligman and Peterson (1986) report some experimental work in this area and provide a useful review of this subject.

There are various biochemical theories of depression and there are no doubt biochemical changes in the brain which correspond to, and indeed are part of, the depressive process. These are to be found in the literature on depression in adults; there has been little research on the biochemical correlates of childhood depression.

As Figure 6.1 shows, depression may be secondary to other disorders. It can accompany other child psychiatric disorders, such as conduct disorders, adjustment disorders, separation anxiety and attention deficit disorders. It is may be difficult to determine which is the primary condition, particularly when conduct disorder and depressive symptoms co-exist.

Depression may complicate physical illnesses such as those listed in Figure 6.1. The use of certain drugs, for example steroid compounds such as cortisone and prednisone, may lead to depression. It is therefore important to enquire about the presence of other illnesses and about drugs being used to treat them. The chronic abuse of drugs, for example barbiturates, cocaine and other 'street' drugs, can also lead to irritable, depressed states.

Description

The essential feature of a depressive disorder is depressed mood, that is a mood of sadness and gloom, often accompanied by tearfulness. The subject usually looks unhappy and may feel miserable or hopeless. There is loss of energy and of interest in the things which usually interest the person. Self-blame and feelings of unworthiness and guilt, of a degree not justified by circumstances, are often present.

Sleep is usually impaired but sometimes there is excess sleepiness. The appetite is usually diminished and weight loss or, in children, failure to gain weight, may follow. In some depressed individuals, however, the appetite may be increased. There may also be slowing of thought processes and of body movements ('psychomotor retardation'). School problems, academic and social, social withdrawal and episodes of aggressive behaviour are common. In severe cases suicidal thoughts occur and these may lead to suicidal behaviour.

Eliciting some of these symptoms in young children can be difficult. Moreover, children are subject to quite rapid changes of mood. They may be crying one moment and laughing the next, so it is important to discover whether they have experienced a sustained depression of mood, rather than a series of brief periods of unhappiness. The limited vocabulary and capacity to conceptualize of younger children may make it hard for them to give clear answers to questions on these points. Sometimes depression is conveyed better in children's play or drawings than in their conversation.

Self-blame and expressions of guilt are common. One depressed 12-year-old said that her 'nervous state' was responsible for her father's difficulties at the office, her mother's anemia and general ill-health and the bad behaviour of her brother and sister. She also had difficulty getting to school and entertained suicidal thoughts.

In adolescents, depression of psychotic intensity, that is with delusions or hallucinations, is encountered more often than in younger children. Well developed delusional systems are uncommon but hallucinations with depressive content are more frequent; they may take the form of voices telling the young person that he or she is a worthless, bad person, responsible for various evil things.

While the onset of depression in adolescents may be acute, it is more often insidious and the signs of depression are not always obvious. There may or may not be a history of family or other stress to which the depression might be attributed. Rather than presenting with depressed mood, the adolescent may present with anxiety (perhaps about going to school), panic attacks or somatic symptoms such as headaches or abdominal pain. The existence of a depressive condition may only come up in conversation, in the course of which the young person may talk about how she or he has been feeling like weeping, can get little or no pleasure out of life and may even have been considering suicide, or perhaps running away. Tiredness, irritability, poor concentration, difficulty in coping with school work which previously presented no difficulty, and sleep and appetite disturbances may also be revealed on questioning.

The term 'anaclitic depression' was coined by Spitz (1946) to describe a condition of misery, crying, withdrawal and failure to thrive in babies and young children suffering from severe deprivation of parental care. This was apparently an environmentally determined reaction to a gross lack of care, such as may be found in large, poorly run institutions (in which in developed countries infants are nowadays rarely placed). It probably has nothing to do with the depressive conditions of later childhood.

George H., the only child of a single mother, was referred for psychiatric assessment at age 11, after he had run away from home and been picked up by police in a town about 100 kilometres away. His chronically depressed mother had had three periods in a psychiatric hospital during the previous two years, each for the treatment of an exacerbation of her depression.

George, his mother and their large dog lived an isolated existence. Ms H. did not mix with the neighbours and said they looked down on her because she was an unmarried mother. She lived on social security payments but from time to time bought George surprisingly expensive presents, such as an electric organ. She and George doted on the dog, for whose affections there was some rivalry between them. George was discouraged from mixing with other children and was frequently warned by his mother against friendships with neighbourhood families. His sleep had been poor and he said he had had difficulty in concentrating. His appetite was unaffected. He denied having entertained any ideas of suicide. At school he was considered a bright pupil, but his work was patchy and unreliable and his concentration often poor. He ran away after leaving a note 'bequeathing' all his possessions, except the few things he chose to take with him, to his mother. On each of the three occasions when his mother had been in hospital George was placed in a foster home.

When first seen George appeared very depressed. He spoke of his longstanding anxiety about his mother, who would from time to time threaten suicide and the restrictions placed by her on his contacts outside the family. He said he ran away with the intention of going to stay with an aunt he knew slightly who lived in another part of the country. Intelligence testing showed him to be of superior intelligence. In tests of attainment in basic school subjects he was performing only at a level about average for a child of his age. In later interviews he spoke of his desire to meet and know more of his father, whom his mother never mentioned.

George was admitted to a child psychiatry unit where his depression rapidly lifted without any drug treatment. It was decided that he would be best discharged to a residential school, a suggestion which he accepted readily. He did well there, returning home to his mother for school holidays. Meanwhile she was supported by visits from a social worker and seemed to benefit from this.

Comment

George had been chronically anxious for many years, but had maintained a precarious adjustment until the approach of adolescence. Following three separations from his mother he became increasingly worried and then depressed. He probably ran away mainly to draw attention to his plight. There were clearly reactive elements to his condition but there was also a strong suggestion of genetic loading. His condition does not meet the DSM-III-R criteria for a major depressive episode but it meets those for dysthymia. The most appropriate ICD-9 diagnosis is neurotic depression.

In assessing children it is important to bear in mind that parents are not always aware of depression in their children. The children tend to be better sources of information than their parents (Moretti *et al.* 1985). Brent *et al.* (1986), in a study of childhood suicidal behaviour, found poor correlation between the reports of the children and those of their parents, though they recommended the more serious report should receive the greater weight.

Probably because the clinical diagnosis of depression in children is not easy, a number of self-report and parent-report scales and some structured and semi-structured interview schedules have been devised to assist in the process. These are valuable in research studies but may be applied to supplement information obtained in the course of clinical assessment. They have been reviewed by Costello (1986).

Associated conditions

The association of conduct disorders and depressive conditions is important and in several studies has been found to be common. It seems that depressive feelings are sometimes 'acted out' in displays of anger or violence towards others, rather than being turned inwards as happens in those who are suicidal.

There is also an important association between eating disorders (see Chapter 13) and affective disorders, chiefly depression. About one-third of the patients with eating disorders present with affective symptoms; in another third they both develop at the the same time. There is also often a history of affective disorders in the families of adolescents with eating disorders.

Suicide and suicidal behaviour

Completed suicide is very rare before the age of 10. Except in certain racial groups it is almost confined to those who have passed puberty (Shaffer and Fisher, 1981; Shaffer, 1986). Suicidal behaviours, such as expressing ideas of suicide, threatening it or even attempting it, occur in prepubertal children but hardly ever lead to death. Pfeffer et al. (1984) studied 101 children aged 6 to 12 (mean age 9.7), randomly selected from the population of a school. They had never been psychiatric patients but 11.9 per cent reported suicidal ideas, threats or attempts, though only 3 had made attempts. The school contained many children from father-absent homes of poor socioeconomic status, so the prevalence of suicidal behaviour would likely be different in other schools.

Shaffer (1974) obtained information about all the recorded suicides in children aged 10 to 14 in England and Wales over a 7-year period. There were no reported suicides below the age of 12 and he cites good evidence that this is not because of under-reporting. Twenty-one boys and 9 girls had died by suicide, an annual rate of 1 child in every 800,000 in the 10- to 14-year age range. The commonest method of suicide was coal gas poisoning (which no longer occurs as natural gas has replaced coal gas), followed by hanging and overdose.

Two personality stereotypes were noted among the children. One was of children who had led a solitary existence, were of superior intelligence and seemed to have been culturally distant from their less well educated parents. Their mothers were mentally ill and before their death they had seemed depressed or withdrawn; some of them had stolen things or had stayed away from school. The second group, which included several of the girls, consisted of children who were judged impetuous or prone to aggressive or violent outbursts; they were also suspicious and both sensitive to and resentful of criticism. In most of the cases there had been prior antisocial behaviour and in 46 per cent previous suicidal behaviour was reported. The commonest precipitant was a disciplinary crisis.

In 1978 the age-specific mortality rate from suicide for children in the age range 10-14 in the United States was 0.81 per 100,000; and suicide accounted for 2.4 per cent of deaths in this group (Shaffer, 1985b). Childhood suicide is thus commoner in the USA than in England and Wales but still very rare. In adolescence suicide is much commoner and in older adolescents and young adults it has been increasing at an alarming rate in many western countries in the last decade or two. The 1978 USA figures for the age range 15-19 show that there were 7.64 suicides per 100,000, or about 8 per cent of all deaths in this age bracket.

Thompson (1987) studied suicides in subjects aged 20 years and younger in Manitoba during the years 1971 to 1982. His findings were similar to those of earlier studies in respect to Caucasian children, but native North American boys and, to a lesser extent Caucasian boys living in rural areas, had rates several times higher than those of other groups matched for age and sex. In the age range 12-14 the rate for native boys was 25 per 100,000.

Most studies of suicidal children have been conducted on clinical populations, especially inpatient ones, and the frequency with which suicidal behaviour is reported in these groups is naturally higher than in the general population. For example Myers *et al.* (1985) reported that 61 (17.5 per cent – 40 boys and 21 girls) of 348 children aged 5-13 admitted to a psychiatric unit had engaged in suicidal behaviour, defined as 'any self-destructive statement or action expressed with explicit desire to kill oneself, and offered either spontaneously or upon interview'. A wish to be dead did not qualify. This is a rather lower percentage than in some other studies. Seven were aged 5-7 and 25 were in the age range 8-10. Most of the suicidal children were diagnosed as having either depressive or conduct disorders; depression was diagnosed in 30 per cent of the suicidal children but in only 3 per cent of the non-suicidal admissions. A conduct disorder diagnosis was made about equally frequently in the two groups.

When the family histories of the suicidal children were compared with those of the non-suicidal admissions, they contained significantly more abused mothers, abusive fathers and reports of suicidal behaviours by other family members. These children had also experienced recent stressful life events more often than their non-suicidal fellow inpatients. Other studies have yielded similar results.

Suicidal behaviour should not be taken lightly. Although it is unlikely to presage actual suicide in a prepubertal child, it is often an indication of serious problems in the family, the child or both. Some young children theaten suicide in imitation of the behaviour of a parent or other family member; while such children may have no intention of killing themselves, living in a family in which suicidal threats or attempts are commonplace may be stressful. In such families children may use suicidal threats as a family-sanctioned way of expressing distress. Suicidal behaviour in any family member often indicates serious family pathology.

In adolescence the risk of suicide is greater. The assessment of suicidal risk is an important part of the psychiatric examination of adolescents and is discussed in Chapter 15. Suicidal behaviour should alert you to the possibility that there may be serious family problems; the suicidal individual may also be in difficulty. The family or the young person may be having difficulty negotiating a step in the life cycle. The subject may, on the other hand, be suffering from a major psychiatric disorder, especially a depressive one. Many adolescent suicides are impulsive rather than planned acts; the availability of a means of suicide, such as a gun or lethal drugs, at the same time as the subject is seized with an impulsive desire to die or to 'get back' at someone, results in the fatal act. Some adolescents kill themselves in the context of the abuse of alcohol or other drugs, which adversely affect their judgment.

Attempted suicide always justifies careful psychiatric assessment of the suicidal individual and the family. The depression which is often present may clear, though perhaps only temporarily, after the attempt; this applies especially if the young person is in hospital and is being treated solicitously by the family and others. The underlying problems may persist, however, and repeated attempts at suicide often occur.

Mania and manic disorders

In mania, and its lesser form, hypomania, the mood disturbance is in the direction of elation. The manic individual may feel excessively happy, though irritability more often predominates, especially in young people. Manic individuals are typically hyperactive, constantly on the go and lacking in judgment. They may spend their money recklessly as if they were millionaires. They sleep less than usual, their self-esteem is inflated and they may engage frantically in many activities, some of them reckless and ill-judged. Their speech is rapid and pressured and may contain many jokes and puns; there may be 'flight of ideas', the rapid movement from one subject to another associated one – though the process may be so fast that others miss the association. The manic subject is readily distractible and often starts things which are never finished. Delusions, usually of grandeur, such as thinking one is the king, or God, or enormously wealthy, or possessed of special powers, are common. Hallucinations, which may reinforce such delusional ideas, sometimes occur.

The term 'hypomania' is used for milder forms of this condition. There is elation and excess activity, often combined with some of the other features mentioned, but the full picture is not present and there are no delusions, hallucinations or psychotic behaviour.

Manic disorders are very rare before puberty, though a few well documented cases are on record. Lowe and Cohen (1980) suggest that three forms of mania, all rare, may occur in young people. These include 'adult-type' mania, which may be genetically similar to the disorder as it occurs in later life; a subgroup of hyperactive children who are born to lithium-responsive manic-depressive parents and whose behaviour problems may improve on lithium; and 'phenocopies', that is cases which are genetically unrelated to adult manic states and may be reactions to drugs such as steroids or phencyclidine (PCP or 'angel dust').

Mania, and especially hypomania, must be distinguished from the hyperkinetic syndrome, or attention deficit disorder with hyperactivity (see Chapter 9). In manic conditions there is usually a history of a marked, and often quite sudden, change in personality; in the other conditions the hyperactivity is a longstanding behavioural trait. It is important therefore to enquire for any *change* in behaviour.

Bipolar affective disorders (manic-depressive psychosis)

Manic or hypomanic states are often episodes occurring in the course of a bipolar affective disorder. The subject has periods of depression alternating with periods of mania or hypomania, often with periods of normal mood in between. A manic or depressive episode may last from a few days to many months but a period of three to six months is typical; the periods of normality may also be just a few days or many months or even years.

Bipolar disorders are very rare before puberty, though some well-documented cases have been reported (Puig-Antich, 1980). They are more frequently encountered in adolescence and many cases are on record with onset before age 16. Hassanyeh and Davison (1980) reported 10 such cases, 5 boys and 5 girls, and reviewed earlier reports. They found that mania was easier to diagnose in the adolescent period than depression, which was sometimes diagnosed retrospectively; but mild cases of mania or hypomania can easily be mistaken for manifestations of conduct disorder. This is especially so when restlessness, hostility, irritability and verbal abuse predominate. In addition to displaying euphoria, hyperactivity, pressure of speech, flight of ideas, grandiosity, sleep disturbance and distractibility, manic adolescents often hurled verbal abuse at their parents and denied that anything was amiss, even in the face of wildly disturbed behaviour. In girls, sexually provocative behaviour, including wandering about the house naked, was common. The manic patients' rooms were in a state of total disorder, which Hassanyeh and Davison called the 'bomb-in-the-room' syndrome. In their depressed phases these patients showed depressed mood, self-depreciation, agitation, sleep disturbance, diminished socialization, changed attitudes towards school, somatic complaints, lack of energy, loss of appetite and/or weight, suicidal ideation and psychomotor retardation. Two of the depressed subjects presented in stupor; others showed severe psychomotor retardation.

Treatment of affective disorders

Depression in young people often appears to be reactive to their circumstances and life events and sometimes the clinical picture meets the criteria for an adjustment disorder (see Chapter 12). Whether or not these criteria are met, however, it is important to look carefully for evidence of stresses which may be contributing. Many depressed children have long been subject to family stress. Apart from general family instability, the stress may include parental alcoholism or drug abuse; physical violence towards the children or between the parents; sexual abuse; emotional rejection; and physical neglect. Any of the mentioned earlier may be operating. The family system may be such that the child plays the role of family scapegoat.

Any stresses that come to light should be the focus of treatment, whether by family therapy; counselling of the parents;temporary removal of the child to a treatment centre or other alternative placement; intervention at school to relieve stress there; or treatment of depression in a parent. In addition, children can often be helped to cope better with such stresses, at least if they are not too severe and chronic, by means of an ongoing supportive relationship with a therapist.

Antidepressant drugs may be helpful in major affective disorders in children (Puig-Antich, 1980; Preskorn *et al.*, 1982). Unfortunately blood levels of the most-studied antidepressant, imipramine, vary widely in children even when standard age- or weight-related doses are given. Periodic estimations of blood levels are therefore necessary to ensure that a therapeutic concentration is present. In adolescents the administration of antidepressant medication is usually indicated in severe cases, in addition to other measures as above. Caution should be exercised in providing adolescents with supplies of medication, since overdoses of tricyclic antidepressants, which may be taken with suicidal intent, are dangerous and sometimes fatal.

When there is severe depression with evidence of serious suicidal intent admission to hospital may be necessary. The decision whether to admit will also depend on the stability of the home and the capacity of the family to care safely for the young person.

In the treatment of mania, medication is often required. In the acute phase the administration of a major tranquilliser, such as chlorpromazine or haloperidol is often necessary. Attention should also be given to relieving any environmental stress which may come to light.

Lithium carbonate is effective in preventing the recurrence of mania and depression in many individuals with bipolar affective disorders. Its use, and that of the other drugs mentioned above, is discussed further in Chapter 19.

Outcome

Affective disorders usually resolve in time, even without treatment, if suicide does not occur; this applies in childhood as well as in adult life. Without treatment, however, they may last many months or even several years. In about one-fifth of cases the response to treatment is not complete and the condition may become chronic, but the outlook for individual attacks is generally good. Unfortunately there is a considerable risk of recurrent attacks occurring and this seems to be even greater in children with primary affective disorders than in adults. When the onset is during adolescence the risk is greater than with onset in adult life but less than when onset is before puberty.

In secondary cases, the outlook depends on the progress of the primary or associated condition(s). If they resolve it is generally good. If the condition is a response to medication with steroids or other drugs, it can be expected to clear up once the medication is discontinued. As a general rule the greater the environmental stress that has appeared to contribute to the disorder, the better the outlook, while the more the disorder seems to be 'endogenous', the worse it is. Heavy genetic loading for affective disorders, alcoholism or antisocial behaviour may be poor prognostic signs.

Chapter 7

Pervasive Developmental Disorders

DSM-III-R uses the term 'pervasive developmental disorder' (PDD) for conditions characterized by:

(A) qualitative impairment of reciprocal social interaction;
(B) impairment in communication and imaginative activity;
(C) markedly restricted repertoire of activities and interests.

It subdivides them as follows:

(1) Autistic disorder. Onset may be in infancy or childhood; if it is after 36 months of age it is specified as 'childhood onset' type.
(2) Pervasive developmental disorder, not otherwise specified.

ICD-9 classifies infantile autism as one subcategory of 'psychoses with origin specific to childhood'. The removal of these conditions from among the psychoses, as in DSM-III-R, seems however more appropriate.

Infantile autism

Leo Kanner (1943; 1944) described a group of severely disturbed children and named the syndrome they presented 'early infantile autism'. For many years this was regarded as a psychotic disorder coming on very early in life; some considered it to be a form of schizophrenia. They argued that, although it differed from schizophrenia in various respects, one could not expect schizophrenia starting before the subject had learned to talk, and while cognitive development was still at an early stage, to present in the same way as in older patients. For example auditory hallucinations would be unlikely in a child who had not started talking.

The results of subsequent research suggest strongly that infantile autism is distinct from schizophrenia (Kolvin *et al.* 1971; Rutter and Garmezy, 1983; see also the discussion of schizophrenia in Chapter 8); and whether it should be regarded as a psychotic disorder at all is in doubt. It seems rather to be a serious disorder of the development of a range of psychological functions, coming on early in life. Psychoses, on the other hand, are characterized by the loss of reality contact in people who previously have maintained a conventional relationship to and understanding of their environment. DSM-III-R's categorization of infantile autism as a 'pervasive developmental disorder' (PDD) is thus a useful step forward. Although these children appear to be out of touch with reality, this is secondary to a gross failure of the developmental process to take its usual course.

Many other names have been used to describe infantile autism and related conditions. These include infantile psychosis, childhood autism, childhood schizophrenia, schizophrenic syndrome of childhood and symbiotic psychosis. These terms are best avoided, particularly those suggesting that the condition is a form of schizophrenia.

Prevalence

British studies by Lotter (1966) and Wing (1980) agree on a prevalence rate of between 4.5 and 5.0 per 10,000 children. In each of these studies rather less than half the children identified were considered as falling into the 'nuclear group', that is those with the full syndrome. The remainder had autistic features but not the full picture. Many of these would probably fall into the DSM-III-R category of 'pervasive developmental disorder not otherwise specified'. Although Lotter's (1966) study suggested that the condition was commoner in higher socioeconomic classes, this was not confirmed by Wing (1980).

Lotter (1978a) also found 'autistic-like' conditions in 2-3 per cent of 300 mentally retarded children in nine African cities, so the condition is not confined to 'western' societies. It seems also that certain autistic features are found more frequently among severely mentally handicapped children; if all such children are included higher prevalence rates prevail.

The condition is about three times commoner in boys than in girls, but there is some evidence that girls tend to be more seriously affected (Tsai *et al.*, 1981; Lord *et al.*, 1982).

Causes and associated conditions

Genetic, organic cerebral, environmental, biochemical and immunological causes have all been suggested for autism. Evidence that genetic factors play some part was provided by a study of 21 pairs of same-sexed twins, one or both of whom had autism (Folstein and Rutter, 1977). Eleven were monozygotic (MZ) and 10 dizygotic (DZ). Four of the MZ but none of the DZ pairs were concordant for autism. Also 6 non-autistic co-twins (5 MZ and 1 DZ) showed some serious cognitive disability, either speech delay, IQ below 70 or scholastic difficulties. Thus there was 36 per cent concordance for autism in MZ twins against none for DZ twins; and 82 per cent concordance for cognitive disorder in MZ pairs, against 10 per cent in DZ pairs. Both differences are statistically significant. The findings could not be explained on the basis of brain damage at birth; it seemed that in some cases the disorder resulted from an inherited cognitive defect plus brain damage.

There are other reasons to believe that genetic factors are involved. The rate of autism in the siblings of autistic children is about 2 per cent, which is about 50 times that in the general population (Rutter, 1967a); and there is a family history of delayed speech development in about 25 per cent (Bartak *et al.*, 1975). Moreover 15 per cent of the siblings of autistic children show evidence of language disorders, learning difficulties or mental retardation, whereas this only applies to 3 per cent of the siblings of children with Down's syndrome (August *et al.*, 1981).

As we saw in Chapter 2 several research reports have suggested a high frequency (20 per cent of autistic boys in the study of Gillberg and Wahlstrom, 1985) of the 'fragile X' syndrome in autistic children. Despite conflicting reports, there does seem to be a connection between the chromosome abnormality and both mental retardation and autism.

Brain damage is certainly present in some children with autism, but most brain-damaged children are not autistic and many autistic children show no evidence of brain damage. Nevertheless many – 29 per cent in one study (Rutter, 1970) – of non-epileptic autistic children develop epilepsy later. This is much greater than the incidence of epilepsy in the general population.

Autistic behaviour is sometimes seen in children with various forms of brain damage and with certain metabolic disturbances (Cohen, 1980). Chess (1977) reported 10 cases of 'the complete autism syndrome' among 243 children with congenital rubella; another 8 showed a 'partial syndrome'. These represent prevalence rates some 200 times those in the general child population. Cohen (1980) has also pointed out similarities between infantile autism and the Gilles de la Tourette syndrome (see Chapter 12).

It seems that brain damage, along with a genetic tendency, may combine to cause some cases of autism (Rutter, 1985a). It is, however, unclear what part of the brain needs to be damaged for this to happen.

Stubbs *et al.* (1985) suggest that some cases may have an immunological basis. They report a study of human leucocyte antigens (HLA) in the parents of autistic children. They found that the parents shared HLAs very much more often than parents of normal children are thought to do. They offer an ingenious explanation of how this might be related to autism in the children; they seek to explain also the occurrence of toxaemia in pregnancy, the male preponderence in autistic children and their frequent ordinal position as firstborns. Kuperman *et al.* (1985) reviewed studies of blood serotonin levels, which are said to be increased in one-third of autistic children; this may, however, be related to the mental retardation that is often present, rather than to the autism.

The immunological and serotonin hypotheses, and others that have been put forward, offer only avenues for further research; none is as yet near to being confirmed. Rutter (1985a) reviewed the evidence from neurophysiological, neuroanatomical, neuropathological and neurochemical studies but found it to be inconclusive. At present we do not understand the physical basis of autism, which may differ in different cases.

Autism has also been attributed to environmental factors, especially family ones. Kanner (1943; 1944) asserted that the parents lacked emotional warmth and were detached and of obsessional personality. There is no firm evidence of this and reported parental attitudes could be reactions to the behaviour of these children, especially their lack of emotional responsiveness. It seems unlikely that adverse parental attitudes or handling could alone be responsible for so severe a condition coming on so early in life. Moreover autism has not been shown to be associated with child abuse or neglect. On the other hand the way autistic children are handled certainly can affect their development. This is the basis of the behavioural treatment of this condition. Given that a child is already autistic, the parents may choose either to accept the withdrawal from contact and the primitive, repetitive play of the child; or they may take active measures to counter such behaviour. The same applies to the reactions of teachers and others.

The association of infantile autism and mental retardation is strong. Most of the autistic children studied by Rutter and Lockyer (1967) had IQs in the 'mentally handicapped' range, though about a quarter fell in the normal range. In most cases the low IQ did not appear to be due to the autistic process; it tended to remain at about the same level even following recovery from the condition.

Other important associations are with impaired language development and epilepsy. Severely impaired language development is a major feature of the condition itself, but language disorders are also present unusually frequently in these children's siblings.

Description

Kanner (1943; 1944) described four main features of 'early infantile autism':

- autistic aloneness;
- delayed or abnormal speech;
- an obsessive desire for sameness;
- onset in the first two years of life.

These have remained the basis for the definition of this syndrome but in DSM-III-R the criteria for making the diagnosis are considerably more sophisticated. Onset in the first two years is not a necessary criterion, even for the type with 'onset during infancy', nor is 'an obsessive desire for sameness' a necessary feature.

The DSM-III-R criteria comprise a number of features under the headings listed as (A), (B) and (C) at the beginning of this chapter, together with onset during infancy or childhood. At least 8 of the 16 items must apply, including at least two from section A, one each from B and C.

Rutter (1985b) summarizes the abnormalities under three headings:

(a) *Abnormal development*, affecting cognition, language and socialization.
(b) *An abnormal style of functioning*, characterized by rigidity, stereotypy and inflexibility.
(c) *Non-specific behaviour problems*. Unlike the first two categories, these are not specific to autistic children but can be very troublesome nevertheless.

(a) The abnormalities of development

Verbal and non-verbal language development are affected. Not only do autistic children fail to develop normal or, sometimes, any speech, but they also fail to communicate effectively by gesture, body movements or facial expression. They differ from children with developmental language disorders (see Chapter 10) who point to what they want, pull people towards those things and generally manage to make their wishes known. And when autistic children do develop speech they fail to use it for social communication in the normal way. They may engage in 'echolalia', the repeating of words or phrases spoken by others; this may be immediate or delayed, the repetition occurring at a later time and resulting in the production of apparent nonsense. These children often acquire stock phrases which they repeat in parrot-like fashion and with little or no relation to what is going on around them. Their speech is often stilted and monotonous, without the usual intonations and inflexions.

The failure to speak is but one manifestation of a profound defect of language function (Bartak *et al.*, 1975). This is often present from the early months, though sometimes speech starts to develop normally and is then lost. This has been found to occur more often in girls than in boys (Kurita, 1985).

The abnormalities of cognitive development are complex and extensive (Rutter, 1983a). A majority of autistic children are mentally retarded but in all of them, whether retarded or not, there is an abnormal pattern of cognitive functioning. Memory may be excellent and visuospatial tasks may be well performed, but these children are very poor at symbolization, understanding abstract ideas and grasping theoretical concepts. They may be preoccupied with mechanical things like train or bus timetables or the different models of cars or aeroplanes. One 11-year-old autistic boy knew the numbers of all the main highway routes in Britain; he spent many hours poring over maps and you had only to ask him how to get from one city or town to another and the road numbers would pour forth instantly and accurately. Abstract or creative thought, however, were beyond him.

The development of social skills is also both retarded and deviant. The parents often report that their autistic children were unresponsive infants who did not seem to want to be kissed or cuddled. They may have failed to assume the posture appropriate for being picked up or nursed. They develop the social smile late and are typically slow to distinguish between parents and strangers, approaching either indis-criminately. A related behaviour is gaze avoidance, the failure to make eye-to-eye contact with people. While autistic children may look at people, they fail to do so when it is appropriate, for example during conversation or when requesting something (Mundy *et al.*, 1986). These children may appear more interested in a person's spectacles or facial contours, than with the individual as a person. 'Indicating behaviours', such as drawing people's attention to things by showing them or by alternately looking at them and making eye contact with the other person, have been found to occur less often than in retarded or normal children at similar developmental levels (Mundy *et al.*, 1986).

In a study of their social interactions (Sigman *et al.*, 1986) young autistic children shared attention with their caregivers and were engaged with them in mutual eye contact, less often than non-autistic children at similar levels of development.

A major problem seems to be impaired capacity for empathy – the understanding and sharing of other people's feelings. The social cues and signals we perceive in others, and make use of in our social relationships, seem to mean nothing to autistic people. Feelings like love and ideas like friendship are hard for them to understand, let alone experience. (In this respect, though this alone, they resemble Spock in 'Star Trek' though he, in 'Star Trek IV', finally learned a little of what emotional feelings are!) In order to enable autistic children to display socially appropriate behaviour, it is often necessary to rehearse them repeatedly in the various things they must do at the event concerned. The able and committed parents of one 14-year-old boy described how they taught their son everything he would have to do at a social event before they took him there; but woe betide them if they missed a step or something unexpected happened, for he could never figure out, from the context, what he should do.

(b) Rigidity, stereotypies and inflexibility

These three features characterize the functional style of autistic children. They resist change; they may wish always to go places by the same routes or to wear the same clothes. Some of them get very upset about minor changes of routine or the moving of furniture in the house, even of books in a bookcase. While they can be taught new skills, they fail to generalize these to new situations or tasks. Their play is also stereotyped and repetitive. It is typically neither symbolic nor imaginative; toys are rarely used as the objects they represent. An autistic child may use a toy telephone to bang on the floor or to swing to and fro, but will probably not imitate adults' use of a telephone as other children do. Lack of symbolic play is, however, also quite common, though less so, in retarded and normal children of similar developmental level (Mundy *et al.*, 1986), so its discriminative value is limited.

Autistic children's use of language shows similar characteristics. Normal children, even those just starting to talk, are constantly making up words and phrases in a creative way (using their creativity to produce words like 'drinked' or 'sheeps', which are logical modifications of words they will have heard). Autistic children do not do this; instead they use stock phrases and stereotyped expressions, often inappropriately.

Ritualistic behaviour is common in these children, for example checking or touching rituals and dressing in a particular way. When these rituals are interrupted they may become anxious or angry. Rocking, twirling, head-banging and similar repetitive movements are often seen, especially in mentally retarded autistic children.

(c) Non-specific behaviour problems

These include overactivity, disruptive behaviour and temper tantrums. Overactivity may alternate with underactivity. Self-destructive behaviours – for example, violent head-banging or biting the arms or wrists – may occur. Other common symptoms are sleep disturbances, fears and phobias, wetting and soiling, and impulsive acts. All these are especially hard to deal with because of the difficulty in communicating effectively with these children.

Elaine was born at full term following a normal pregnancy. Her birth weight was 2.5 kg. She appeared a healthy baby but feeding her was difficult. Breast feeding was abandoned after two weeks but even on the bottle she was difficult and fractious. She was an active baby and slept only for short periods. Her motor development during the first year was if anything a little advanced. She was reported to have said her first words at 10 months and was reciting nursery rhymes by 18 months. She was very musical and by this age could sing several songs. When just over 12 months Elaine had several breath-holding attacks; one of these was followed by a major convulsion. She was given phenobarbitone but reacted badly to it. She was taken off it after a few weeks and had no more seizures.

When aged about 21 months, towards the end of her mother's second pregnancy, Elaine's behaviour began to cause the parents concern. She repeatedly and often inappropriately made remarks like, 'I don't like Mummy poorly', and expressed dislike of various people.

Her condition deteriorated following the birth of her sister when she was 23 months old. Her speech regressed further and she started repeating people's questions instead of giving replies. She no longer talked to people, took little notice of them and spent long periods rocking. Episodes of severe temper and screaming developed but she retained her musical skill. At 2 years 6 months a neurologist diagnosed her as autistic.

At age 3 Elaine was taken to a child guidance clinic but 12 weeks of weekly attendance brought no benefit. She had by this time lost most of her speech. She remained hyperactive and difficult to manage at home.

When Elaine was seen for consultation at 4 years 6 months her parents described her as being hyperactive, impossible to communicate with, obsessed with food and unpredictable in mood, quiet periods being succeeded by severe tantrums. She would not go on her own to the toilet as she had done at one stage. She often wet and occasionally soiled herself. But she was considered intelligent, had a good memory and knew where everything was. She now had no speech. Her hearing had been tested and pronounced normal. She was agile and good with her hands.

Elaine was an attractive, overactive child. She ignored the examiner and engaged in a manneristic dance from time to time. At other times she moved restlessly and apparently aimlessly about the room. She did not play with any toys in a conventional way; instead put them into her mouth. She made no response to speech. She vocalized a few sounds but produced no recognizable words. She laughed once or twice for no obvious reason. Otherwise she showed little emotional reaction. The presence in the room of three unfamiliar adults did not seem to affect her behaviour.

Elaine's parents were university graduates, father a university lecturer, mother a school teacher. Both were deeply concerned about Elaine and were prepared to go to great trouble to help her and obtain treatment for her. The family appeared stable and there was no family history of psychiatric illness.

Comment

Elaine's condition fits the DSM-III-R criteria for an autistic disorder. Onset was during the second year after a period of apparently normal development. It seemed to the parents initially to be a reaction to the mother's pregnancy and the birth of the second child, but the birth of a sibling is a common event in the second year of life and this may have been coincidence. Well developed musical ability is often reported in these children, some of whom can retain and reproduce long musical pieces.

Infantile autism, residual state

This category appeared in DSM-III but it has been omitted from DSM-III-R. It is, however, useful as a category for the disorders of individuals who once had a disorder that met the criteria for infantile autism and who still have some features but no longer meet the full criteria. These 'post-autistic' children and adults have partially recovered but they often display strange personality characteristics. They may appear emotionally distant and aloof, and the lack of empathy with others and social awkwardness are usually still evident. Speech and communication skills are seldom normal and their capacity for abstract thought and creative thinking is usually limited. Thinking is 'concrete', that is concerned with facts, mechanical matters, putting things in order and the like. They may be a rather different group from subjects whose disorders never met the full criteria for an autistic disorder.

Pervasive developmental disorder not otherwise stated

This rather clumsy DSM-III-R term is provided for use when the diagnostic criteria for an autistic disorder are not fully met but 'there is a qualitative impairment in the development of reciprocal social interaction and in verbal and nonverbal communication skills'. Such disorders are less distinctive and less generally recognized entities than infantile autism. They are probably quite a large group, however, and in DSM-III were classified as 'atypical pervasive developmental disorder'. Many partially recovered autistic children come into this category, in addition to those who have never displayed the full autistic clinical picture.

Differentiating PDDs from other conditions

Pervasive developmental disorders require to be distinguished from deafness, various forms of mental retardation, developmental language disorders and the various psychotic disorders discussed in the next chapter.

There is usually good evidence from the history and the clinical examination, that the child's problem is failure to respond to people, rather than inability to hear. Nevertheless it is usually wise to arrange audiometry to ensure that there is no hearing defect. These children can be hard to test, however, and in difficult cases the measurement by electroencephalography (EEG) of the evoked responses in the cerebral hemispheres to auditory stimuli may be helpful.

While mental retardation and PDD may co-exist, retarded children usually relate freely with people, are not preoccupied with sameness, and are more generally retarded; the retardation of children with autistic disorders and other PDDs is more patchy and confined to the particular functions we have discussed above. The language structure of children with PDDs is particularly characteristic.

Developmental language disorders are described in Chapter 10. Children with such disorders are not usually emotionally withdrawn; they respond to people normally and communicate freely by non-verbal means. Echolalia and pronominal reversal are much less common than in autistic children. Bizarre behaviours, rigidity, stereotypies and lack of symbolic and imaginative play are not features of developmental language disorders.

Some of the forms of disintegrative psychosis, discussed in Chapter 8, may mimic PDDs. Emotional withdrawal of an intensity rivalling that seen in autistic disorders, is often encountered in children who have had infantile myoclonic epilepsy and, as we have seen, in some with congenital rubella. The distinction between these conditions and PDD can usually be made by means of careful history taking and neurological assessment.

Treatment

Infantile autism

We do not have available any effective means of remedying the ill-understood basic causes of autism, although some of the behaviours of autistic children can be changed using behaviour therapy techniques (Currie and Brannigan, 1970; Lovaas *et al.*, 1973). Speech can also be taught by similar means but progress is usually slow and intensive, long-term treatment is needed.

Treatment should aim to promote healthier and more normal development. An excellent summary of how this task may be approached is that of Rutter (1985b). He deals with the various developmental delays seen in autistic children, in each case suggesting means whereby development may be promoted. Educational and behavioural methods are the mainstays of treatment.

Rutter (1985b) considers, in the case of each developmental problem, what the child's need is and how this need can be met in respect of each of the specific problems the child faces. A basic principle is that children (and adults too) generally learn more from doing things than from having them done for them.

Rutter starts with the need all children have for 'active, meaningful experiences'. He then considers what particular experiences are needed to counter the various problems autistic children have in the area of cognitive development. Thus for 'self-isolation' planned periods of interaction are needed; for 'impaired understanding', simplified communication and individual teaching; for specific cognitive defects, learning tasks which capitalize on the skills the child does possess while helping develop those that are weak; and for lack of initiative, a more structured and direct teaching approach than is used with normal children. He then considers language skills, social skills and the capacity to learn, all of which can be promoted using similar principles.

Some of the implications of this approach are that the treatment plan should aim to counter social isolation by ensuring periods of interaction; it should break learning down into small steps specifically suited to the child's progress to date; teaching should take place in structured, individualized situations; and personalized caretaking should be enhanced by the avoidance of residential care in early childhood. The treatment, which means largely the teaching, of autistic children is a complex and challenging undertaking. The article by Rutter (1985b) provides an excellent introduction to the concepts on which programmes should be based. A sound knowledge of behaviour therapy principles, which are outlined in Chapter 19, is also needed.

The teaching of communication skills, principally speech and language, is an important but usually long and difficult task. It has been suggested that 'nonvocal' methods – that is, the use of sign language or of symbols – may have a useful part to play in teaching autistic children to communicate. Kiernan (1983) reviewed the literature on this subject but found much of it of poor quality. Although these children often have as much difficulty with nonverbal as with verbal communication, a combination of the two may promote faster development than either alone. It may be especially helpful with the more severely retarded. While autistic children can learn to use signs to communicate their needs, the part sign language should play in treatment plans is unclear.

Some general points about treatment are that this should be a joint venture of the planners of the programme, the professional behaviour therapists, the speech therapists and teachers concerned and the parents. Treatment is best located in the home and a neighbourhood school, preferably in a special small class or group, with increasing opportunities for the autistic children to mix with their non-autistic peers as their condition improves. Residential placement is to be avoided; these children are particularly susceptible to institutionalization because of their tendency to withdraw from social contacts, and their communication difficulties. Some parents become highly skilled behaviour therapists themselves. Their children are at a great advantage; the amount of treatment they receive may be much greater than it otherwise would be, since it can continue at home when no professionals are available.

Other treatment measures which may be helpful include the use of drugs to control certain behaviours. Haloperidol has been reported to reduce stereotyped behaviour and it may help some children become more susceptible to behaviour therapy (Cohen et al., 1980). It may also be helpful in modifying hyperactive behaviour. Medication may also be indicated for severe sleep disturbances, especially when these are seriously interfering with the sleep of other family members. It is doubtful whether any drugs affect the autistic process itself. There has been a suggestion that fenfluramine may have some such effect but this is based on only three cases (Geller et al., 1982).

Help for the families is often needed, since the presence in a family of a severely disturbed child can have great repercussions on the family system as a whole. Some parents also experience feelings of guilt about having an autistic child. It should be made clear to them that PDDs are not caused by the handling or upbringing children have received, though the parents can do much to help promote more normal development. The experience of being 'co-therapists' can itself help guilt-ridden or despairing parents gain new hope and more positive attitudes towards their children's problems. There are also, in most areas, organizations of parents and others interested in the problems of, and services for, autistic children. Many find it helpful to become active in such societies.

Treatment of other pervasive developmental disorders

The literature on the treatment of PDDs other than those that fit the criteria for autistic disorders is scant, perhaps because these are less well-defined conditions. Approaches similar to those outlined for autistic children are usually needed. Treatment programmes must be designed to deal with the specific developmental problems of the particular child. These other PDDs are a more varied group of disorders than those which fit the DSM-III-R criteria for autistic disorders. Some are less severely disturbed in their development. They may be able to attend normal school classes or classes for children with learning difficulties, if given additional help.

Outcome

Many autistic children show a measure of improvement, sometimes quite a marked one. This may start at about age 4 to 6, sometimes later. Much depends on the child's level of functioning early on. Those with IQs below about 50 (assuming that they co-operated in the testing), and those who have acquired no speech by age 5, mostly remain severely handicapped. A normal non-verbal IQ and some speech at age 5 are hopeful signs.

According to a review by Lotter (1978b) about two-thirds of all autistic children remain severely handicapped in adult life. Most of these end up in institutions. Fewer than one-fifth are working and surviving in the community; some of these are likely to be found in sheltered occupations or situations. Well-planned long-term active treatment, constructive care in a concerned family and avoidance of residential care (except for very short-term admissions to give the family a break or deal with crises) all probably improve the outlook. Some useful speech is acquired by about 50 per cent of autistic children but few achieve normal language skills. Epilepsy often appears during the course of the disorder, especially during adolescence. Deykin and MacMahon (1979) reported its appearance in one-fifth of 183 autistic subjects.

As adults, autistic subjects almost always show residual signs of their disorder. They tend to be emotionally cold and aloof and lack the capacity to show empathy with others. Their social life is limited and they seem to have no idea how to make friends. They show continuing evidence of their language disorder, with poor comprehension of abstract concepts and the use of stilted, repetitive, mechanical or echolalic phrases.

Rumsey *et al.* (1985) report a detailed study of 14 men, with a mean age of 28, who had well-documented histories of autism. In half the cases the diagnosis had been made by Leo Kanner. They were a predominantly high functioning group, 12 having performance IQs in the normal range. Social relationship difficulties, concrete thinking and stereotyped repetitive movements were particularly common. Language skills 'ranged from normal to complete mutism', but the report does not make it clear how many of the men had completely normal language.

Rutter (1985a) provides an excellent summary of the course and outcome in infantile autism. Little systematic data is available concerning the outcome in other PDDs but since these are often milder disorders it may be better than when the child has displayed the full autistic syndrome.

Chapter 8

Schizophrenia and Other Psychoses of Childhood

The essential feature of psychotic disorders is altered contact with reality. The psychotic person is attempting to adapt to a subjectively distorted concept of the world. Individuals with neurotic/anxiety disorders, on the other hand, are adapting in morbid ways to their real-life situations.

It can be hard to know whether young children are psychotic because of their limited verbal skills. Their concept of the world has to be inferred from their behaviour. Another difficulty is that psychoses arising in childhood seriously distort personality development and learning processes. Intelligence, at least as it is assessed by many tests, is manifested largely through such learned behaviours as verbal and motor performance skills. Children who have failed to learn such skills because of preoccupation with their psychotic world cannot give evidence of their intelligence in the usual ways. As time passes and the psychotic process continues, a child's intellectual performance may gradually fall off; it can then be hard to know what level of cognitive functioning the child might otherwise have achieved.

We will consider psychotic disorders under the following headings:

(a) schizophrenia;
(b) disintegrative psychoses, including those due to organic disease of the brain;
(c) reactive psychoses;
(d) toxic confusional and delirious states.

Childhood schizophrenia

Research during the last two decades has clarified somewhat the nature of the major psychiatric disorders of childhood. A clear distinction between autistic disorders and schizophrenia is now generally accepted. Autism is probably best regarded as a severe distortion of development rather than as a psychotic condition. It is also generally agreed that schizophrenic psychoses such as occur in adults can afflict children. Such disorders have been reported in children as young as 5 years, though the condition is very rare before about age 7 (Tanguay and Cantor, 1986). Whether schizophrenia occurs before the age of 5 is open to question.

Several studies, such as those of Kolvin *et al.* (1971) and Green *et al.* (1984), provide good evidence that autism and schizophrenia are distinct entities. Autistic children do not develop schizophrenic clinical pictures as they grow older; and even when they develop speech they do not become hallucinated. Indeed the symptoms of schizophrenia are quite different from those of autism. Genetic studies also fail to provide support for the idea that autism is an early developing form of schizophrenia.

The prevalence of schizophrenia

Prepubertal schizophrenia is rarer than infantile autism, occurring at perhaps seven-tenths the prevalence rate of the latter condition (Tanguay and Cantor, 1986); there is no preponderance of boys, as opposed to girls, as there is in autism. After puberty schizophrenia occurs more frequently and late adolescence is a very common time for it to appear.

Causes

The causes of schizophrenia are not fully understood. Genetic predisposition plays a role in both adults and children. In adults environmental factors seem to play their part, certainly in predisposing to relapse in schizophrenics discharged from hospital and perhaps in precipitating the disorder. There is evidence that a high level of expressed emotion (EE) in families leads to a higher relapse rate. (The research on EE is described in *Expressed Emotion in Families* (Leff and Vaughn, 1985) and is summarised in *Basic Family Therapy* (Barker, 1986, Chapter 11).) Whether similar processes operate in childhood schizophrenia is not known but it has been suggested that another combination of behaviours, known as 'communication deviance' (CD) (Singer *et al.*, 1978; Wynne, 1981), may contribute to the development of schizophrenia.

CD consists of various forms of vague, ambiguous, wandering, illogical and idiosyncratic language, in some ways similar to, though less severe than, schizophrenic thought disorder. It may be present in the parents' language patterns for some years before the onset of schizophrenia in their offspring. It does not invariably lead to schizophrenia but Wynne, Singer and their colleagues believe it increases the likelihood of it occurring.

Clinical picture

Despite the possibility that schizophrenic processes starting in childhood might reasonably be expected to present in a different way to those starting in adult life (Tanguay, 1984), many investigators have chosen to use the diagnostic criteria developed for adults. This has the advantage of making it more likely that the children diagnosed as schizophrenic are suffering from the same condition. Beitchman (1983), however, argues that there are differences between childhood and adult-onset schizophrenia and suggests retention of 'childhood schizophrenia' as a distinct category. A later section will consider abnormalities that may be found in children who develop schizophrenia later.

The principal symptoms of schizophrenia are:

(1) Disorders of thought content, expressed as delusional beliefs. These may include delusions of persecution by persons known or unknown; delusions of reference (for example, that items in advertisements or newspapers, or on television, refer to oneself); the belief that thoughts are being put into, withdrawn from or broadcast from one's head (thought insertion, withdrawal and broadcasting); and the belief that one's thoughts are controlled by some external force. 'Delusional perceptions' arise fully fledged on the basis of a genuine perception which would be regarded as commonplace by others.

(2) Thought disorder. Associations become loosened, so that the subject's thoughts move from one subject to another apparently unrelated or distantly related one; sometimes the process resembles the 'knight's move' in chess. Although these patients may talk a lot, it is hard to grasp what they are saying. Poverty of thought, that is to say the existence of little content, may co-exist with the copious production of speech. In extreme cases talk may become completely incoherent.

(3) Hallucinations. These typically occur in clear consciousness and are most often auditory. They may consist of voices repeating the subject's thoughts out loud or anticipating them; or two or more hallucinatory voices may be discussing or arguing about the patient who is referred to in the third person; or voices may comment on the subject's thoughts or behaviour.

(4) Disorders of affect. The subject's emotional reactions are often blunted, flattened or inappropriate. Thus painful experiences may be described with a smile and there may be sudden, apparently inexplicable changes of mood.

(5) Volitional disorders. These patients may feel that their impulses,

acts and emotions are under external control. They may say they feel like robots or as if they have been hypnotized. Lack of interest and drive, with failure to initiate activities or follow them through, often leads to a falling off in school or work performancé.

(6) Disorders of motor behaviour. These include overactivity and underactivity; repetitive, stereotyped and often bizarre movements; and the assumption of inappropriate or bizarre postures, which may be maintained for long periods (catatonia).

(7) Other features. These include social isolation, often combined with preoccupation with fantasy or with delusional or illogical ideas; and loss of one's sense of identity. These patients may be puzzled about who they are, the meaning of their existence, and the nature of the world around them.

Many of these symptoms can be difficult to elicit in children, especially withdrawn ones; their limited cognitive skills make it hard for them both to understand what they are being asked about and to describe accurately their subjective experiences.

The onset of these disorders is usually insidious and it can be hard to say when the child actually developed schizophrenia. Developmental and other problems may have been present previously (see below). At the onset, however, there is a change of personality and an alteration in the quality of the contact the child makes, on an emotional level, with the environment. There may be progressive withdrawal from people, with violent reactions if attempts are made to counter this; the degree of withdrawal is however less marked than that seen in infantile autism, certainly in the early stages. Gradually other symptoms in the above list appear, in various combinations, with differing severity and at differing rates. Once the condition is established there are usually delusions, hallucinations, disorders of the form of thought and marked changes in the child's emotional reactions.

The behaviour of schizophrenic children is often changeable and unpredictable. Impulsive and overactive behaviour may alternate with withdrawn and underactive periods. Psychosocial development is delayed or halted and there may also be regression to earlier stages of development, with the return of long-abandoned behaviours such as wetting, soiling and infantile mealtime habits.

Most schizophrenic children are of normal intelligence, though the condition can occur in the mentally retarded. They may continue to perform in intelligence tests at or even above the average level long after the onset of their illness, but they usually fall behind in their school progress because in their disturbed state learning is impaired.

Paranoid schizophrenia, in which the patient falsely believes he or she is being persecuted, is seldom seen in childhood; it is commoner in adolescence.

Precursors of schizophrenia

There is reason to believe that individuals who later develop schizophrenia, whether before or after puberty, may show a variety of abnormalities long before a diagnosis of schizophrenia is warranted (Kolvin *et al.*, 1971: Green *et al.*, 1984). While this may be no more than another way of saying that the onset is often insidious, Green and his colleagues report that 9 of 24 autistic children they studied (37 per cent) had developed 'general abnormal behavioural symptoms' by the age of 4 years 11 months. Yet none of the children developed a schizophrenic disorder before age 5 and only 3 before age 7; and in only 5 (21 per cent) was there 'an acute onset of psychotic symptoms from a relatively normal premorbid adjustment'.

The point at which a diagnosis of schizophrenia is made is to some extent arbitrary, depending on the criteria used and how these are interpreted. It really marks but one stage in an unfolding process. When this has started is often hard to tell.

Barbara Fish has long believed that schizophrenia may occur in infancy and early childhood (Fish, 1977). Recently she described the early history of a patient who developed an acute schizophrenic illness at age 19 (Fish, 1986). He was the son of a chronic schizophrenic woman and had been studied from birth as part of a research project. Fish states that 'on the research observations he had deviate development from his first day'. He was late smiling, and rocked 'endlessly' on his rocking horse when young. By 6 years of age there was 'much more severe psychopathology', with difficulty in social relationships. When 9 years 7 months he was diagnosed as having 'a severe personality disorder with schizoid and paranoid traits'. While single case studies must be regarded with caution, the onset of this young man's schizophrenic illness seems to have been the culmination of a long, perhaps lifelong, period of abnormal development. This may apply to other cases.

Nuechterlein (1986) reviews the literature on childhood precursors of adult schizophrenia. These may include attentional and information processing abnormalities; neurological 'soft signs' (minor neurological abnormalities not indicative of structural lesions of the nervous system, which would be within normal limits if the child were younger); abnormalities of the autonomic nervous system; defects of social functioning; and other factors such as the familial emotional styles and communication patterns mentioned above.

Treatment of schizophrenia in childhood

According to Cantor and Kestenbaum (1986) treatments that have been used include 'parentectomy, psychoanalysis for both child and parents, behaviour therapy, milieu therapy, family therapy, educational therapy, and a variety of psychotherapeutic techniques such as movement and paraverbal therapy'. These have been offered, 'with or without psychopharmacological intervention and alone or in combination with other approaches'.

This situation no doubt reflects our lack of knowledge about what is most effective in treating schizophrenic children. Furthermore, the needs of schizophrenic children differ, depending on their ages, developmental levels and symptoms.

Systematic studies of the treatment of childhood, as opposed to adult, schizophrenia have been largely lacking (Beitchman, 1983). In adolescence approaches similar to those used with adults are often productive. The main features are:

- family intervention;
- the use of antipsychotic drugs;
- the long-term support of the patient by a therapist who also coordinates the work of a multidisciplinary team.

'Family intervention' is distinct from family therapy. Traditional family therapy techniques have not proved effective (McFarlane, 1983a) and techniques designed to achieve such specific objectives as reducing expressed emotion or communication deviance appear likely to be more helpful. The book *Family Therapy in Schizophrenia* (McFarlane, 1983b) addresses these issues. Leff *et al.* (1983) describe a socio-educational project which was designed to educate relatives about schizophrenia and reduce EE where this was high. How effective these measures would be in prepubertal schizophrenia is not known.

The role of antipsychotic drugs, principally phenothiazine compounds and haloperidol, is well established in the treatment of adults. The same drugs are also used with adolescents; they are probably indicated also in most children with schizophrenia. Caution is advisable in the use of these drugs and doses should be kept as low as possible because the long-term use of these drugs can lead to serious side-effects. Drug treatment is discussed further in Chapter 19.

Long-term support by a therapist is a must. It is doubtful whether dynamic psychotherapy, or indeed any specific form of psychotherapy, affects the basic schizophrenic processes. As these children grow up, however, they inevitably encounter difficulties in various areas of their lives. These may be educational, social or vocational, or they may concern the child's individual development and relationship to the world and the people in it. Cantor and Kestenbaum (1986) discuss the various ways in which therapists may help these children with such problems. They suggest that the therapist should be prepared to function as 'auxiliary ego, as facilitator of sensory perceptions, and as coordinator of a multidisciplinary treatment team'.

Outcome

Schizophrenia is a serious disorder at any stage of life but in childhood its implications are particularly grave. Occurring in a personality which is still incompletely developed, it may stunt or block completely the normal processes of psychological growth, in addition to causing the symptoms described above. For this reason the outlook tends to be better the later the age of onset. Sudden onset in a child or adolescent whose personality development and relationships have previously been normal tends to carry a better prognosis. Complete remission occasionally occurs.

The short-term response to medication may be gratifying, but it is not always maintained and lifelong medication has serious drawbacks. A major need in most cases is to help the young person handicapped by schizophrenic symptoms make the best possible adjustment in society. Many of these children and adolescents become chronic schizophrenics in adult life. At some point, often when their families are no longer able or willing to care for them, they may require admission to an institution for care.

Disintegrative psychoses

ICD-9 defines disintegrative psychoses as those in which 'normal or near-normal development for the first few years is followed by loss of social skills and of speech, together with a severe disorder of emotions, behaviour and relationships'. The loss of speech and social skills usually occurs over a period of a few months. Overactivity and repetitive, stereotyped behaviour are common; intellectual impairment is a frequent but not invariable part of the clinical picture.

DSM-III-R does not use the term 'disintegrative psychosis', suggesting instead that these disorders should be classified as dementias. Evidence of a dementing process is not however invariably present.

Causes

Disintegrative psychoses are often due to organic brain disease, though sometimes no evidence can be found for any organic disorder

(Evans-Jones and Rosenbloom, 1978). Such evidence may, however, emerge much later, sometimes at post-mortem examination (Creak, 1963).

Disintegrative psychoses may be divided into two groups:

- Progressive cases, usually due to a progressive neurological condition (Corbett *et al.*, 1977).
- Non-progressive cases, due either to neurological damage which is not progressive or to unknown causes.

Some of the neurological conditions which may be responsible are mentioned below.

Description

The clinical picture is quite varied. The condition most often develops over a period of a few weeks or months. Speech and language, and the capacity to comprehend language, deteriorate. Other features commonly seen are relationship difficulties, usually withdrawal; ritualistic and manneristic behaviour; delusions; hallucinations; deterioration of social behaviour; and a marked falling off in school performance, if the child is able to attend school.

The symptoms of the causative neurological disorder may appear first, followed by disturbed, overactive, irritable or otherwise uncharacteristic behaviour. In other cases there is some family disturbance or other psychosocial stress, followed by behavioural symptoms.

Intellectual function deteriorates. The performance, as opposed to the verbal, sections of intelligence tests are usually affected first. Neurological signs indicating focal lesions in the nervous system may appear. Psychotherapy and behaviour therapy are usually either ineffective or only briefly effective.

The EEG often becomes abnormal and serial examinations may show deterioration. Other special investigations such as computerized axial tomography (CAT Scan) may reveal evidence of brain damage or degeneration.

The history and clinical picture vary according to the cause.

(a) Non-progressive causes

Encephalitis, which may be associated with measles, mumps, influenza or other acute infectious diseases, may be followed by psychotic symptoms such as those described above. If the condition is associated with one of the common infectious diseases, there will be a history of this disease, often with a high fever, followed by loss of consciousness, seizures and various neurological signs. Sometimes encephalitis presents simply as a febrile illness with signs of cerebral involvement. Examination of the cerebrospinal fluid in the acute stage usually provides evidence of involvement of the central nervous system. The worldwide epidemic of encephalitis after the 1914-18 war led to many cases of severe post-encephalitic psychotic disorders;most of the early children's psychiatric inpatient units in the USA were opened primarily to treat children with such disorders (Barker, 1974a). Since then cases have been mainly sporadic.

Infantile myoclonic seizures (infantile spasms, salaam attacks) are a form of epilepsy occurring in children aged 3 to 18 months. The attacks consist of sudden flexion of the arms while the head simultaneously drops forward. At the height of the disease there may be scores or even hundreds of attacks each day. The EEG shows a characteristic pattern known as hypsarrhythmia. The attacks usually cease during the second year of life, leaving a severely mentally retarded child, but some of these children present with a psychotic picture. The degree of emotional isolation may resemble that seen in autism, though the history usually distinguishes the conditions.

The 'West syndrome' comprises infantile spasms, developmental regression and hypsarrythmia; it has many known causes, including brain damage at or before birth, reactions to immunization, tuberous sclerosis (see below), various inborn errors of metabolism and cerebral agenesis (Gomez and Klass, 1983). Treatment with adreno-corticotrophic hormone (ACTH) seems to lessen the chance of the child being left with severe brain damage.

Lead encephalopathy results from the ingestion of excessive amounts of lead. It is often associated with pica, the eating of substances not normally regarded as edible. (Pica is discussed in Chapter 12.) Old lead paint, car batteries and lead plumbing are among the commoner sources of ingested lead. Lead poisoning may occur in children living in deteriorating old buildings and in those who play in such buildings or on rubbish (garbage) dumps. Lead can be absorbed through the skin and lungs as well as the gastrointestinal tract.

In mild cases there may be a behaviour disorder with irritability, restlessness, inability to concentrate and apathy. Loss of appetite, vomiting and pallor due to anaemia may accompany these symptoms. In severe cases the psychiatric symptoms may be of psychotic intensity. Acute encephalopathy occurs with blood lead levels of about 150μg/dl or higher; its features are impaired consciousness, coma and seizures.

Lead poisoning should be investigated and treated in a specialist centre. All sources of lead in the environment should be removed; in severe cases chelating agents, which promote the removal of lead, should be administered.

'Idiopathic' cases of non-progressive disintegrative psychosis also occur, such as those reported by Evans-Jones and Rosenbloom (1978).

(b) Progressive causes

Tuberous sclerosis (epiloia) is a rare condition due to a dominant autosomal genetic trait. Sporadic cases also occur. Multiple tumours and malformations in the brain are associated with epilepsy and mental deterioration. There may also be behavioural symptoms and emotional withdrawal of psychotic intensity.

Hepato-lenticular degeneration (Wilson's disease) is inherited as an autosomal recessive trait and is a disorder of copper metabolism. Various parts of the body are affected; the damage to the brain may cause a psychotic syndrome or milder psychological symptoms. Involuntary movements, emotional lability, seizures and a dementing process are characteristic features. Restriction of copper intake and the use of chelating agents to increase copper excretion help some of these children.

Disorders of sphingolipid metabolism (lipidoses) are conditions which are mostly due to inherited recessive genes. Fatty substances (sphingolipids) accumulate in the brain and other parts of the body. Various neurological symptoms occur, for example blindness and seizures. Onset may be at any time during childhood, with progressive deterioration leading eventually to death. Sometimes the presenting picture is that of a progressive disintegrative psychosis, or it may resemble infantile autism. Deterioration may be quite slow. Tay-Sachs disease ('amaurotic family idiocy') and metachromatic leukodystrophy are particular forms that may present with psychiatric symptoms, leading ultimately to dementia and death.

Diffuse cerebral sclerosis (Schilder's disease) describes a group of conditions in which the white matter of the brain degenerates. Some forms are genetic in origin. The myelin sheaths of the nerve fibres are lost (demyelination) and this is followed by the growth of fibrous tissue (gliosis). Several forms have been described, with onset from infancy onwards. In the early stages there may be bizarre, unpredictable and variously disturbed behaviour, often with apparent loss of contact with the environment. Cortical blindness or deafness, in which the brain is unable to make use of the nerve impulses reaching it, may be present. A deteriorating performance at school may be the presenting symptom; other early features may be labile and inappropriate emotional responses. The course is progressive and the early symptoms are followed by profound dementia.

Subacute sclerosing panencephalitis (von Bogaert's disease or SSPE) is a rare disease believed to be due to the measles virus entering the brain cells during an acute attack of measles. Occasionally it follows immunization against measles. Onset is most often between 8 and 14 but may be as young as 2 years. It may present with a psychotic picture or as deteriorating performance at school. Personality change, intellectual decline, memory loss, generalized myoclonic jerks and withdrawal may be followed by epilepsy, leading to a state of profound dementia and ultimately death. The EEG findings are characteristic and diagnostic.

Dementia infantilis (Heller's syndrome) was the term used by Heller in 1930 to describe a dementing process, with disturbed, restless, psychotic behaviour, starting at about age 3 or 4 (Heller, 1954). These were probably cases of progressive disintegrative psychosis. The term is little used nowadays.

Acquired immune deficiency syndrome (AIDS) has recently emerged as a cause of neuropsychiatric symptoms in both children and adults. It seems that most AIDS patients suffer from brain damage as part of the disease (Wortis, 1986); such damage may be even commoner in children with AIDS than in adults with the condition. Atrophy of the brain occurs, leading to regression of language and motor functions and dementia (Barnes, 1986). AIDS in children is usually due either to infection *in utero* or during birth, or to the transfusion of infected blood.

Other rare neurological conditions may cause similar clinical pictures. The organic brain conditions mentioned above, and other rare ones, are described more fully in textbooks of paediatrics and neurology.

Treatment of disintegrative psychoses

It is rarely possible to reverse the underlying disease process, though palliative measures are possible in some cases. In lead poisoning, for example, the lead present in the body can be removed, sometimes with clinical improvement. Treatment is, however, mainly symptomatic.

Non-progressive cases often benefit from treatment methods similar to those used in pervasive developmental disorders. Epilepsy may complicate the clinical picture and anticonvulsants should be used to achieve as complete control as possible. Restless or hyperactive behaviour may be improved by administration of a phenothiazine drug or haloperidol (see Chapter 19).

Help for the families of children with these devastating and often fatal disorders is usually a major need. The assistance of support groups and professional social workers can be invaluable. Sometimes psychotherapy for the parents or the family is needed also.

Outlook

The outlook in the progressive disorders is generally poor. In many cases a state of severe dementia eventually develops, leading to death, though this may not occur until well into adult life. In non-progressive cases much depends on the severity of any brain damage there may be. Social and language skills may improve with maturation, especially if an appropriate educational programme and suitable behavioural management are provided. Considerable recovery may occur after encephalitis; this may continue for up to a year, sometimes even longer.

Reactive psychoses

DSM-III-R distinguishes 'brief reactive psychoses', in which psychotic symptoms appear in response to a psychosocial stress such as would be 'markedly stressful to almost anyone in similar circumstances'. The clinical picture involves emotional turmoil presenting in a person who previously was functioning well, together with at least one of the following:

- incoherence or loosening of associations;
- delusions;
- hallucinations;
- behaviour that is grossly disorganized or catatonic.

The symptoms last for a few hours or days but clear up within two weeks. The condition may occur in adolescence or middle childhood. It does not seem to be common in young people in western cultures. In Africa it occurs as a complication of school anxiety (the 'brain fag' syndrome – see Chapter 5) and its presentation can be quite dramatic. It may be exacerbated by the subject's belief that he or she has been bewitched.

Short-term administration of major tranquillisers such as phenothiazine drugs or haloperidol, together with reassurance and nursing in calm and quiet surroundings, usually leads to rapid improvement and resolution within a few days. The nature of the causative stress should then be investigated and if possible steps should be taken to remove or alleviate it. Therapy with child or family, and sometimes liason with the school, may be needed to guard against recurrence. The longer-term outlook is usually good.

Toxic confusional and delirious states

In these conditions there is diffuse, general impairment of brain function with a state of delirium or confusion. In delirium consciousness is clouded and the subject's awareness of the environment is altered. Orientation for time, place and person is impaired. Attention is ill-sustained and the stream of thought is disordered. Illusions, the misinterpretation of sensory stimuli (as, for example, when an inanimate object is perceived as a monster about to attack one); bizarre or frightening fantasies; and hallucinations, often visual, may occur. In severe cases the subject appears completely out of touch with reality.

Confusional states are milder degrees of disorientation and confusion, without the full picture of delirium.

These conditions may be acute, coming on quite suddenly, or subacute, starting gradually over the course of a few hours. The causes include:

- systemic infections, especially when there is high fever;
- metabolic disturbances, for example hypoglycaemic reactions in diabetics;
- acute brain injury and infections;
- some rare forms of epilepsy;
- chemical intoxication by drugs.

Children, especially in their first few years, are particularly prone to develop delirious reactions during acute febrile illness such as measles, pneumonia and other childhood infections. The advent of antibiotics, in those parts of the world where these are freely available, has greatly reduced the frequency of these reactions.

Chemical intoxication is a frequent and important cause. It occasionally results from the use of drugs medically prescribed for specific conditions, but in adolescence a more important cause is the abuse of prescription drugs and the use of 'street' drugs. Prescription drugs which may be responsible for confusional states if abused include sleeping tablets of various sorts, codeine-containing analgesics, tranquillisers such as diazepam and other benzodiazepines and many others. Among the 'street' drugs used by young people are marijuana, lysergic acid diethylamide (LSD or 'acid'), mescaline, phencyclidine (PCP or 'angel dust'), 'magic mushrooms', amphetamine drugs, cocaine (which can cause a severe psychosis with paranoid delusions) and heroin. This list is not exhaustive. We have mentioned, in Chapter 4, the glue, petrol (gasoline) and solvent sniffing which occurs in younger children as well as in adolescents. It, too, can cause transient confusion.

The *Handbook of Abusable Drugs* (Blum, 1984) is a good source of information on the wide variety of drugs that may be abused and their properties. Virtually all of them have been known to be abused by young people.

The *treatment* of delirious and confusional states is primarily the treatment of their causes. Medical conditions should receive the appropriate therapy, the use of any causative drugs should immediately be stopped and any necessary treatment given to deal with drug overdoses. These patients should be nursed in a quiet environment with a minimum of sensory stimulation.

Drug abuse is discussed further in Chapter 16.

Chapter 9

Hyperkinetic and Attention Deficit Disorders

Definition and prevalence

Activity level was one of the features found by Thomas and Chess (1977) to distinguish between the behavioural styles of the infants they studied (see Chapter 2). Some children are so active that they present major challenges to those caring for and attempting to educate them. Some of these represent one end of a continuum of activity level, perhaps with a normal distribution, but others may be suffering from a specific disorder, though the nature of this is not fully understood.

The 'hyperkinetic syndrome of childhood' is the term used in ICD-9 for a condition of short attention span, distractibility and 'disinhibited, poorly organized and poorly regulated extreme overactivity'. ICD-9 subdivides hyperkinetic disorders into:

- simple disturbance of activity and attention, in which the above symptoms are not accompanied by disturbance of conduct or delayed development of specific skills;
- hyperkinesis with developmental delay. In these cases there are associated delays in the development of speech, motor skills, reading or other specific skills;
- hyperkinetic conduct disorder, in which there is an associated 'marked conduct disturbance' but no developmental delay;
- 'other' and 'unspecified' categories, which are not defined.

The authors of DSM-III chose to emphasize the 'attention deficit' aspects of this syndrome. They also distinguished attention-deficit disorders with and without hyperactivity. The validity and practical usefulness of this distinction have, however, been questioned and in DSM-III-R we find only two categories:

- attention-deficit hyperactivity disorder (ADHD);
- undifferentiated attention-deficit disorder.

These disorders are characterized by inattention, impulsivity and hyperactivity. But while many disturbed children undoubtedly have difficulty sustaining attention, it is unclear whether this should be the basis for a diagnostic category. The findings of Shekim *et al.* (1985), for example, suggest that attention-deficit disorder with hyperactivity (ADDH), as it was defined in DSM-III, is rarely encountered on its own. They surveyed 114 9-year-old children using two diagnostic interview schedules, one administered to the children, the other to the parents. Not only did the two diagnostic schedules identify mainly different children as having ADDH (only two out of 18 who were given the diagnosis by one or other instrument were given it by both), but in only one case was the ADDH diagnosis the only diagnosis given. Even if we disregard co-diagnoses of 'transient tics' and enuresis there were only two 'pure' diagnoses of ADDH.

Prior and Sanson (1986), in a wide-ranging review of 93 articles and books, pointed out that attention is 'a diffuse and wide ranging ... concept involving ... at the very least, concentration, search, set, selective attention, activation and vigilance'. They considered that it had not been properly defined in relation to ADDH. They suggested that, even if one overlooks the problems of defining attention deficits, ADDH lacks 'a clearly distinguishable symptomatology', sharing symptoms with, in particular, conduct disorders and learning disabilities. Attention deficits are also found in autism, developmental delay, epileptics on medication and schizophrenics. The additional diagnoses in the study of Shekim *et al.* (1985) included, in at least two cases each, overanxious disorder, oppositional disorder, dysthymic disorder, conduct disorder and separation anxiety. In 12 of the ADDH cases associated conduct or oppositional disorders were diagnosed.

The usefulness of the concept of the 'hyperkinetic syndrome' has also been questioned. Shaffer and Greenhill (1979) argued that this diagnosis tells little about etiology, response to treatment or longer-term outcome. Nor, they say, does it permit generalizations to be made about clinical state. Yet there seems to be evidence for the existence of relatively 'pure' syndromes of hyperactivity. Trites and Laprade (1983) surveyed over 9000 Canadian children, using the Conners Teacher Rating Scales, a widely-used means of rating children's behaviour in school (Conners, 1969). They subjected the responses to factor analysis and found evidence of the existence of a group of children who 'might best be labelled as hyperactive', and who show neither symptoms of conduct disorder nor are 'emotionally over-indulgent' (their term for the features of another factor identified in the study). These 'pure hyperactives' comprised 1.6 per cent of the population. Using their criteria, 3.2 per cent of the children were hyperactive but not conduct disordered and a grand total of 5.75 per cent were hyperactive, regardless of what other symptoms they showed. In other words there were some children with hyperactivity, some with conduct disorders and some with both. Although there has been some criticism of this study, the findings accord with clinical experience.

Prevalence figures naturally depend on the criteria used to make the diagnoses and the characteristics of the populations studied, especially the children's ages. Rates of hyperactivity as high as 40 per cent have been reported (Safer and Allen, 1976) but these have been based on parent or teacher reports. More rigorous studies yield lower prevalence rates such as those mentioned above. Rates reported from Britain tend to be lower than those reported from North America. This is probably because British psychiatrists usually require hyperactivity and other symptoms to be present in a variety of settings, including the clinical assessment interview. In North America reported symptoms are given more weight.

More boys than girls are affected, the ratio probably being about 3:1 or 4:1, though in the DSM-III-R manual a ratio of from 6:1 to 9:1 is quoted (down from 10:1 in DSM-III).

'Undifferentiated attention-deficit disorder' is one of DSM-III-R's 'residual' categories. It is characterized by 'developmentally inappropriate and marked inattention that is not part of another disorder'. Thus it would not be applied to disorders which meet the criteria for ADHD. Many of the conditions that met the DSM-III criteria for attention-deficit disorder without hyperactivity (ADDWO) would now fall into this category. The validity of this DSM-III category is however doubtful. Thus in one study (Lahey *et al.*, 1984) the behaviour of 625 elementary school children was rated by teachers, using a scale different from that used by Trites and Laprade. According to the criteria used in this study, 10 (1.6 per cent) of the children had ADDH, and 20 (3.2 per cent) had ADDWO. They also found evidence that ADDH and ADDWO 'are dissimilar disorders, and perhaps should not be considered subtypes of the same disorder'. ADDH children tended to show aggressive conduct disorders and bizarre behaviour, and were lacking in guilt feelings and unpopular with peers and teachers. ADDWO children were found to be anxious, shy, socially isolated, unpopular (but less so than the ADDH children) and poor in sports. Both groups performed poorly at school, showed evidence of depression and had poor self-concepts.

In a later paper, Lahey and his colleagues (1985) presented data suggesting that ADDH and ADDWO also differed in their core attention deficits. ADDH children were found to be 'irresponsible, distractible, impulsive, answering without thinking, and sloppy', while ADDWO children were described as 'sluggish and drowsy'. Similar results were reported by King and Young (1982) and by Edelbrock *et al.* (1983).

Causes

Simple motor overactivity, as distinct from the 'hyperkinetic syndrome' (HS) described above, may be no more than one extreme of the range of activity levels that exists in any population. In the same way, children may be unusually tall without having anything wrong with them. Using Chess and Thomas' (1984) concept of 'goodness of fit', however, normal children who are unusually active could get into difficulties in families in which the parents are temperamentally unsuited to handling very active children. Secondary problems, including family systems dysfunction, might then arise. Clinical experience suggests that this sometimes happens. Yet in many cases the problem is more than just a poor 'fit' between temperaments.

Adoption studies (Morrison and Stewart, 1973; Cunningham et al., 1975) and twin studies (Willerman, 1973; Torgerson and Kringlen, 1978) suggest that genetic factors are involved. Brain damage, food additives and allergies, raised blood lead levels, psychological stress and family systems problems have also been invoked as causes.

The concepts of 'minimal brain dysfunction' (MBD) and 'minimal brain damage', once popular, have now largely been discarded. At one time 'hyperkinetic syndrome' and 'MBD' were used almost synonymously by many but the relationship that was believed to exist between minor brain abnormalities, as manifested by 'soft' neurological signs, and hyperactivity, has not been satisfactorily demonstrated. MBD, as a clinical entity, was probably a myth (Schmitt, 1975) and use of the term is better avoided. There is no good evidence that hyperactivity is specially associated with brain damage and most brain damaged children are not hyperactive.

Claims have been made that diets such as that of Feingold (1975) are effective in reducing hyperactivity and related problems, but their results may be due in part to the faith of those who believe in them. There is, however, some evidence that they are effective in certain cases (Conners, 1980). Egger et al. (1985) studied 76 severely overactive children, some of whom had neurological, allergic or other physical symptoms. They were given an 'oligoantigenic' diet and 62 (81.5 per cent) improved, 21 (28 per cent) achieving 'a normal range of behaviour'. Twenty-eight of the responders completed a double-blind, placebo-controlled trial of the suspected food; the results strongly suggest that the children's behaviour was better on the placebo diet. The authors seem justified in their conclusion that 'the suggestion that diet may contribute to behaviour disorders in children must be taken seriously'. Whether the primary effect is on activity level seems less clear.

We have seen, in Chapter 8, that exposure to lead can cause

psychiatric symptoms; these may include restlessness and impaired attention but in most hyperactive children there is no evidence that lead is involved. Investigation of blood lead levels is, however, a sensible precaution.

The role and importance of psychological factors and the family environment in contributing to these disorders are also unclear, but the focussing and sustaining of attention are probably to some extent learned skills (Taylor, 1980). The learning processes are likely to be impaired in disorganized and unstable families, but there has been little research into exactly how this happens.

There are also biochemical theories concerning the etiology of hyperactivity which may be associated with 'perturbations in brain neurotransmitter function' (Shaywitz *et al.*, 1983). Research findings concerning this and other aspects of these disorders are discussed in a series of chapters in *Developmental Neuropsychiatry* (Rutter, 1983b).

Description

The research findings outlined above suggest that children with attention deficits and hyperactivity may not comprise a distinct clinical entity. ADDH and ADDWO may be different in their nature, and Prior *et al.* (1985) report research which casts doubt on the proposition that hyperactive children show attention deficits! 'Hyperkinetic syndromes' certainly exist but they have variable manifestations; hyperactivity may present in relatively pure form, or along with other symptoms or disorders, especially behaviour problems (conduct/ oppositional disorders in the terminology of DSM-III-R) and poor school progress.

From a clinical point of view it is important to recognize that there is a group of children who present with motor hyperactivity, restlessness, impaired attention and impulsivity. Many of them are readily distractible but they usually attend only briefly to the distracting stimuli. Onset is usually before age 3 but some children may not come to professional attention until they start school. The hyperactivity may be manifest in infancy; it may even be reported by the mother while the child is still *in utero*. In many instances, though, it first becomes evident when the child starts to walk. Serious management problems may then arise. Typically these children are constantly on the go, concentrate poorly, and may interfere with furniture, ornaments, the contents of drawers and other items, to an unusual extent. Sleep disturbance is often reported in younger children, but some sleep well, apparently because their daytime activity has exhausted them by bedtime, though they may waken early in the morning.

The symptoms often become more troublesome when the child first enters school. Some parents seem able to manage hyperactive children well at home; in the case of first children they may not even realize that the level of activity is abnormal. In such cases entry into school may precipitate a crisis. The child does not respond to the disciplinary measures used by the teacher, disrupts the class and may show other behaviour problems, such as non-compliance to instructions, aggression towards other children, and noisy, overtalkative behaviour. These children do not attend to their work and normal methods of control are ineffective; in due course many of them fall behind in their academic progress.

The early chapters of the book *Hyperactive Children Grown Up* (Weiss and Hechtman, 1986) contain excellent descriptions of hyperactive individuals at the different stages of childhood, adolescence and young adult life.

Assessment and treatment

The treatment plan should be based on a careful assessment of the type of motor activity and/or attention problems present; the situations in which these are more, or less, prominent; any associated learning difficulties, or perceptual or behaviour problems; and the family and school situations. Depending on this assessment, any combination of the following may be needed.

Medication

Among child psychiatric symptoms, hyperactivity is one of the few which respond to medication. Methylphenidate, a cerebral stimulant, in suitable doses usually improves concentration and classroom behaviour, decreases impulsivity and makes purposeless activity more goal-directed. It has been found to improve on-task behaviour, test-taking attitudes, the organization and sustained deployment of effort, accurate and efficient information processing and the correction of errors the subjects make (Douglas *et al.*, 1986). Other stimulants, such as amphetamine drugs and pemoline, have similar effects. The longer-term effects of these drugs seem to be less satisfactory; children receiving medication may still fail at school, develop antisocial behaviour and experience social ostracism (Weiss, 1981).

The action of these drugs is probably not specific to hyperactive children, since dextroamphetamine has been shown to reduce also the activity levels of normal prepubertal boys (Rapoport *et al.*, 1978). Tranquillisers such as chlorpromazine, thioridazine and haloperidol may also reduce activity levels, but often at the cost of sedating the child. A recent trial suggests that clonidine, an unrelated drug, may be of value (Hunt *et al.*, 1985). The dosage, side-effects and other aspects of the use of these drugs are discussed in Chapter 19. Useful as medication can be in these disorders, it alone is seldom an adequate treatment.

Behaviour modification

Behaviour therapy techniques may be helpful when there are marked attention deficits, impulsivity or other behaviour problems. Operant conditioning (see Chapter 19) may improve attention and cognitive behavioural methods may help children displaying poor impulse control (Kendall and Braswell, 1985). Teaching children behaviours that are more adaptive is to be preferred to symptomatic treatment using medication but is more difficult.

Parental counselling

The parents of these children often need help and support in managing them. This may range from advice concerning the arrangement of the home, so that breakable objects and items that might be dangerous to the child are out of reach, to behaviour therapy regimes designed to modify specific behaviours.

Intervention in the school

Counselling and support for these children's teachers and other school staff may be needed. The cooperation of the staff in the application of behaviour therapy and in the assessment of treatment effects using, for example, the Conners Teachers' Rating Scale, is also important. Remedial education may be needed by children whose academic progress has been impaired as a result of their attention problems and hyperactivity.

Outcome

Hyperactivity tends to lessen with increasing age but other features of these disorders may persist well into adult life. The most comprehensive long-term study of the progress of individuals with this condition is that reported in *Hyperactive Children Grown Up* (Weiss and Hechtman,

1986). This book is also a mine of information about hyperactive children. It reports the progress of a group of children studied by the authors and summarizes the findings of other researchers.

Weiss and Hechtman consider the 'core features' of the syndrome to be inappropriate restlessness, attentional difficulties and impulsivity. When hyperactive children reach adolescence the core symptoms are still present though they may be less marked and frequently are no longer the presenting complaints; these tend now to be poor school performance, relationship difficulties and antisocial behaviour – which affects about 25 per cent. Hyperactive adolescents have lower self-esteem and poorer social skills, and are more impulsive than normal controls.

By the time these individuals reach adult life, about one-third to one-half, depending on the study, become 'indistinguishable from normal adults'. But in all studies a higher percentage of hyperactives than control subjects have been found to have a history of antisocial behaviour. They have also used alcohol or cannabis products more often and/or more heavily. However, drug addiction or alcoholism have not been identified as adult outcomes. Hyperactives report more malaise, score lower on self-rating scales and have impaired social skills, compared with controls. Some 20 per cent or more display the features of 'antisocial personality disorder', as it was defined in DSM-III. Most are economically self-sufficient and gainfully employed, but as a group they hold jobs for shorter periods, are laid off or quit more often and have lower status jobs than control subjects; and their work performance is rated as inferior by employers.

The children studied by Weiss and Hechtman (1986) and most of those in the other studies they reviewed were not treated by the methods currently advocated. It is therefore uncertain how the use of contemporary approaches may alter the longer-term outlook.

A notable feature of *Hyperactive Children Grown Up* (Weiss and Hechtman, 1986) is a chapter entitled 'Looking back: reminiscences from childhood and adolescence,' by Ian Murray, a subject in the authors' 15-year follow-up study. He gives us a rare insight, from the perspective of adulthood, of what it is like to to be a hyperactive child and adolescent, subject over the years to the ministrations of mental health professionals (Murray, 1986).

The Overactive Child (Taylor, 1986a) contains contributions by various authors on different aspects of these disorders and is a good source of further information.

Chapter 10

Specific Delays in Development

Both the multiaxial scheme based on ICD-9 (Rutter *et al.*, 1975) and DSM-III-R place specific developmental disorders in Axis II. In DSM-III-R they share this axis with personality disorders and other developmental disorders, whereas in the ICD-9-based scheme they alone comprise the second axis. The ICD-9 categories are:

(1) specific reading retardation;
(2) specific arithmetical retardation;
(3) other specific learning difficulties;
(4) developmental speech/language disorder;
(5) specific motor retardation;
(6) mixed developmental disorder.

The DSM-III-R categories are:

(1) developmental arithmetic disorder;
(2) developmental expressive writing disorder;
(3) developmental reading disorder;
(4) developmental articulation disorder;
(5) developmental expressive language disorder;
(6) developmental receptive language disorder;
(7) developmental coordination disorder;
(8) specific developmental disorder not otherwise specified.

Any of the above may affect a child without there being a general psychiatric disorder. The conditions are, rather, specific delays in the development of particular functions. All occur more frequently in boys than girls. Although the terms and definitions used in the two schemes differ somewhat, they cover essentially the same disorders.

Reading problems

Some children experience particular difficulty learning to read, while their development in other areas is normal. In technologically advanced societies, in which a high level of formal education is necessary for performance of the better-paid jobs, failure to achieve literacy is serious and handicapping.

Prevalence

This depends on the age group and population studied and the criteria used to define reading retardation. As a general rule, attainment of reading skills is related to intelligence level; intellectually brighter children learn to read faster than those whose IQs are lower. While the reading quotient cannot be expected always to equal the IQ (for definitions of these terms see Chapter 3), the expected reading age can be calculated from a child's age and IQ (Yule, 1967). By this means it can be determined whether children have *specific* reading retardation (Rutter and Yule, 1975); this is distinct from *general reading backwardness*, which simply describes the situation of children who are reading below the level expected of children of their chronological ages. General backwardness may be associated with below average general ability and the reading problem may thus be but one feature of generally delayed development.

In the Isle of Wight epidemiological study of 9- and 10-year-olds (Rutter, Tizard and Whitmore, 1970) a prevalence of specific reading retardation, defined as a reading level 28 months or more below that expected for age and IQ, was found to be about 4 per cent. The boy:girl ratio was 3.3:1. The prevalence of reading backwardness (28 months or more behind the level expected on the basis of age alone) was about 6.5 per cent, with a boy:girl ratio of 1.3:1. The Isle of Wight is a mainly rural area, and reading problems are generally commoner in big cities, especially poor inner city areas. A study in inner London, using the same criteria as in the Isle of Wight, revealed specific reading retardation in 10 per cent of 10-year-olds and general reading backwardness in 19 per cent (Berger *et al.*, 1975).

A study of 952 9-year-olds in New Zealand (Silva *et al.*, 1985) showed that 40 (4.2 per cent) had specific reading retardation, defined as being at least 24 months below the expected level; 35 were boys and 5 girls (a boy:girl ratio of 7:1). The prevalence among boys was 7 per cent, and among girls it was 1.1 per cent.

Causes

The predominance of boys, especially among those with specific reading retardation, suggests biological susceptibility, perhaps genetically determined. Boys with a 47,XXY chromosome complement have deficiencies in reading and/or spelling skills and impaired development of language, especially expressive language. (See Walzer, 1985, for references to the original studies.) The great majority of children with such reading and language problems have normal chromosomes however. Yet in both groups of reading retarded boys (the XXY boys and those with the normal number of chromosomes), there are the same specific deficits in processing auditory stimuli at an adequate rate and in auditory memory (Tallal, 1980; Walzer, 1985). The association of reading problems, delayed language development and current speech difficulties (Rutter and Yule, 1975) suggests that there may be underlying biological deficits, which may have genetic causes. A recent study of 13-year-old twins suggests that genetic factors may be important in the etiology of spelling difficulties, but it gave little support to the proposition that they are important in reading retardation at this age (Stevenson *et al.*, 1987).

How well children learn to read and write depends also upon how they are taught, their motivation to learn and the regularity of their school attendance. Frequent changes of school, teacher or teaching methods may adversely affect progress. (DSM-III-R suggests that when the problem is due to 'inadequate schooling' a diagnosis of developmental reading disorder should not be made, but in clinical practice it is hard to assess the adequacy of children's schooling, except in extreme cases. When the child's performance is in line with that of others of the same age in the school, however, the problem is probably the school's, not the child's.)

Cultural factors affect the learning of reading skills. Children from homes in which books and written materials are much valued and used are more likely to be motivated to read than those from homes where this is not so. Such factors, combined with biological vulnerability, may lead to reading delay.

Description

The clinical picture is that of a child, more often a boy, with a history of serious delay in learning to read. This may have been preceded by delay in the acquisition of speech and language skills, while development in other areas has been relatively normal. Writing and spelling are usually also poor. The spelling difficulty may persist after the child has learned to read.

Secondary emotional problems may be present, usually in children who have been subjected to parental or other pressure to perform at a level beyond them, but the most common association is with antisocial behaviour. This was evident in the Isle of Wight study (Rutter, Tizard and Whitmore, 1970), and has been confirmed in other studies (McGee *et al.*, 1986). Evidence that the reading problems are the cause of the antisocial behaviour, or *vice versa*, is lacking (Sturge, 1982).

McGee *et al.* (1986), in a longitudinal study of over 900 children, found significant associations between both specific reading retardation and general reading backwardness, and problem behaviour. The teachers of the children with reading problems reported behaviour problems from the time of school entry, principally hyperactive and aggressive behaviours. It may be that when these children enter school they already have both poor 'pre-reading' skills and poor social adjustment. On entering school they are liable to experience failure both in reading and in making the necessary social and behavioural adjustments, exacerbating their overall difficulties.

The term 'developmental dyslexia' has been used for the problems of children with specific reading difficulties. It is probably best avoided, however, because it may suggest that the condition is a 'disease'. There is no objection to describing a child as dyslexic, though this is only using a Latin word to say that the child has a reading problem. Better than bestowing a label is the making of a comprehensive functional diagnosis, taking into account all contributory and associated factors.

Assessment and treatment

These are the special province of the educational psychologist and remedial teacher. Appropriate tests of cognitive function and academic attainment should be performed. If behavioural or other problems are also present, child and family should be assessed, as set out in Chapter 3. The assessment should lead to a plan to provide the child with appropriate remedial help in school and to deal with any co-existing behavioural problems, using the principles discussed in Chapter 4. Gittelman (1985) summarized the results of research studies into ways of remedying reading problems. The family may need advice, support or family therapy, especially when there are associated behavioural or family problems.

Outcome

This depends on the severity of the disorder and the help available to the child in school and at home. Many children overcome their reading problems, often with extra help. Some seem eventually to reach a state of 'reading readiness' but if reading problems are not detected, assessed and treated in good time, both behavioural and emotional difficulties may develop, along with progressive failure at school. The ability to read is necessary for success in other school subjects; the inability to read may lead to general, chronic school failure. This in turn is damaging to the child's self-esteem, with all the unfortunate consequences that follow.

Arithmetic problems

Both ICD-9 and DSM-III-R have a diagnostic category for 'specific' (ICD-9) or 'developmental' (DSM-III-R) arithmetical disorders. These are conditions in which the child has particular difficulty with arithmetic. Slade and Russell (1971) described four cases of 'developmental dyscalculia', as they called the condition. They were adolescents who had all had severe difficulty with arithmetic from an early age, such as could not be accounted for by generally low intelligence. All four basic arithmetical processes were affected, multiplication most severely.

Specific retardation in mathematics generally, or arithmetic in particular, has been studied less than reading problems. Lansdown (1978) suggests a multifactorial etiology and offers a 'tentative description of mathematical retardation'.

Arithmetic difficulties are less handicapping than reading problems, though they may lead to secondary emotional problems. The advent of portable, low-priced electronic calculators has, I believe, lightened the burden of children who have difficulty learning mathematics.

Speech and language problems

Language can be either verbal or non-verbal. Non-verbal language consists of gestures, facial expressions, voice tones and inflections, and various forms of 'body language'. DSM-III-R and ICD-9, however, confine themselves to defining and categorizing disorders of verbal language; the latter will be the focus of this section.

Language development

A baby's first sounds are undifferentiated crying. By two months this has become differentiated, varying according to the circumstances, be they hunger, pain or cold. Within a month or two the baby starts to babble. Then the variety of sounds produced, consonants and vowels, increases. Babbling comprises a succession of spontaneously produced sounds, many of which will be incorporated into words when speech develops.

By about nine months the use of consonant-vowel combinations takes on a communicative function. Various combinations are used for calling, responding and expressing intentions.

The development of language is a complex process. The child must learn to observe objects and events before coming to understand them and express them in language. Language development is thus closely related to cognitive, that is thinking, development. Similarly the learning of the meaning of words depends on the development of the relevant concepts. Subsequently the child has to understand and learn sentence forms (syntax) and the skills necessary to request, protest, label and express other intentions (pragmatic abilities).

The first spoken words usually appear around the age of one, though most children attempt to communicate by simple vocalizations and gestures before that. The first words are often ones like 'dada' or 'mama', which may simply be pieces of babble reinforced by the attention and approval given them by the parents. The subsequent acquisition of vocabulary is closely tied in with the child's perception, for example, of shape and the words heard and used in relation to that perception. Thus at first all round objects may be labelled 'ball'. At the same time the child is trying actively to work out how language is put together, so that every attempt at communication is, in a way, a testing of an hypothesis. This applies to the acquisition of words, phrases and sentences.

Even very young children make up 'new' words using rules they have inferred, as when they say 'sheeps' or 'gived', which they will not have heard used by others. Such errors are often corrected by parents and others with whom the child talks. Much the same applies to phrase and sentence construction and the learning of syntax starts almost from the acquisition of the first words. When a child says something that is not properly understood it is necessary to try again, perhaps after receiving some help or instruction from the person being addressed. It is largely by such give-and-take that children learn to master the complexities of verbal language. For all this there must, of course, be a background of neurological readiness.

During the second year an increasing, but quite small, number of words is acquired, many of them the names of objects. Short phrases appear about the middle of the second year, sentences and simple questions by about age two. At first small groups of words, mainly nouns and verbs, are produced, for example 'mummy come'. 'No' and 'yes' are often incorporated into phrases like 'apple no' or 'Johnny apple no', which express their meaning quite well in a sort of verbal shorthand. Phrases of this type are often acquired during the second year; gradually sentences with more normal structures replace them. Adjectives are used increasingly to qualify nouns, and pronouns are used with greater correctness. Subsequently the finer points of syntax are gradually mastered, though this is a process which continues well into and through the child's primary school days. The use of adverbs, prepositions and conjunctions appears relatively late, though normally by about age 5.

There is a rapid increase in vocabulary in the third and fourth years.

At the same time articulation, the accuracy with which words are pronounced, improves. At first the child's attempts at many words may be poor. Parents usually understand them before outsiders do.

Vocabulary and sentence structure are culturally determined. In many countries there are both regional and social class variations, as well as differences related to educational level. Thus 'normal' speech development in a labourer's child is likely to differ from the 'normal' for a university professor's child, as regards both vocabulary and syntax. For example in some English-speaking cultures the double negative ('I don't want no more of that') is accepted usage and the child growing up in such a culture will learn to use it. In other cultures this would be considered incorrect.

Between the ages of about 2 and 7 there are important changes in children's capacity to comprehend spoken language. Comprehension is also learned in an organized way. At first children interpret sentences by assuming that the first noun is the subject/actor of the sentence. The sequence subject-verb-object is taken to represent actor-action-recipient. This strategy works well in phrases like 'the boy chases the girl', but later the child must learn to refine and change such strategies to deal, for example, with 'the boy is chased by the girl'. Children gradually develop the skills to deal with sentences of increasing complexity, as they hear these used.

A more detailed and comprehensive account of language development is to be found in the book *Language Development: Structure and Function* (Dale, 1976).

Abnormalities of speech and language development

Language disorders may involve non-verbal comprehension, verbal comprehension and verbal expression. (We are excluding from consideration here non-verbal expression, important as it is.) The division of these disorders into receptive and expressive types, as in DSM-III-R, is overly simplistic. Martin (1980) points out that various types of language disorder are possible, depending on the presence and extent of difficulties in the three main functions mentioned above. More important than attaching a diagnostic label, though, is the definition of precisely which language functions are lacking, and to what degree.

As a general rule verbal expression cannot be better than verbal comprehension, nor verbal comprehension than non-verbal. Occasional exceptions are encountered, as when totally deaf children are taught verbal expressions through lip reading and highly specialized teaching methods.

Prevalence of language disorders

Prevalence figures depend on ascertainment criteria, the population studied and the age of the children concerned. In the Isle of Wight study of 9-, 10- and 11-year-olds (Rutter, Tizard and Whitmore, 1970), 6.2 per cent of 147 'controls', that is children without intellectual retardation or specific reading retardation, showed 'poor complexity of language'. Similar language problems were present in 15.1 per cent of those with specific reading retardation and in 63.2 per cent of those who were intellectually retarded.

Cantwell and Baker (1985), reviewing the findings of various studies reported since 1930, state that 'as many as 6 per cent of children may have disorders of language development'.

Causes

Children may fail to develop language because of impaired hearing, mental retardation or severe environmental deprivation. While total deprivation of verbal language experiences is rare, relative deprivation may occur in large, badly run orphanages or other institutions, and in some poorly endowed, underprivileged families. In such families the language development of all members may be retarded. Failure to develop language normally, or at all, is also a feature of infantile autism (Chapter 7).

When one of the above conditions is considered responsible for delayed language development, the terms 'specific' or 'developmental' language disorder are not usually applied. These terms are reserved for cases in which the problem appears to be one of delayed neurological maturation, and in which other specific causes are absent. But when there is delayed neurological maturation, a mild degree of deprivation of language experience may have a disproportionate effect. In reality these disorders, like so many others, usually have multiple causes and their classification on the basis of supposed etiology is somewhat arbitrary. The causes of the postulated delayed neurological development cannot usually be discovered, though sometimes there is a history of cerebral trauma at or soon after birth. We have seen also that language development is impaired in boys with a 47,XXY chromosome complement, who have problems in processing, storing, retrieving and/or expressing linguistic information (Walzer, 1985). These facts; the predominance of these disorders in boys; and the existence in many cases of a family history of late speech development, other speech problems, and reading and spelling problems, suggest that genetic factors may be important.

Description

The main feature of this disorder is delayed development of speech. The first words, except perhaps for 'dada' and similar items of babble, are acquired late, sentence construction is delayed and when words are produced they are abnormal. The extent to which these children understand speech varies and in severe cases there is little or no understanding of it, a condition which used to be called 'congenital auditory imperception'.It is invariably associated with an expressive disorder.

There is a close association between reading disorders and language disorders; there may be persisting reading problems even when these children have developed good language skills. There is also an association between language problems and behaviour problems – not surprising in view of the known association between reading difficulties and behaviour problems. A study of 3-year-olds showed a strong association between language delay and behaviour problems even at this age (Stevenson and Richman, 1978); and a follow-up study of the 3-year-olds showed that those with a low score on a measure of language structure at age 3 had a high rate of 'neurotic deviance' at age 8. This relationship existed even when behaviour at age 3 was taken into account (Stevenson *et al.*, 1985).

Diagnosis

Consideration of the processes illustrated in Figure 10.1 assists in the understanding of the problems of children with language and reading problems. Any of the processes shown may be affected, but language disordered children have difficulties in the decoding-encoding areas.

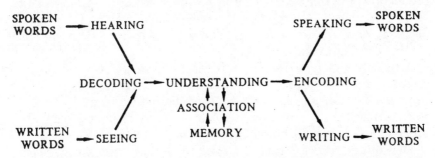

Figure 10.1 The comprehension and expression of language.

Hearing should always be carefully tested. Impairment involving only certain frequencies, which may not be apparent during clinical interview, can cause delay in the development of speech. The child's general level of ability should be assessed to discover whether the delayed language development is specific or a feature of generally delayed development. Many special tests of language function are available. These can help pinpoint the problems and assist in the planning of remedial measures.

Treatment

The treatment of children with language disorders is usually carried out by speech therapists, working in cooperation with neurologists, psychologists and/or psychiatrists. The treatment plan should be based on a comprehensive assessment of the child's abilities. When receptive language is adequate and the difficulty is mainly with expressive functions, concentrated training, perhaps using operant conditioning techniques (see Chapter 19) often yields good results. Receptive difficulties, especially when they are severe and involve non-verbal as well as verbal comprehension, are harder to treat. Fortunately many cases are relatively mild and seem to be the result of delayed neurological maturation. These children develop speech in due course, and can be helped by speech therapy (Lahey and Bloom, 1977).

Articulation problems

Developmental disorders of articulation are given their own category in DSM-III-R, according to which they occur in about 10 per cent of children below age 8 and about 5 per cent of those over 8.

Abnormal articulation may be a consequence of neurological conditions affecting control of the muscles responsible for the production of speech sounds; it may be due to structural abnormalities of the larynx, palate or tongue; it may be a 'developmental' condition; or it may have emotional causes. The latter two groups are the main ones of psychiatric importance.

Articulation is invariably affected when there is a severe language disorder and the problems of articulation may persist after the language disorder has disappeared. Developmental disorders of articulation, in the absence of language problems, are characterized by the undue persistence of infantile modes of articulation.

The clinical picture is that of a child who speaks freely and appears to understand speech normally (unless there is also a language disorder), but is hard to understand because of the use of ill-formed words. Longer words are more affected than shorter ones, parts of words (often the ends) may be missed out and consonants are more affected than vowels. The later acquired speech sounds (t, sh, f, z, l and ch) are most affected. Family members usually understand the child better than outsiders do. Sometimes the severity of the speech problem may not be evident to the parents, who have become used to the child's way of pronouncing words.

Treatment is primarily the sphere of the speech therapist. The outlook is generally good. Milder cases often recover spontaneously.

Emotionally determined immature articulation may occur in children showing other evidence of delayed emotional maturation. Such children may be overprotected by their parents and may use 'baby talk' when with them. Severe emotional stress may cause regression to infantile speech patterns, along with regression in other behaviours, especially in children who have only recently started talking. In these cases the diagnosis depends on a general assessment. There is usually a history of normal, or at least better, articulation previously or in certain circumstances, as well as other evidence of emotional immaturity. Some of these disorders may be classified as adjustment reactions (see Chapter 12). Treatment depends on the nature of the stress the child faces. Counselling for the parents, psychotherapy for the child or family therapy may be needed. When the stress is acute and time-limited, the problem may clear up without treatment.

Specific motor retardation

This ICD-9 category is probably the same as DSM-III-R's 'developmental coordination disorder'. These are disorders in which the main feature is a serious impairment in the development of motor coordination, not explicable in terms of general intellectual retardation. The condition has also been called 'developmental dyspraxia' (Walton *et al.*, 1962).

Children with this disorder are characteristically late developing motor skills such as dressing, feeding and walking. They experience difficulty in writing, drawing and copying. They perform badly at ball games, tend to break crockery and are poor at handicrafts. In severe cases the clumsiness may be so great that it interferes with the child's school work, games and physical education. Intelligence is normal when assessed using verbal tests, though the child tests at a lower level on non-verbal tests. In verbal tasks these children usually function well but because of their inability to write, or because they can only write legibly if they go extremely slowly, they may be thought to be intellectually dull or even retarded. In other instances they are regarded as lazy and the view is taken by others that they could do better if they tried.

'Clumsy children', as these are often called, do not usually show evidence of an abnormality in their ability to carry out voluntary movements; their problem is in coordinating them to perform particular tasks. The condition is analagous to developmental reading disorder, in which the subject can see the writing but cannot organize it into the meaning it represents.

Children with this disorder may present at psychiatric clinics or offices, sometimes with secondary disorders and sometimes because the nature of the problem has not been recognized; instead of being regarded as a developmental disability it may have been thought to be a manifestation of emotional disorder or negativistic refusal to do school work. Careful history taking usually indicates the true state of affairs. This can be confirmed by asking the child to write and draw. The results are then compared with the child's verbal productions. These children usually read better than they write.

Treatment involves explaining the nature of the child's disability to child, family and school staff. Special teaching and training to develop motor skills should be provided. Modification of the school routine may be needed, along the lines of relieving these children of motor tasks that are beyond them, for instance in games, other physical activities and classroom activities like writing and drawing. They should be given opportunities to demonstrate their knowledge verbally when their motor disability prevents them from expressing it in writing. Some clumsy children learn to use typewriters or computers better than pens or pencils.

A fuller account of this disorder, including the results of two population surveys and information about neurological disorders which may cause clumsiness, is available in *The Clumsy Child* (Gubbay, 1975).

Mixed Specific Developmental Disorders

Mixed developmental disorders comprise combinations of the various disorders discussed above. The coexistence of developmental reading and language disorders is one of the commoner manifestations.

Chapter 11

Enuresis and Encopresis

Enuresis and encopresis appear as 'special symptoms not elsewhere classified' in ICD-9, and as 'functional enuresis' and 'functional encopresis' in a category entitled 'elimination disorders' in DSM-III-R. These conditions may exist on their own or as part of another psychiatric disorder.

Enuresis

Bedwetting, otherwise known as nocturnal enuresis, often occurs as an isolated delay in the development of nocturnal continence. Less often it is accompanied by daytime wetting (diurnal enuresis). Less commonly still, daytime wetting occurs on its own. Most children achieve day and night continence by about four years of age, some earlier; they are usually dry by day before they are dry at night. DSM-III-R arbitrarily defines 'functional enuresis' as the voiding of urine during the day or at night into bed or clothes, occurring at least twice a month between the ages of 5 and 6, and once a month for older children. For the diagnosis to apply the child must have a mental age (see Chapter 3) of at least 4.

Prevalence

Prevalence figures vary according to the population studied and the criteria used to define enuresis. Very roughly, 10 per cent of 5-year-olds wet their beds and 5 per cent of 10-year-olds; 1-2 per cent continue into their teen years, but there are wide variations from country to country. Thus in Australia and North America the rate is three times that in Sweden. The British rate is nearer the Swedish one, rather than that of what have been called the 'bed-sodden states of America' (British Medical Journal, 1977).

Verhulst et al. (1985) report the prevalence of nocturnal enuresis in boys and girls between the ages of 4 and 16, based on a study of 2600 Dutch children. At age 5, 17.9 per cent of boys and 10 per cent of girls wet the bed at least once a month, while 14.1 per cent of boys and 6.7 per cent of girls were wet at least twice a month. At nearly all ages the prevalence in boys was greater than that in girls; prevalence declined more rapidly between the ages of 4 and 6 in girls than it did in boys. Bedwetting was rare in girls from the eleventh year onwards and in boys from the thirteenth year. These finding are in general agreement with those of other studies (DeJonge, 1973).

Daytime wetting is less common than nocturnal wetting and occurs in girls more than in boys. About 2 per cent of 5-year-olds are wet by day once a week or more, though about 8 per cent are wet at least once a month (DeJonge, 1973). In the 7- to 10-year-old age range diurnal wetting occurs in about 1 per cent of children.

Causes

Most cases of enuresis are not associated with any demonstrable physical cause, though in girls with diurnal enuresis urinary tract infections are common. In a group of 35 girls treated by Halliday *et al.* (1987), 21 had had previous infections and 12 had one or more episodes of infection while being treated. It seems that diurnal enuresis predisposes to infection, which in turn may exacerbate the enuresis. Rarer causes are physical abnormalities of the urinary tract, nocturnal epilepsy and excessive production of urine (as in diabetes). Most physical causes lead to diurnal as well as nocturnal wetting.

The bladders of enuretic children tend to be functionally, though not anatomically, smaller than those of non-enuretics. As a group, enuretic children pass urine more frequently than non-enuretics but this does not seem to be related to their functional bladder capacities (Shaffer *et al.*, 1984).

Enuresis tends to run in families and genetic factors may be involved. A study of twins by Bakwin (1971) showed monozygotic twins to be concordant for enuresis about twice as often as dizygotic twins. Delay in achieving bladder control is a feature of mental retardation; it is marked in cases of severe retardation.

Unusually deep sleep has been suggested as a cause of enuresis but satisfactory evidence that enuretic children sleep more deeply than non-enuretics is lacking. There is an association between enuresis and emotional disorder, though most enuretic children are not emotionally disturbed. Enuresis may be a feature of regressive behaviour appearing in situations of emotional stress. It may also be present in children with conduct disorders, neurotic conditions or psychoses. Diurnal wetting is probably more often associated with psychiatric disorder than is bedwetting (Berg, 1979).

In most cases no specific cause can be found for the enuresis. It is often ascribed to delayed neurological maturation, to which genetic factors may contribute. If family disorganization is combined with such delayed maturation and the child receives inconsistent toilet training, delayed achievement of bladder control may be even more probable. Other anxiety-producing stresses might also contribute.

Enuresis and its causes are discussed more fully in the book *Bladder Control and Enuresis* (Kolvin *et al.*, 1973).

Description

In most cases enuresis is 'primary', that is to say the child has never become dry. In nocturnal enuresis the only symptom, initially at least, is the passing of urine while asleep. The child has never learned to control micturition while sleeping. About one bedwetter in five also has increased frequency of micturition by day but without daytime wetting. In other, but fewer, cases there are both increased frequency and wetting by day.

Enuresis may later be complicated by feelings of anxiety or guilt, especially if the child is blamed or punished for the enuresis. Much depends on the family's attitudes towards the problem; enuresis causes great unhappiness and distress to some children, though if handled sensibly it need not do so.

Secondary enuresis is defined as enuresis starting after the child has achieved continence for a certain period – 3 months in the study of Shaffer *et al.* (1984), 1 year in that of Starfield (1967). It has been suggested that secondary enuretics, like daytime enuretics, more often have psychiatric disorders than primary nocturnal enuretics, though the findings of Shaffer *et al.* (1984) do not support this. These authors did, however, find an association between psychiatric disturbance and functional bladder volume; anxiety during testing might have been responsible for this.

In summary, functional enuresis (that is enuresis in the absence of demonstrable organic cause) may be nocturnal or diurnal, or both; it may have been lifelong or it may have started after a period of continence; and it may or may not be associated with evidence of psychiatric disorder. (There does not seem to be any reason to regard uncomplicated enuresis as evidence of psychiatric disorder.)

Investigation and treatment

In cases of primary enuresis, carefully taken histories from child and parents will establish that lifelong enuresis is the main problem. If anxiety or other psychiatric symptoms have arisen in response to family members' attitudes towards it, this also should become clear as the history is taken and the current family situation is assessed. It is important to adopt an optimistic outlook while taking the history; you should let the family know that the problem is a common one and not too serious, despite the inconvenience it may cause. Many parents and children are unaware of the frequency of the complaint and any self-blame should be dispelled as far as possible.

The history should be reviewed for evidence of an underlying physical cause, such as an abnormality of bladder or urethra or infection of the urinary tract. It is important to ascertain that the child has conscious control over micturition, that is to say that the muscles responsible for preventing micturition are functioning, even though control lapses from time to time. With some anatomical abnormalities urine is constantly leaking and control is never complete. Urinary infections are often accompanied by painful micturition as well as increased frequency.

A physical examination should be carried out and the urine examined for evidence of infection or diabetes. In some clinics X-ray examination of the urinary tract is routinely carried out. It is probably only necessary if there is evidence to suggest a physical cause, which is unlikely if the enuresis is purely nocturnal. If an associated physical problem is suspected, paediatric consultation is advisable.

Three treatment approaches are available for uncomplicated enuresis: conditioning, medication and hypnotherapy. Whichever treatment is used, support and reassurance for child and family are important. The symptom is best referred to as a 'delay in learning to control the bladder while asleep' (or 'when excited', etc.), rather than as a serious disease.

(a) *Conditioning* is often used as the treatment of first choice. Various devices are available.

The 'pad and buzzer' or 'bedbuzzer' is illustrated in Figure 11.1. Nowadays many enuresis alarms have a single pad which is placed in the bed between a rubber sheet (underneath) and a cotton or flannellette sheet, on which the child lies. The 'Nytone' alarm* uses metal terminals similar to press fasteners; the child wears underpants, the material of which is clamped between these metal terminals. Headingly Scientific Services** manufacture alarms using plastic sensors. (Figure 11.2). They also make a remote alarm which can sound in another room, for example the parents'; and a 'silent alarm'. Instead of a buzzer the latter uses a low frequency vibrator mounted in a flat case which is placed under the pillow. This can be useful when

---

* Nytone Medical Products Inc., Salt Lake City, Utah 84119, USA.
** 45 Westcombe Avenue, Leeds LS8 2BS, England.

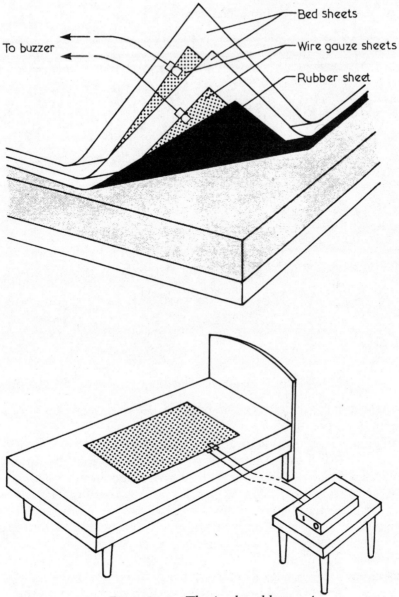

To buzzer

Bed sheets

Wire gauze sheets

Rubber sheet

Figure 11.1 The 'pad and buzzer'.

bedrooms are shared and in institutions. Extra loud, two-tone and intermittent alarms are also available.

The apparatus is set up so that when the material concerned gets wet a low power electrical circuit is completed, setting off the buzzer or bell. The alarm may be placed beside the bed or the 'Nytone' buzzer can be strapped to the wrist. It is switched on at bedtime. When it goes off, the child should get out of bed, switch the alarm off, pass urine and

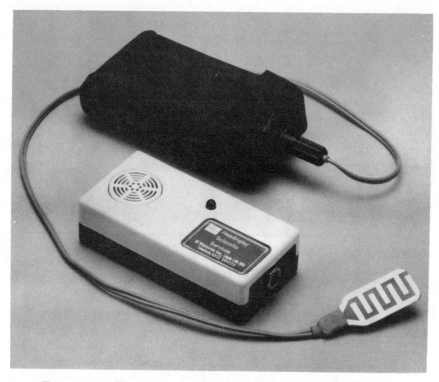

Figure 11.2   Enuresis alarm (Headingly Scientific Services).

re-set the apparatus. In the initial stages the buzzer may sound two or three times per night.

The apparatus is used until the child has been continuously dry for three weeks. If relapse occurs, a further course of treatment is indicated. It is best if the child, whose cooperation is essential, sets up the apparatus, switches it on and keeps the record of dry and wet nights. Adequate explanation, demonstration and preparation are necessary; some children are frightened or suspicious of the apparatus. They can easily sabotage its use, so any such feelings must be explored and dealt with before treatment starts. If after a few discussions the child does not wish to use the buzzer, there may be an associated emotional or family systems disorder. The amount the child drinks should not be restricted; doing so may delay the conditioning process. The apparatus can seldom be used effectively in children much below the age of six.

Over 80 per cent of enuretics who use the pad and buzzer properly become dry. Some of these later relapse and not all relapses respond to further treatment, though most do. Dische *et al.* (1983) reported initial arrest of wetting (42 successive dry nights) in 95 (84 per cent) of 113 children but 40 relapsed, of whom only 31 were retreated; of these 31,

16 became and remained dry, giving a long-term success rate of 63 per cent.

The use of conditioning in the management of diurnal enuresis has been studied by Halliday *et al.* (1987). A flat plastic wetting sensor was attached to the underpants, connected by wire to the alarm which can be worn on a belt, in a pocket or strapped on the back. Figure 11.2 illustrates this apparatus, which can also be used at night as a bedbuzzer. Figure 11.3 shows an alarm worn on the back.

This device was found to be effective in about two-thirds of the children who used it. Interestingly, the results were as good whether a contingent alarm (one that sounded only when the sensor became wet) or a non-contingent one (an alarm that went off from time to time regardless of whether the underclothes were wet) was used. In either case the child was to go to the toilet and pass urine when the alarm sounded and then re-set the alarm.

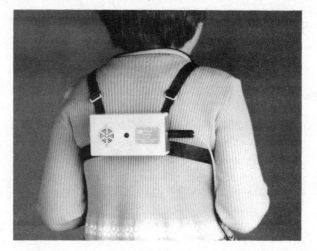

Figure 11.3

(b) *Medication*, using the antidepressant, imipramine, reduces the frequency of enuresis but the relapse rate is high. Doses of 25 to 50 mg of imipramine at bedtime are usually required; if there is no response blood levels should be assessed since these may not be dose-related in children. Medication should be continued until the child has been continuously dry for a month, then gradually reduced over several months. Other tricyclic antidepressants may also be used, but in view of the high relapse rate, medication is of limited value in enuresis.

(c) A recent study of *hypnotherapy* suggests that it may achieve results comparable to those of the pad and buzzer (Edwards and van der Spuy, 1985), though further study of it is required. Formal trance induction is apparently not necessary, which is in keeping with the experience of other contemporary hypnotherapists (for example, Araoz, 1985).

Outcome

As the prevalence figures indicate, most enuretic children will grow out of the symptom in time but the spontaneous recovery rate does not justify therapeutic inaction. Treatment is successful in well over half the cases but sometimes secondary emotional disorders or family disorganization prevent the consistent use of conditioning methods. Children from impoverished homes and dysfunctional families may be difficult to treat.

Encopresis

Encopresis, or fecal soiling, is the passing of feces in the clothes rather than in the toilet. It may occur by day or by night. Children usually achieve fecal continence by about age three; soiling after the age of 4 is abnormal, except in the mentally retarded.

Prevalence

A study in Sweden (Bellman, 1966) revealed a prevalence of soiling at age 7 of 2.3 per cent in boys and 0.7 per cent in girls, a ratio of 3.4:1. In the Isle of Wight study of 10- and 11-year-olds the prevalence rates were 1.3 per cent in boys and 0.3 per cent in girls (Rutter, Tizard and Whitmore, 1970). By age 16 the prevalence has fallen almost to zero.

Causes

Figure 11.4 illustrates the various ways in which soiling can arise.

Encopresis may be retentive or non-retentive, depending on whether or not feces have accumulated in the colon and rectum in abnormal quantities. Retention of feces may have physical or emotional causes. Physical ones include anal fissure, which causes severe pain on defecation, and Hirschprung's disease, a rare condition in which the nerve ganglia are congenitally absent from a section of the colon; the smooth muscle of this section does not contract properly, so that feces are not moved on as they should be.

The emotional state most frequently associated with fecal retention is anger, though encopretic children may also harbour much repressed anxiety. The problem usually arises in the context of a disturbed parent-child relationship (Anthony, 1957; Pinkerton, 1958). Toilet training may have started early, even within the first few weeks of life,

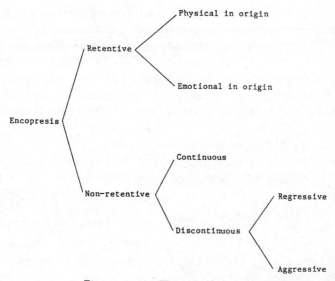

Figure 11.4   Types of encopresis

and success surprisingly early, though short-lived, may be reported. The subsequent negativistic refusal to defecate may be a reaction to coercive, rigid toilet training by parents who have a high regard for order and cleanliness, and overvalue early bowel and bladder control; they may also have obsessive personalities. These children are believed to be expressing their unconsciously felt anger towards their parents by soiling; they choose this method of expression because issues of bowel control are matters of special concern in these families. The mothers often have a fear of constipation and may use laxatives to excess. Their preoccupation with bowel function may date back to their own childhood experiences.

As these children continue to resist defecating, feces accumulate in the large intestine. This becomes distended and the feces in it ultimately become hard and impacted. Liquid feces may pass round these masses and leak out of the anus, the child no longer having control over the process. The end result may be indistinguishable from that occurring in encopresis resulting from physical causes. Retentive soiling in the context of the above type of parent-child relationship now seems less common than it was in the 1950s when the papers by Anthony and Pinkerton were written. This may be because attitudes to toilet training have become more relaxed and permissive; rigid and coercive methods are now widely recognized as inappropriate.

Non-retentive soiling may be 'continuous', that is present from birth, or 'discontinuous', the child never having been successfully toilet trained.   Continuous soiling tends to occur in children who are poorly cared for in ways other than having lacked proper toilet training. They may be dirty and badly dressed and show other evidence of ineffective social training. They may play truant from school and their academic progress tends to be below average. Their families usually have other problems such as unsatisfactory housing, a burden of debt, unemployment or criminal records. The child's soiling may thus be but one feature of a family pattern of immature behaviour.

Moderately and severely mentally retarded children are late achieving bowel control or may never do so, but they are readily distinguished by their generally retardated development.

Discontinuous non-retentive soiling may be either 'regressive' or 'aggressive'. Regressive soiling is usually a reaction to an acute or continuing stress; it may be accompanied by regression in other spheres of behaviour. There may be other symptoms of anxiety but if so these are understandable in the light of the stress the child is facing. (If they were disproportionately severe, a diagnosis of an anxiety or neurotic disorder might be appropriate. Some short-lived episodes of regressive soiling reactive to acute stress are appropriately classified as adjustment reactions – see Chapter 12). Regressive soiling is closely akin to the diarrhoea some adults experience before examinations, important interviews and the like.

Aggressive non-retentive soiling has a similar psychopathology to that of psychogenic retentive soiling except that instead of refusing to defecate at all, the child refuses to do so at the place and time desired by the parents. In these cases, too, there is an ongoing battle between child and parent(s) over control of the child's bowels – something described graphically in Anthony's (1957) paper.

Description

The main clinical feature is the passing of feces in the clothes. The symptom may be lifelong or it may have started after a period of fecal continence. In severe cases of retentive soiling the rectum is found, on digital examination, to be enormously dilated and packed with feces; around these liquid or semi-liquid fecal material is leaking from the anus, the child having no voluntary control over this. In such circumstances the constipation and fecal retention must be dealt with first.

The soiling itself may vary from the regular passage of all feces in the clothes, to staining of the underwear or nightclothes. It may occur daily or as little as once or twice a week. In some cases it does not occur when the child is at school, yet it is reported to be frequent at home, suggesting a connection with family relationship difficulties.

The history given by child and family will vary according to the type of encopresis. There may have been either coercive or lackadaisical, or even absent toilet training; but very relaxed and 'laid back' training, in a stable family in which the children feel secure, may be effective. It is in the chaotic, disorganized families that inconsistency and the lack of proper training seem to lead to encopresis. Careful enquiry about past and current toilet training methods is important.

Aggressive soilers, whether retentive or non-retentive, are often clean, indeed too clean, well-dressed, inhibited children who do well at school. They may seem ashamed of their soiling, and may try to conceal it, for example by hiding or destroying underclothes – though this also can infuriate the parents and may be but another means whereby their aggression is expressed. They are often reluctant to discuss anything related to bowel function, but may allude to it in play or drawings. In about half of this group associated food refusal is reported by the parents, though these children are usually adequately nourished. They may not engage in rough play and be self-assertive to the extent usual in their their age group, their aggressive feelings being expressed instead through refusal to conform in the spheres of bowel and, often, eating behaviour. Typically the aggressive soiler is a bright, successful pupil at school, in contrast to the 'never properly trained' continuous soiler, who usually is not. A clear history of a period of fecal continence is not always obtained in these cases.

Regressive soiling is distinguished by the presence of other regressive behaviours such as clinging to mother, 'baby talk', infantile feeding behaviour, refusal to sleep or go to bed alone or a return to immature patterns of play. There is usually a history of a recent or continuing stressful experience.

The clinical picture is not always as clear cut as the above account might imply. Mixed forms of encopresis can occur. Some 'aggressive' soilers, whether retentive or not, have never achieved fecal continence; and aggressive soiling can occur in socially disorganized, poorly functioning families as well as in rigid, obsessional, materially success-ful ones. Sometimes there are both aggressive and regressive features as, for example, when the child feels both anxiety about the family or some other situation and hostility towards the parents.

Soiling may be a feature of pervasive developmental disorders, and conduct disorders, adjustment reactions and mental retardation. In such cases the other disorder is usually the primary focus of clinical attention, the soiling being but one feature of a wider clinical problem. For purposes of diagnostic categorization the other disorder should take precedence.

Investigation and treatment

It is important to establish whether or not there is retention of feces and if so whether the soiling is due to overflow incontinence. If there has been longstanding fecal retention it can be difficult to discover how the problem first arose. If it was originally physical, emotional difficulties may have developed as secondary phenomena. If it was emotional, the child's negativistic refusal to defecate may have been complicated by longstanding constipation and dilatation of the large intestine.

Abdominal and rectal examinations, and if necessary X-rays of the abdomen, usually establish whether there are accumulations of feces in the large intestine. In Hirschprung's disease, a barium enema examination typically shows a length of narrow, undilated colon with a great increase in the size of the colon proximal to it. In psychogenic cases the whole length of the colon is dilated.

Severe fecal retention must be treated. The long-term administration of a laxative such as Senokot may be sufficient, even in quite severe cases. If it is not, rectal suppositories (such as Dulcolax) may be used, or enemas may be necessary. Severe cases of fecal retention are best treated in hospital, especially if physical treatment other than oral laxatives is required (Pinkerton, 1974). Even then, enemas and suppositories should only be administered after a good relationship with the child has been established by the nurse, and after due explanation of the treatment to the child. Otherwise the child may feel that the treatment is another aggressive attack. Physical measures should always be part of a wider plan of treatment dealing also with the emotional problems.

Most children who soil become clean within two or three weeks of admission to hospital if they are treated appropriately and any fecal retention is relieved. If the encopresis continues it may be because the hospital staff are dealing with it in a punitive or hostile way, or because the dysfunctional interaction between child and parent(s) is continuing. For example, one boy for several weeks handed his mother soiled clothes to take home to wash, unknown to the hospital staff.

If there is no retention of feces, physical treatment is not required. If toilet training has not been provided, the child usually responds to a period of consistent, firm and kind training, using behaviour modification principles (Sluckin, 1975). This is best carried out at home by the parents, though it may also be done in a day hospital or residential setting. The administration of a laxative along with the behaviour modification programme does not seem to help in cases in which there is no constipation (Berg *et al.*, 1983).

Treatment specifically for the soiling may not be necessary in regressive soiling. Attention should be directed to removing or alleviating the stress that is responsible for the child's anxiety. If this cannot be done, psychotherapy for the child may be needed.

Family therapy or counselling for the parents is often needed. When the encopresis is but one of many family problems, therapy to improve family functioning may be needed before the parents can effectively apply behavioural or other treatments for the soiling.

Sometimes the attitudes of the parents towards bowel function generally and soiling in particular need attention, especially in cases of aggressive soiling in over-controlled children. The mother is often the parent most involved in the battle with the child. Once a trusting relationship with her has been established, bowel function and constipation and its dangers may be discussed. Some people who have been brought up to be very bowel conscious find it hard to get this in perspective. They believe it is vital for their children to pass feces at least once a day. They overrate the importance of bowel regularity and function. Not until these fears and anxieties have been put to rest, as explained by Pinkerton (1958), is it useful to go on to discuss the child's symptoms. The parents must be led to understand the soiling as a means of self-expression or protest in a child who is unable to express angry feelings in other ways. They also need to see that the open expression of aggression is a sign of improvement. Simple explanation of these points is seldom sufficient. Discussion over a period of time, in the context of a trusting relationship with the therapist, is required. Group therapy may also help (Hoag, 1971).

Psychotherapy with the encopretic young child may not be needed if the above approaches are used. Older children (those over about 8 or 9 years of age) with chronic symptoms are sometimes less sensitive to changes in parental attitudes and may need individual therapy.

Outcome

Progress and response to treatment depend on the type of encopresis and the openness of the family to change. Regressive soiling generally disappears quite quickly, once the stress to which it is a response is resolved. Aggressive soiling, especially when it is of long standing and accompanied by fecal retention, is harder to treat. When soiling is a feature of a disorganized family system, the outlook depends on the skill of the therapist in engaging these sometimes very difficult families and the responsiveness of the family.

Soiling has usually ceased by the mid-teen years but some children subsequently express their unresolved aggressive feelings in other ways.

Chapter 12

Other Clinical Syndromes

Adjustment reactions

Adjustment reactions are defined in ICD-9 as 'mild or transient disorders ... without any apparent pre-existing mental disorder'. The term is applied to circumscribed or situation-specific disorders which are generally reversible. They are usually related to major stresses, and may last a few days or as long as several months. The following subtypes are listed:

- Brief depressive reaction.
- Prolonged depressive reaction.
- With predominant disturbance of other emotions.
- With predominant disturbance of conduct.
- With mixed disturbance of emotions and mood.
- 'Other' and 'Unspecified'.

DSM-III-R defines 'adjustment disorder' as a 'maladaptive reaction to an identifiable psychosocial stressor or stressors' and arbitrarily sets a limit of 3 months from the onset of the stressor to that of the disorder. It lists 8 subtypes, these being characterized respectively by 'anxious mood', 'depressed mood', 'disturbance of conduct', 'mixed disturbance of emotions and conduct', 'mixed emotional features', 'physical complaints', 'withdrawal' and 'work (or academic) inhibition'. There is also a 'not otherwise specified' category.

In the case of both ICD-9 and DSM-III-R the use of these subcategories does no more than draw attention to the predominant symptoms. Since adjustment disorders are defined by their reactive and time-limited nature there is no typical clinical picture. The following are examples.

Susan was referred at age 14 by a juvenile court. She was born in Jamaica. Her parents migrated to England when she was 3 but she remained with her grandmother in Jamaica, joining her parents when she was 12.

Susan was said to have had no problems while in Jamaica, where she had a warm relationship with her grandmother and progressed well in school. She was unhappy, however, from the time of her arrival in England. She said this was partly because she found the work and atmosphere at school different from that she was used to, but mainly because of her home situation. Her parents had been strangers to her when she arrived to live with them but they had expected love and obedience from her, which she found it hard to produce on demand. She said of her mother, 'She treats me different, she don't like me, she treats me like a dog'. She believed she was brought over just to look after the four younger children born in England, who seemed to have secure, warm relationships with the parents.

After months of increasing unhappiness and failure at school, Susan ran away and was missing from home and school for 2 months. It was then discovered that she had been living with a 17-year-old distant cousin. Psychiatric assessment revealed no evidence of a current disorder, though Susan described graphically how unhappy she had been at home. Her parents reported unfavourably on her behaviour when she had been at home, but did not seem to feel she had been particularly unhappy.

Susan refused to return to live with her parents and was placed in a group home. There she settled down well, behaved normally, showed no signs of psychiatric disorder and said she was happy.

Comment

Susan's was a reversible, though prolonged, reaction to migration from one culture and family situation to another. In her new home she did not get the support, security and understanding she needed but her symptoms subsided quickly with a change of environment. This was an adjustment disorder 'with prolonged depressive reaction' (ICD-9) or 'with depressed mood' (DSM-III-R, although Susan did not run away until more than 3 months after coming to England and might therefore be held not to fit the DSM-III-R criteria, depending upon when the 'stressor' was considered to have been operative).

Selina, aged 2 years 6 months, was brought by her Anglo-Indian father and Swazi stepmother because for two weeks she had been sleeping poorly, clinging to her stepmother whenever strangers were present, eating little and crying a lot. These were unusual behaviours, for she had previously seemed a happy, well-adjusted child. She had lived with her father and stepmother for 18 months, but had been with her mother for about two months after her parents separated when she was 10 months old.

The symptoms were reported to have started on Selina's return from a visit with her mother. The latter was supposed to take her for the afternoon, as she had done a few times previously, but instead kept her overnight and most of the next day. The father suspected that Selina had been left on her own for at least part of the night, though the mother denied this.

The father and stepmother were advised that the symptoms would resolve within a few weeks at most, provided Selina was subjected to no more unexpected stresses of the sort that appeared to have precipitated this reaction. They did indeed clear up within three weeks, though some further work with the two natural parents was needed.

Comment

This is an example of an adjustment reaction 'with disturbance of emotions' (ICD-9) or 'with mixed emotional features' (DSM-III-R).

Quentin was referred at age 5 after his mother had been told by the school principal that he would not respond to discipline and therefore could not attend school. The school staff complained that, among other things, Quentin went into the girls' toilets in spite of being told not to and had repeatedly climbed a wall, which was forbidden because there was a busy road on the other side and the teachers feared for his safety.

Quentin was the only child of an unmarried mother. He had apparently led an isolated life with little company except that of his mother and maternal grandparents, before starting school. He had a slight speech defect and was mildly hyperactive. It seemed that he had been much indulged and overprotected by his mother and especially his grandparents, who had undertaken the lion's share of his care. He had had no preschool experience away from the three doting adults with whom he had lived and had grown up – apparently – with the expectation that he would always get his way.

Quentin was admitted briefly to an inpatient unit where he showed only mild, transient behaviour problems. He was discharged to attend a different school, the family were counselled on his management and he did well subsequently.

Comment

This was an adjustment reaction with disturbance of conduct, arising when an indulged only child who was accustomed to getting his own way was admitted to a school with strict rules and demanding standards.

Treatment

When the stress to which the disorder is a reaction is short-lived little treatment may be needed beyond support and reassurance for all concerned. If the stress is continuing, efforts should be made to remove it; if this is impossible, continuing psychotherapeutic help may be needed by child and/or family. Occasionally the temporary removal of the child to a different situation may be necessary.

Children's reactions to stress

Children's reactions to stress vary greatly, depending on the nature, severity and duration of the stress; their personality strengths, temperaments and previous experiences; and the social and emotional supports available to them during and following stressful experiences. There may be no detectable disturbance of functioning; adjustment disorder syndromes such as those outlined above may develop; or more serious and prolonged disorders such as post-traumatic stress disorder may follow.

The latter condition, classified under anxiety disorders in DSM-III-R, is characterized by episodic re-experiencing of the traumatic event in dreams or the waking state; diminished involvement with the external world, with feelings of detachment or constricted emotional reactions; sleep disturbance; hyper-alertness or exaggerated startle responses; impaired memory; and avoidance of activities or places which remind the child of the event, together with intensification of symptoms in such situations. There may also be guilt feelings about having survived the event if others, perhaps family members or friends, did not.

The May 1986 issue of *The Journal of the American Academy of Child Psychiatry* (Volume 25, No. 3) contains papers dealing with children's reactions to such stresses as witnessing parental murder; being attacked by a psychotic parent; a school disaster; the Three Mile Island nuclear power station accident; a devastating earthquake; the situation of American embassy children in Afghanistan and Pakistan in 1978 and 1979; and the events of the Pol Pot regime in Cambodia. Garmezy (1986) provides an overview and reviews previous literature on the subject.

Personality disorders

Many psychiatrists are rightly reluctant to use the term 'personality disorder' in young people whose personality development is far from complete. Yet some children show such seriously maladaptive personality characteristics from an early age that the diagnosis is justified.

A diagnosis of personality disorder implies that the individual has developed inappropriate ways of dealing with daily tasks, interpersonal relationships or the handling of stressful situations. The problems are severe and well-established, and affect a number of areas of the person's life.

Causes

Serious distortions of the normal processes of personality development have been attributed to constitutional, including genetic, causes and to environmental ones. The etiology probably varies from case to case and disorder to disorder.

Extremely unfavourable experiences during early life are often blamed for personality disorders. Barbara Dockar-Drysdale (1968; 1973) and Richard Balbernie (1974), influenced by the work of Donald Winnicott (1960), suggested that many children with personality disorders have lacked 'primary experience'. Balbernie (1974) writes, 'The mother in nurturing and care, provides regular, ordered, complete experiences of well-being through which a child learns that it does survive separation'. Lacking this experience, children act out their anxiety, do not feel guilt, lack regard for others' feelings and fail to value themselves. To quote Balbernie again, 'The basis of well-being is the experience of a basic sense of natural order that is internalized'. This has not been provided for children who lack primary experience. They are described as 'unintegrated'.

Among the categories of unintegrated children are 'frozen children', whose primary experience has been interrupted when they and their mothers should be starting to separate out. They survive 'without boundaries to personality, merged with their environment and unable to make any real relationships or feel the need for them'. 'Archipelago children' are those who have achieved the first step towards integration, but whose 'ego-islets' have 'never fused into a continent', that is a whole person.

Two other categories are 'false-selves' and 'caretaker-selves'. Describing the 'false-self', Winnicott (1960) wrote:

> 'The false-self sets up as real and it is this that observers tend to think is the real person. In living relationships, work relationships, and friendships, however, the false-self begins to fail. In situations in which what is expected is a whole person the false-self has some essential lacking.'

Winnicott describes types of false-selves approaching more closely a state of health. The 'caretaker-self' is built upon identifications. Inside the caretaker is the child's 'little self', carefully concealed. There may then, for example, be a delinquent 'caretaker' stealing, without conflict, on behalf of the 'little self'.

These ideas are based upon clinical experience, rather than on a firm body of scientifically established evidence. Yet such experience makes it hard to avoid the conclusion that seriously deviant early rearing, and repeated changes of parent figures, can have unfortunate effects on children's personality development. It may be, however, that a combination of these experiences with constitutional susceptibility is necessary for the development of a personality disorder. When personality disorders do develop in such circumstances, they are likely to be of the 'antisocial' or 'sociopathic' type.

A genetic cause has been suggested for 'schizoid personality disorder', also known as Asperger's syndrome (van Krevelen, 1971). In the study of 17 cases of this condition by Wolff and Barlow (1979), the children's histories revealed no adequate cause for the disorder. Much work remains to be done on the genetic and other factors which may lead to personality disorders in children.

Table 12.1 Categories of personality disorder.

ICD-9	DSM-III-R	Main features
Anankastic	Obsessive–compulsive	Rigid, inflexible, obsessive, ritualistic, perfectionistic.
Hysterical	Histrionic	Over-dramatic, flamboyant, labile mood, suggestible, drawing attention to self, egocentric, dependent.
Asthenic	Dependent	Helpless, clinging, passively compliant, lacking vigour.
Sociopathic/asocial	Antisocial	Lacking feeling for others, disregarding social norms and obligations, failing to plan ahead or learn from failure, poor work and parenting record.
Schizoid	Schizoid	Distant, cold, aloof, detached, introspective, unresponsive, few or no close friends.
—	Schizotypal	Social isolation, ideas of reference, 'magical' thinking, recurrent illusions, odd speech, suspiciousness, hypersensitivity.
Paranoid	Paranoid	Suspicious, jealous, sensitive to slight or imagined insults, affective responses restricted.
Explosive	—	Readily express anger, violence, hate, affection, either verbally or physically. May relate in shallow fashion. Demand immediate gratification.
Affective	—	Show lifelong mood deviation or alternation.
—	Narcissistic	Grandiosely self-important, with fantasies of success, power, brilliance or ideal love. Require attention and admiration, resent criticism, lack empathy and take advantage of others.
—	Borderline	Impulsive, unpredictable, with unstable but intense interpersonal relationships. Identity uncertain, mood unstable, fearful of being alone, self-damaging.
—	Avoidant	Hypersensitive to rejection, avoiding relationships, socially withdrawn, desiring affection and acceptance. Low self-esteem.
—	Passive–Aggressive	Resisting social and work demands, procrastinating, dawdling, stubborn, intentionally inefficient.
'Other' and 'Unspecified'	Not otherwise specified	—

Description

Both ICD-9 and DSM-III-R list various types of personality disorder but these categories are based mainly on work with adults. Table 2 lists the categories with their main features. While some appear with similar (though not always identical) descriptions in both schemes, others are found in one only. This empasizes that, in the present state of knowledge, the combinations of personality characteristics chosen to describe personality 'disorders' are largely arbitrary.

Caution is advisable in applying these labels in childhood; the younger the child the greater the caution that is in order. Only serious, longstanding disorders, especially those that persist regardless of environmental circumstances, should qualify. In DSM-III-R three of them are defined as applying only over age 18. Below the age of 18 there is a 'corresponding diagnostic category', as shown in Table 12.2

Table 12.2   Corresponding disorders in DSM-III-R.

Disorders of childhood and adolescence	Personality disorders
Conduct disorder	Antisocial personality disorder
Avoidant disorder of childhood or adolescence	Avoidant personality disorder
Identity disorder	Borderline personality disorder

Although setting age 18 as the lower age limit for the development of certain personality disorders is arbitrary, there are advantages in avoiding the use of personality disorder diagnoses in children and young people; children's personalities are less fixed than those of adults and there is a greater potential for change as maturation continues.

Two categories of personality disorder that merit further discussion here are schizoid personality and antisocial (or sociopathic/asocial) personality.

Schizoid personality

Asperger (1944) described what he called 'autistic psychopathy of childhood'. He seems to have been referring to children with personalities described as 'schizoid' in both DSM-III-R and ICD-9. Wolff and Barlow (1979) described 17 such children and reported a study which compared them with intelligent autistic children and with normal children. Schizoid children are distant, aloof and lacking in empathy. They find group activities, especially rough games, stressful.

Other features are obstinacy and aggressive outbursts when under pressure to conform, often at school; preoccupation with their own systems of ideas and beliefs, for instance electronics, dinosaurs or space travel; emotional detachment; rigidity, which may be of obsessional proportions; sensitivity, sometimes with paranoid ideas; learning problems which may be present despite above-average IQ; and bizarre antisocial behaviour in a few cases. The condition is much commoner in boys than girls (the ratio being 9 or 10 to 1). Referral is most often because of school adjustment problems. Presenting problems include school refusal, running away, temper outbursts, suicidal threats, stealing and elective mutism (described below).

This seems to be a distinct group of children who are in many respects intermediate in their clinical features between autistic children and normal ones. Like autistic children they show stereotypies and tend to impose patterns on their environment, and they have linguistic handicaps and lack perceptiveness for meaning. Yet they lack the repetitiveness and the motivation for tasks of cognition and memory of autistic children. It has also been suggested that there may be a relationship between this disorder and schizophrenia (Wolff and Chick, 1980), though this is far from proven.

Thomas had always been a difficult child, his mother said. His first weeks of life were disrupted by an operation for pyloric stenosis and he was a difficult, negativistic baby and toddler. More serious, however, was his lonely, asocial behaviour. As he grew up he would not talk to other children or to strangers. He violently resisted going to school at age 5, kicking and screaming and refusing to do anything he was asked. Transfer to a school for slow-learning children, and then a year in a children's convalescent hospital under the care of a psychiatrist, did little to help him.

At age 9 Thomas was a well-dressed, good-looking boy, but timid and anxious. He failed to respond to most questions. The few answers he did give were either very short verbal ones or consisted of nodding or shaking his head.

During subsequent inpatient and daypatient treatment Thomas made little progress. He remained quiet, isolated and passively resistant, though he could become acutely physically and verbally aggressive, for example when attempts were made to take a sample of blood from him. He persistently resisted participating in psychological testing.

The family situation was difficult in that there was much marital strife, Thomas being the focus of parental disagreements. The parents were divorced when Thomas was 11 and soon afterwards his mother remarried. Thomas, however, remained a passive, non-communicative, friendless boy without social contacts outside his home.

Comment

Thomas' personality had been odd, and his relationships with his family unusual, from infancy. By the time he was seen for psychiatric assessment a gross, longstanding disorder was well established. This conformed to the picture described in schizoid personality disorder. He also showed features of elective mutism, but his disorder involved his whole personality and his social and educational development, not just verbal communication. His early experiences,, the family relationship difficulties and inborn biological factors may have combined to produce the clinical picture.

Antisocial or sociopathic personality disorders

ICD-9 defines these as characterized by disregard for social obligations, lack of feeling for others and impetuous violence or callous unconcern. The subject's behaviour is grossly at variance with society's norms and is not readily modifiable by experience, including punishment. These individuals are often emotionally cold and may be unduly aggressive or irresponsible. They have low frustration tolerance, blame others and/or offer plausible rationalizations for their antisocial behaviour. They may engage in a wide range of crimes, drug and alcohol abuse and prostitution. They do not hold jobs for long and tend to be neglectful parents.

ICD-9 recognizes that personality disorders, defined as 'deeply ingrained maladaptive patterns of behaviour' may be recognizable by the time of adolescence or earlier. It allows a diagnosis of a 'sociopathic/ asocial' personality disorder to be made during childhood. On the other hand DSM-III-R recommends that the category of 'antisocial person- ality disorder' be used only for subjects over 18, though the onset of some of the features has to be before 15. Below the age of 18 the 'corresponding' childhood diagnostic category of conduct disorder is to be used. This may obscure the fact that some children with conduct disorders have serious underlying personality problems, while others do not.

Children meeting the above description, and in whom the personal- ity traits described are well established, are encountered as early as late childhood or early adolescence. The following is an example.

Laura was first seen at age 13, at which time her mother said she could no longer cope with her. She was stealing money both in the house and outside it, lying, staying out late and associating with delinquent 'friends' her mother had forbidden her to see. When asked to mind her two younger half-siblings she acted irresponsibly. She had twice run away, each time for a few days.

Laura had had many changes of home. For her first few months she lived with her mother and father. When they separated she was placed with an aunt who was later convicted of child abuse; the charges related to her own children, but Laura said she too had been beaten repeatedly. At age 5 Laura returned to live briefly with her mother, who was now divorced. For the next 8 years she lived an unstable existence. At times she was in the care of child welfare agencies, at others she was with her mother, who had a number of brief relationships with different men.

These men would live in the home for periods of a few days to a few weeks, before the relationship broke up.

Laura was admitted to a residential centre for assessment and treatment. She proved a difficult child to get to know. She was emotionally cold and aloof, so that staff never felt they knew what she was thinking or feeling. At various times she ran away, sometimes to her father. She played truant from school, stole money and other children's property and told lies. She was also suspected of having clandestine meetings with boys with whom she had been told not to associate. Staff found the biggest problem in helping Laura was making emotional contact with her. She seemed always to give the response that seemed most expedient, which often involved lying. It seemed impossible to get to the real Laura. Her life seemed to be like a store front, with little or nothing behind it - or at least nothing that could be discovered. She did, however, from time to time reveal fantasies about her family, especially her father. She said he loved her and that only circumstances beyond his control stopped him having her to live with him. In fact he had only had about half-a-dozen contacts with her in the previous 10 years, but on 2 or 3 occasions when she had run away to him at his place of work he had given her a friendly reception and had even bought her lunch.

While it proved possible to modify Laura's behaviour using behaviour therapy techniques, the changes did not persist when the treatment was stopped. Changes in Laura's ways of relating to people were not apparent.

Comment

The central feature of Laura's disorder seemed to be an inability to form warm, loving, trusting relationships with people. Instead she treated people in an exploitative fashion, stealing from them, lying to them and trying to manipulate them to meet her immediate wants. Her unstable early life and lack of a secure and consistent relationship with her mother (who shared many of Laura's personality character-istics and was a regular abuser of marijuana and alcohol), were probably important etiological factors. Genetic factors may also have been involved.

A DSM-III-R diagnosis of conduct disorder would have been appropriate, but Laura appeared also to have a serious disorder of personality development. A conduct disorder diagnosis does not fully do justice to this. Using ICD-9 a diagnosis of sociopathic/asocial personality disorder was probably appropriate.

Borderline personality disorder

'Borderline' states or disorders (see Table 12.1) are so named because of the tenuous hold on reality these individuals have; they border on being psychotic, though frankly psychotic behaviour is not evident (Masterson, 1972). They are often complicated by symptoms of other types of personality disorder, for example schizotypal, histrionic, narcissistic and antisocial disorders.

Treatment and outcome

The treatment of children and adolescents with personality disorders presents great challenges. One of the biggest is establishing a trusting relationship with the young person. These subjects are adept at arousing therapists' despair, anger, disgust or other negative emotions. They are usually reluctant or downright unwilling to enter therapy. Young people with asocial or borderline personality disorders may need to be treated in residential settings where their environments are tightly structured, so that they cannot manipulate them.

A excellent account of what may be involved in the treatment of a personality-disordered adolescent who has had adverse early experiences is that of Rossman (1985). This paper illustrates the vicissitudes of the process in a particularly graphic way; the severity of the psychopathology that may emerge is also well illustrated.

Psychosexual problems

Both ICD-9 and DSM-III-R have categories for disorders of psychosexual development. In DSM-III-R the term 'gender identity disorder of childhood' is used to describe conditions in which a child has 'persistent and intense distress ... about his or her assigned sex and the desire to be, or insistence that he or she is, of the other sex'. Such individuals persistently repudiate their own anatomical attributes and wish to belong to the opposite sex. Onset is before puberty.

ICD-9 has a category, 'disorders of psychosexual identity', the criteria for which are less stringent, in that 'identification with the behaviour and appearance of the opposite sex is not yet fixed'.

There is a continuum of children ranging from those who are completely identified with their anatomical sex, to those who totally reject it. The DSM-III-R criteria mentioned above single out the latter group. The ICD-9 criteria cover a rather broader one. In its extreme (DSM-III-R) form gender identity disorder is rare but milder forms of effeminacy in boys and 'tomboyishness' in girls are quite common. The term 'transvestism' describes persistent dressing by males in female clothes (DSM-III-R), or by individuals of either sex in the clothes of the opposite sex (ICD-9), to obtain sexual excitement. It may occur in both childhood and adolescence.

In child psychiatric practice parents who express concern that their sons are overly effeminate are met with more often than those who are worried about masculine behaviours or attitudes in their daughters. Society is more accepting of 'tomboyish' behaviour in girls than of effeminate behaviour in boys. Girls may wear masculine clothes and play boys' games without causing concern, but boys who wear girls' clothes and engage in 'feminine' behaviour are less readily accepted (Williams *et al.*, 1985).

Causes

Biological, especially genetic, factors and environmental ones combine to produce a child's sense of sexual identity, as explained in Chapter 1. Just how they do this, and the relative roles of each group of factors, are not fully understood. Social learning theories have been advanced to explain the process but the child's biological substrate surely limits what social learning can do. The sexual identity assigned to a child in infancy, and the consequent experience of being raised as a member of that sex, used to be considered the most important factors. This now appears to be an over-simplification and it is recognized that the process involves a more complex interaction of factors than was realized. The nature and concentration of the hormones produced as boys and girls grow, approach puberty and become adolescent, differ and clearly also play their parts in the process (see Green (1985a) for a summary of research findings).

Effeminate boys tend to be overinvolved with their mothers from an early age and for well into middle childhood (Sreenivasan, 1985). This may help cause the effeminacy but it could also be a result of biologically determined behaviour in the child.

There is less information on the development of 'tomboy' girls but Williams *et al.* (1985), in a longitudinal study of 50 such girls and a control group of 'nontomboys', found that tomboys are more likely to take their fathers as favoured parent and model, rather than their mothers. Tomboys had less physical contact with their mothers during the first year of life than the 'nontomboy' controls, though father-daughter interaction did not differ in the two groups. These investigators found that the mothers of the tomboys dressed in 'masculine' clothing significantly more than the 'control' mothers; they were also reported to have more often been tomboys themselves as children, suggesting a possible genetic influence.

Description

Sreenivasan (1985) assessed 100 consecutive referrals of boys aged 6 to 12 to a child psychiatric clinic. She found that 15 showed a high measure of 'effeminacy', though none met the DSM-III criteria for gender identity disorder and none was referred because of a gender identity problem. There was, however, a relationship between high effeminacy and paranoid (or 'hypersensitive') personality disorder.

Anxiety, dysthymic and somatoform disorders were also significantly associated with high effeminacy. Sreenivasan (1985) describes a 'composite picture of the effeminate boy'. He is born to, or adopted by, a woman who sees him as not very manly; is a cuddly baby; clings to his mother as a toddler; and continues to wish to do so. His mother does not discourage this. He sleeps in his mother's bed well into late childhood, even though his father lives at home; has personality traits of hypersensitivity and insecurity; and may develop a neurotic disorder. Antisocial behaviour may develop later when he feels rejected by those who previously accepted his cross-gender activities and peers stigmatize him. In Sreenivasan's series, only 1 of the 29 boys living in a traditional nuclear family showed high effeminacy; the presence of the father in the household seemed to be more important in promoting masculine attitudes than the quality of the father-son interaction.

Gender identity disorders, as defined in DSM-III-R, are much rarer. Boys with this condition have a strong and persistent desire to be female or even insist that they are. They may like to dress in girls' clothes, participate in girls' games and play with dolls as girls do. They may disclaim their penis or testes or believe they will disappear. Onset of cross-dressing is usually before the fifth birthday.

Girls with gender identity disorders show a desire to be or believe that they really are boys. While they prefer boys' clothing and games, this usually causes less concern.

It appears that extreme boyhood feminity is usually not an isolated phenomenon; it is often accompanied by other behavioural or emotional symptoms, particularly separation anxiety disorder (Bradley *et al.*, 1980; Coates and Person, 1985).

Sexual Identity Conflict in Children and Adults (Green, 1974) was a pioneering publication; it, and subsequent publications by Green and his colleagues (listed by Zucker *et al.*, 1985), are good sources of further information on these disorders.

Treatment

Green (1985a) raises ethical issues concerning what the treatment of children with atypical psychosexual development should aim to do. In severe cases of gender identity disorder it may not be realistic to try to reverse the child's sexual identity; to try might be traumatic or at least less helpful than other approaches. Yet the parents usually seek treatment for these children, who may be socially ostracised and suffer much unhappiness, especially the boys.

Psychotherapy for child and parents is usually the treatment employed. It should aim to increase the child's comfort in being anatomically male or female, reduce sex-role behaviours which peers will regard as inappropriate, strengthen the child's relationship and contact with the same-sex parent, and identify and facilitate the child's involvement with a same-sex peer group which will accept him or her. As well as individual therapy for the children and therapy for the parents as couples, behaviour modification, group therapy or family therapy may sometimes be helpful.

Outcome

A study of 44 boys aged 13 to 23 (mean 18.5), who had previously shown extensive cross-dressing behaviour found that 30 were bisexually or homosexually oriented, while this applied to none of a comparison group of 34 boys (Green, 1985b). Data on the longer term outlook are lacking. Zucker *et al.* (1985) reported one-year reassessments of 44 'cross-gender-identified' children, and found that they had either maintained or reduced their cross-gender behaviour. Improvement seemed to be related to the amount of therapy received, the number of parent sessions apparently being more important than the number of child sessions.

Other psychosexual problems

Other psychosexual problems are sometimes encountered in young people. These include voyeurism, in which the subject spies on unsuspecting people who are undressing, naked or engaging in sexual activities; and exhibitionism, the exposing of one's genitals to strangers to achieve sexual excitement. The causes are not properly understood but some of these children have had unstable childhood experiences, with long periods of institutional care or deviant rearing. Individual psychotherapy, counselling for the parents, family therapy or behaviour therapy may be helpful, but severe, established cases present difficult treatment challenges.

Tics and the Gilles de la Tourette syndrome

Tics, sometimes known as habit spasms, are repeated, sudden movements of muscles or groups of muscles, not under the voluntary control of the subject and serving no obvious purpose. They most often affect the muscles of the face and eye-blinking tics are one of the commoner forms. Various facial contortions may occur and muscle groups in other parts of the body may be affected. Thus the head and neck may be suddenly and briefly moved in one direction or contorted.

210 Basic Child Psychiatry

There may be similar movements of trunk or limbs. The same movements tend to occur repeatedly, in severe cases scores or hundreds of times a day; the involuntary movements in the various forms of chorea, on the other hand, are more varied and less predictable. Tics, especially when they involve large movements of trunk or limbs, can be seriously handicapping.

DSM-III-R distinguishes three varieties of tic disorder:

• Tourette's disorder;
• chronic motor or vocal tic disorder;
• transient tic disorder.

Tourette's syndrome is defined as the combination of motor tics, as described above, with one or more vocal tics. The latter may be sounds such as grunts, yelps, barks, sniffs, coughs or words. In about 60 per cent of cases the words consist of obscene utterances (or 'coprolalia').

In 'chronic motor or vocal tic disorder' there are either motor tics or vocal ones but not both. The features of 'transient tic disorder' are single or multiple motor and/or vocal tics occurring many times a day for at least two weeks but for no longer than 12 months.

ICD-9 does not subdivide its category labelled 'tics'. This diagnosis appears under 'special symptoms or syndromes not elsewhere classified'. Whether there is any fundamental difference, other than one of severity, between DSM-III-R's three categories is uncertain.

Prevalence

Studies suggest that between 10 per cent and 24 per cent of children will experience tics at some time (Corbett and Turpin, 1985), but many have the symptom only briefly and the prevalence at any one time is lower. Tourette's syndrome is much less common. Tics are commoner in boys than in girls, the ratio being at least 2:1. Onset is usually between 2 and 15 years of age.

Causes

Genetic factors are important. Evidence exists for an autosomal dominant pattern of transmission of Tourette's syndrome, chronic tics and obsessive-compulsive disorder (Pauls and Leckman, 1986). It seems that there is a spectrum of disorders which are inherited, with a sex difference in the expression of symptoms. Tics are more common in males with the gene concerned and obsessive-compulsive symptoms in females. It is unlikely that all obsessive-compulsive disorders are inherited this way, and some individuals with Tourette's disease (perhaps about 10 per cent) may be phenocopies (non-genetically determined cases). But in certain families this genetic pattern seems to prevail.

What other factors are involved is uncertain. Emotional tension, brain damage, developmental deviation and adverse learning experiences have been suggested, but the roles, if any, of these factors are not established. Biochemical theories have also been put forward, but so far are no more than hypotheses (Devinsky, 1983).

Description

A review of the cases of 100 ticquers seen at the Maudsley Hospital, London (Corbett *et al.*, 1969), revealed that they comprised 7 per cent of the children seen in the child psychiatry department. Only about half had been referred for their tics, which were often associated with symptoms of emotional disturbance. The tics started most commonly at about age 7. The face was the most frequently affected part of the body. Isolated tics of other parts were less common. The ticquers showed certain emotional symptoms significantly more often than the general clinic population of disturbed children. These were 'gratification habits, speech disorders, disorders of defecation (including encopresis), and obsessional and hypochondriacal symptoms'. By contrast, temper and aggression, truancy, fighting and depression occurred less often in ticquers. These findings might mean that tics and the symptoms that go with them represent expressions of anxiety and aggression in individuals who have difficulty expressing such emotions directly. The genetic association of obsessive-compulsive disorder with tic disorders might be held to support this notion. Moreover many of the ticquers were found at later follow-up to be anxious even though the tics had improved.

Tourette's syndrome is probably just a severe form of tic disorder, though it is a generally more chronic and socially disabling condition.

Treatment

A supportive attitude is important in the management of these children and their families. Any possible sources of anxiety should be removed or alleviated, as far as possible. The tics may be explained as somatic manifestations of anxiety, and appropriate treatment should be provided for any co-existing psychiatric problems. The tics themselves should be made light of since nothing is gained, and the child's anxiety may be raised, if attention is focussed on them.

Many specific treatments, including individual psychotherapy, behaviour therapy and various forms of pharmacotherapy have been described and recommended, but the most effective seems to be the drug haloperidol. Doses up to 6 mg per day may be required (Greenberg and Stephans, 1977) and higher ones have been used. Unfortunately this drug may cause side-effects (see Chapter 19) and long-term use should be avoided if possible. An alternative drug that may be helpful is pimozide. Behavioural treatments can also play a useful part in the treatment regime and have been reviewed by Turpin (1983).

Outcome

The results of the Maudsley study (Corbett *et al.*, 1969) suggest that most children's tics improve, and 40 per cent had recovered at follow-up 5 years after psychiatric consultation. There seemed to be a tendency for anxiety and neurotic symptoms to be present in the patients followed up. Tourette's syndrome presents a more challenging treatment problem, but the combination of behaviour therapy and medication often keeps the symptoms in abeyance and in some instances they remit in due course.

Stuttering

Stuttering is listed as a diagnostic category in both ICD-9 and DSM-III-R. Sometimes called stammering, it is the repeated interruption of the flow of speech by repetition, prolongation or blocking of sounds. In children aged 2 to 4 there are often hesitations, repetitions of the first sounds of words or phrases and irregularities of the rhythm of speech. This is known as 'clutter' and sometimes precedes true stuttering, though more often it gradually disappears and the child then speaks normally.

Stuttering may appear after speech has been acquired but onset is usually before age 10. It occurs in about 4 per cent of boys and 2 per cent of girls; about 1 per cent of children continue stuttering in adolescence, more of them being boys than girls. Its causes are not fully understood, but there is often a positive family history of the symptom and mutifactorial inheritance may play a part (Kidd *et al.*, 1978); so also may anxiety and stress (Greiner *et al.*, 1985). Other psychological factors are probably involved, and some stutterers can sing fluently or speak normally while acting on stage, but stutter in ordinary conversation. Some children speak fluently at home but stutter at school. Some are worse when anxious, while others are not. Disturbed parent-child relationships may affect the learning of fluent speech.

The severity of stuttering varies from occasional repetition of speech sounds to severe blocking of speech which seriously interferes with communication. Anticipatory anxiety may be present, leading to avoidance behaviour. At first a few letters or sounds may be avoided; later many places and social situations may be shunned. This can drastically affect the subject's life. Stuttering may cause children to become isolated and impair their ability to take part in school activities.

Stuttering is not usually part of a general psychiatric disorder. The causative role of emotional disorder is in most cases small, though anxiety may either complicate or exacerbate the condition. Stuttering was well described in *The Syndrome of Stuttering* (Andrews and Harris, 1964).

Treatment is usually undertaken by speech therapists. The psychiatric contribution is limited. Techniques designed to relieve anxiety, promote relaxation and encourage self-confidence may help. Specific techniques such as 'syllabic speech' may be used; stutterers are taught, usually in a group setting, to speak slowly and deliberately, syllable by syllable. Psychotherapy should be reserved for cases in which there is associated emotional disorder in child or family. Treatment approaches and other aspects of stuttering are discussed by Wingate (1976).

Stuttering is often mild and transient and most children outgrow it by the mid-teens. In a few cases it persists into adult life. It may be reinforced by 'secondary gain', being used, perhaps unconsciously, to gain control of or avoid certain situations or to evoke sympathy or attention.

Elective mutism

In elective mutism the child refuses to talk in certain situations, such as school, yet talks in others, usually at home.

Prevalence

Brown and Lloyd (1975) surveyed 6072 5-year-old children starting school in Birmingham, England. They found that 42 were still not speaking in class after 8 weeks in school, a prevalence rate of 7.2 per 1000. During the following four terms the number of mute children fell steadily, so that after 64 weeks only one child remained silent in school. The condition is thus fairly common as an initial reaction to school but rare as a persisting problem. Bradley and Sloman (1975) found 26 electively mute children among 6865 Canadian kindergarten children, with a highly significant excess being children from immigrant families (who were also over-represented in Brown and Lloyd's sample).

The prevalence rate in 7-year-olds is probably about 0.8 per 1000 (Kolvin and Fundudis, 1981) but it depends on the diagnostic criteria used. Elective mutism, unlike most child psychiatric disorders, is as common in girls as in boys, possibly a little commoner.

Causes

Genetic factors are suggested by the high prevalence of shyness that has been found in parents, in whom there seems also to be an unduly high incidence of psychiatric illness. Electively mute children are themselves often considered shy. Kolvin and Fundudis (1981) reported several 'subsidiary' patterns of behaviour: 'submissive'; 'sensitive and weepy'; and 'moody-aggressive, sulky and stubborn'. The last-named was the commonest. These children tend to be late talking, have speech abnormalities when they do start to talk and are enuretic and encopretic more often than controls. They come from a wide variety of socioeconomic backgrounds.

Elective mutism is probably a complex disorder to which genetic, personality, emotional and family factors all contribute.

Description

The main feature is the child's failure to talk in most situations, such as school, public places, clinics, doctors' offices and consulting rooms, in fact anywhere but at home with the family. Brown and Lloyd (1975) found that children who were mute at school showed other behaviour patterns which distinguished them from children who spoke. They were more likely to stop an activity when the teacher approached and to avoid playing with other children; they were less likely to draw, go to the toilet or approach the teacher's table.

In the doctor's office or therapist's playroom these children usually behave as negatively non-verbally as they do verbally. They may passively decline to sit down or to play when invited to do so. Some will nod or shake (usually shake) their heads in reply to questions, others deny the examiner even this response. At the same time they are usually looking around the room, apparently taking everything in. They can be extraordinarily stubborn, remaining silent for session after session. Yet given the right conditions (for them) they can speak freely. One girl who was making good, if non-verbal, progress at school was observed on closed-circuit television to be talking freely and in a relaxed way when alone with her family; but as soon as a member of the clinic staff entered she became silent and remained so until that person left.

Various subtypes of electively mute children have been described. Haydon (1980) distinguished 'symbiotic', 'reactive', 'passive aggressive' and 'speech phobic' varieties. Wright *et al.* (1985) suggest that Hayden's 'symbiotic' and 'reactive' cases are what Kolvin and Fundudis (1981) called, respectively, 'elective' and 'traumatic' mutism. Haydon's 'passive aggressive' group seem rather different, with a later age of onset, often in adolescence. In practice it is hard to categorize cases of elective mutism. This seems rather to be a syndrome with varying manifestations, occurring in children from many different types of families. There are, however, certainly some children in which anxiety seems to dominate the picture and others in which negativism does. Immigrant children seem particularly prone to mutism, though it is usually transient.

Kolvin and Fundudis (1981) report a mean IQ of 85 in their 24 elective mutes, while the mean IQ of speech-retarded comparison subjects was 95 and that of normal control subjects was 101.

Treatment

Many treatments have been proposed for electively mute children, but the established, severe case often presents a considerable therapeutic challenge. Brown *et al.* (1975), in a review of treatments reported, list the following: suggestion, persuasion, coercion, psychodynamically orientated play therapy, speech therapy, family therapy and behaviour therapy. Wright *et al.* (1985), reviewing reports of 81 cases, found that behavioural intervention was used most often (in 27 cases), with 'psychodynamic' intervention second in 15. They also report three cases, all with onset at age 3, which presented in the preschool period and were treated in a diagnostic nursery with good results. They suggest that early treatment may prevent the condition becoming chronic and less responsive to later treatment measures. They thought that important factors contributing to their good results were early intervention, the expectation that the children would speak and the conjoint family work that was done.

Because of the varied circumstances of these cases, it is likely that the treatment needs vary also. While many children do grow out of the symptom, this does not justify inaction since we know that some do not do so for a very long time. In the case of the child who fails to speak on first entering school, it may be justifiable to wait a month or two, especially if there are no other psychiatric symptoms.

A small group setting with speaking peers and adults, treatment staff who expect the child to talk and do not accept the mutism as inevitable, and family intervention, as described by Wright *et al.* (1985), seems helpful. For older children combinations of behavioural interventions, family therapy and, in some cases, play therapy may offer the best prospects of success.

Outcome

The mutism is usually self-limiting and total mutism seldom persists into adult life, though in severe cases it may be present for much of childhood and even into early adolescence. Little data are available on the general adjustment of these children once they do start to speak, but it seems they are inclined to be shy, retiring individuals. The outlook is good for the child whose mutism is a reaction to starting school and who has previously communicated normally.

The Kleine-Levin syndrome

This disorder of unknown origin consists of episodes of disturbed mental function, greatly increased appetite and excessive sleepiness (Orlosky, 1982). The episodes last from a few days to several weeks. The onset is usually in adolescence but may occur before puberty (Ferguson, 1986). The psychiatric symptoms often consist of mood disturbance – depression, unwarranted anxiety or mania – but other delusional ideas, including erotic ones, have been reported. No specific treatment has been shown to be effective, but the condition usually resolves spontaneously in time.

Epilepsy

Although in some parts of the world, for example much of Africa, epilepsy is considered a psychiatric disorder, in western countries specialist help for epileptics is usually provided by paediatricians and neurologists. Nevertheless, the psychiatric importance of epilepsy is considerable, for the following reasons:

(a) Epileptic seizures may have major repercussions in a child's life (Bagley, 1971). Repeatedly losing consciousness or displaying abnormal behaviour in school or other public places may lead others, especially the child's peers, to become frightened, anxious or hostile. Depending on the attitudes of family, friends and others, epileptic chidren themselves may feel imperfect or stigmatized, so that their self-esteem suffers. Anxiety or depression may follow.

(b) Symptoms which are due to epilepsy may be erroneously regarded as psychogenic. Thus 'absence seizures', lapses of consciousness which last 5 to 15 seconds and which may occur hundreds of times a day, may be mistaken for inattention of emotional origin. This applies also to 'complex partial seizures', in which there is an aura (a subjective experience the child is aware of briefly before the seizure itself commences), then loss of consciousness for 30 seconds to 2 minutes. There may be automatisms in both types of seizure but they are more complex in the latter (Stores, 1987).

Epileptic discharges arising in the temporal lobes can cause abnormal behaviours which may not be recognized as epileptic. The behaviour may appear purposive and complex – for example, running about, screaming and shouting. It sometimes takes the form of aggressiveness and temper attacks. Children showing such behaviours are sometimes wrongly diagnosed as suffering from conduct disorders.

'Non-convulsive status epilepticus' is a condition in which epileptic discharges continue for periods which may be as long as several months, but without typical seizures appearing. As well as neurological symptoms such as ataxia, dysphasia, myoclonic jerks and atonic attacks, there may be disorientation, fluctuating responsiveness, developmental regression and aggressive behaviour (Manning and Rosenbloom, 1987).

(c) Epileptic seizures and 'pseudoepilepsy' may occur in the same individual. Pseudoepilepsy includes certain manifestations of conversion and dissociative disorders (see Chapter 5), as well as behaviours due to other non-epileptic processes. Distinguishing the seizures that are epileptic from those which are not can be difficult. The EEG is useful but recordings taken between epileptic attacks may be normal, unless they are done very soon after an attack. Detailed study of the circumstances in which the attacks occur and careful observation of the attacks themselves (observations which often have to be made by relatives, teachers and others and reported to the professionals concerned), are necessary to unravel these complex cases.

Nowadays equipment is available in many centres for the continuous monitoring of the EEG while patients go about their activities. The recording is done by telemetry, using a radio transmitter, or by means of a cable running from the child to whom the electrodes are attached, to the EEG laboratory; but the subject has to be near the laboratory, which normally means being in hospital during the recording. 'Ambulatory' EEG monitoring at home, in school or elsewhere is possible using small cassette recorders worn by the subject (Stores,

1985). These devices can help distinguish epilepsy from other types of seizure.

'Secondary gain', such as the experience of increased attention and solicitude, or special consideration when family activities are planned, may be part of the unconscious motivation behind 'pseudoepileptic' seizures, especially when the 'organic' ones are controlled by medication. In some cases the child has other emotional problems or there are contributory family systems problems.

(d) 'Pseudoepileptic', or 'hysterical' seizures may masquerade as epileptic ones in children who do not have epilepsy at all. These children may have had contact with epileptics and witnessed seizures. Such experiences serve as unconscious models of disturbed or 'sick' behaviour; these may be used as part of the symptomatology of a neurotic disorder. Careful history taking, a full psychiatric assessment, EEG examination perhaps with continuous monitoring, and paediatric consultation usually lead to the correct diagnosis.

(e) Epilepsy may be a complication of certain psychiatric disorders, notably infantile autism (see Chapter 7). It can also be a feature of some of the conditions causing disintegrative psychoses (Chapter 8).

(f) The side-effects of some of the drugs used in the treatment of epilepsy include depression, irritability and various forms of behaviour disorder. Phenobarbitone and phenytoin, both valuable anticonvulsants, are particularly liable to cause such problems.

In all the above clinical situations, close collaboration and communication between psychiatrists and other mental health personnel concerned on the one hand, and the paediatricians and/or neurologists on the other, are essential if these often difficult cases are to be managed properly. Paediatrics and child psychiatry are closely related specialities but there is perhaps no area in which the fields come closer than in the management of seizure disorders. In addition, teachers, psychologists, social workers and other professionals may have important roles to play in the management of these families.

The papers by Goodyer (1985) and Stores (1985) are valuable sources of information on the assessment and investigation of seizure disorders, particularly those in which both organic and emotional factors play a part. Goodyer (1985) includes case reports of 5 adolescents with various forms of 'pseudoepileptic' seizures, including a 12-year-old girl whose lapses of consciousness were eventually thought to be due to hypotensive attacks and blackouts related to solvent abuse. This reminds us that seizures may be due to neither epilepsy nor a conversion or dissociative disorder, and illustrates how important it is to make a comprehensive assessment of every case.

The treatment of epileptic children usually combines anticonvulsant medication with suitable general care and management of child and family. Stores (1987) emphasizes that there is no such thing as the 'epileptic personality'. He points out that 'the typical psychological problems of people with epilepsy are depression and anxiety caused by unhelpful and uninformed social attitudes' (page 90). Drug treatment can contribute too. In dealing with epileptic chidren it is important to be neither too restrictive nor too permissive, though striking the right balance can be difficult, especially for anxious parents. Excellent communication between the members of the team treating child and family is a prerequisite for good results. In a minority of cases, but in many of those in which there are pseudoepileptic seizures, psychotherapy for child and/or family may be required.

Chapter 13

Mind-Body Relationships

There is evidence that both physical and emotional factors are important in most, if not all, illnesses. Thus the division of diseases into 'organic' and 'non-organic' (or 'physical' and 'psychological') varieties is artificial and may be misleading. It is also questionable whether the conceptual division of mind and body makes sense. The brain, a part of the body, is the organ of the mind. Changes in a person's emotional state or behaviour must have their correlates in brain activity, whether these are chemical, electrical, physical or structural, just as changes in the blood electrolytes have their correlates in the activity of the kidneys, lungs and other organs.

Unfortunately the dynamic relationships between, for example, electrolyte levels and renal activity (each of which affects the other), are better understood than those between brain activity and emotional state or behaviour. This is partly because the brain is an immensely complex organ and singularly difficult to study during life. Nevertheless, our ignorance is lessening and the advent of non-invasive techniques, such as positron emission tomography (PET) scanning and nuclear magnetic resonance (NMR) imaging, open up the prospect of our learning much more about brain function

For the time being we must regard mind and body somewhat separately, but this is an artificial dichotomy, necessary because of our ignorance of the connections between the two.

The influence of the body on the mind

It is well known that being diagnosed as having a serious physical disease may affect a person's mental state. Discovering that one has cancer, or acquired immune deficiency syndrome (AIDS), causes emotional repercussions, though these vary from person to person. Chronic diseases such as diabetes, cystic fibrosis, asthma, rheumatoid arthritis, congenital heart disease or eczema influence the self-images, development and emotional states of affected children. So also may congenital deformities, dwarfism, cerebral palsy and other physically obvious and handicapping conditions.

In these disorders the effect of the bodily condition on the mind can be explained as due to the subject's conscious awareness of the condition, the handicap it causes and the effect it has on the attitudes of others. The body can also affect the mind in other ways. Apart from obvious examples like brain tumours and diseases, many physical illnesses influence people's emotional states, thinking processes or behaviour. In diabetics, for example, fluctuations in the blood sugar level, and the accumulation of ketones in the blood, affect the mental state. Hypoglycaemia from other causes has effects similar to those seen when diabetics have insulin reactions. Raised or lowered levels of thyroid hormones also lead to changed mental states.

These relationships are not necessarily one-way processes. Minuchin *et al.* (1978) have shown that unstable diabetes in children may be related to emotional and family factors, alleviation of which improves the control of the children's diabetes. The effective severity of a physical handicap also depends on emotional factors. Some people make little effort to overcome their disabilities and choose to remain dependent on others, while the mental attitudes of others lead to their making vigorous efforts to overcome their handicaps. The results may be remarkable, as in the case of Douglas Bader who continued flying planes as a Battle of Britain fighter pilot after having both his legs amputated; or Helen Keller who was remarkably successful in overcoming the dual handicaps of blindness and deafness.

The effects of the mind on the body

The effects of the emotions on bodily functions are familiar to all and are subsumed in phrases such as 'scared stiff' and 'shaking with laughter'. When people are frightened or anxious they may lose their appetite or feel the urge to urinate or defecate. Some peptic ulcer patients suffer exacerbations when they are worried or under stress and many other conditions are stress-related.

Despite the above examples the extent of the influence of the mind on the body is too often overlooked or underestimated. Rossi (1986a) reminds us of the significance of phenomena such as voodoo deaths and the placebo response. In certain cultures some people die because they believe a spell has been cast over them. Similar processes also promote recovery from illnesses. The culture of the western world is that of the vitamin pill, antibiotic, sleeping tablet or cold cure, rather than of the witchdoctor's spell, but the mechanisms involved may be the same. We know that inert medication may promote recovery in 30 per cent to 40 per cent of patients with certain disorders, presumably because their faith in the medication they take is as great as that which people of other cultures have in their traditional healing methods.

In *The Psychobiology of Mind-Body Healing*, Rossi (1986a) reviews the current state of research into mind-body mechanisms. There is good evidence that nerve impulses arising in the hypothalamus in response to emotional changes, affect the functioning of the autonomic, endocrine and immune systems.

The phenomena of hypnosis also provide evidence of the influence of the mind on the body. During hypnotic trance many subjects can induce anaesthesia in specific parts of the body, alter skin temperature and modify a variety of symptoms. At hypnotherapy workshops it is a commonplace to see hypodermic needles being passed painlessly through skin folds; and individuals maintaining arm levitation for periods so long that they would have suffered intolerable discomfort and muscle fatigue if not hypnotized. Major abdominal, dental and other surgery has been done on subjects with no anaesthetic procedure other than hypnosis. Painless and haemorrhage-free dental extractions are carried out under hypnosis, even in haemophiliacs, who can be taught to control the blood flow to the dental sockets concerned.

Swirsky-Sacchetti and Margolis (1986) investigated the results of a comprehensive self-hypnosis training programme for haemophiliacs. They found that during an 18-week follow-up period the amount of Factor VIII concentrate used to control bleeding by the subjects was significantly less than that used by control subjects. (Haemophiliacs bleed because of a lack of Factor VIII.) These authors seem justified in their claim that self-hypnosis is both an effective and a cost-effective treatment for haemophilia.

Psychosomatic considerations in child psychiatry

What do the above considerations mean for the clinical management of children's disorders? Their most immediate practical implications are that in formulating the case of a child patient, and in treatment planning, consideration should be given to:

- organic factors, whether inborn or acquired;
- emotional/psychological factors;
- family interrelationships;
- the interplay of all three.

We should no longer regard some disorders as psychosomatic, while the majority are looked upon as either 'organic' or 'psychological'. In a sense every disorder is psychosomatic, in that both physical and psychological factors are involved in some degree. This applies even to a condition as 'organic' as a fracture of a leg bone. We have seen, in Chapter 2, that some children are accident-prone and that predisposition to injury may be characteristic of certain families; conversely there is always some emotional reaction to an injury involving a fracture. Some families overprotect their members and this can make such members unduly susceptible to stress and promote invalidism.

Graham (1985) suggests that one can construct a hierarchy of conditions on the basis of the relative importance of physical and psychological components in their etiology and treatment. He proposes that, among conditions commonly dealt with by paediatricians, psychological factors might be ranked in the following ascending order of importance: congenital malformations, cancers, metabolic disorders, infections, epilepsy, failures of growth, bronchial asthma, enuresis/encopresis, accidents and emotional/behavioural disorders. This is a more realistic approach than labelling some conditions psychosomatic and others not, but it suggests a static relationship between physical and psychological factors. In reality, the relative importance of these factors varies. As an example, we may take anorexia nervosa. Initially this may be a predominantly emotional disorder but it may progress to become a mainly physical and even fatal one. Furthermore, the etiology of some conditions, growth failure for example, varies from case to case, the problem sometimes being mainly physical, as in Down's syndrome, sometimes mainly psychological, as in cases of severe psychosocial deprivation.

A word of warning about linear thinking: in practice we are often dealing with circular causative processes, rather than linear ones. Consider the example of retentive soiling. We have seen, in Chapter 11, how coercive bowel training may lead to fecal retention. But fecal retention may cause the parent to increase the coerciveness of bowel training, leading to more determined fecal retention and ultimately to gross constipation with impaction of large fecal masses. Parental despair and demoralization of the child may then follow. In such cases a circular process has been present all along. It can be hard to determine whether the constipation or the coercive training came first or the two developed together, but by the time the family presents for treatment a circular process may have long been established.

Many examples could be cited to illustrate the interrelation of mind and body; in fact almost any disease could be used but in some the interplay of emotional and physical factors is particularly clearly evident. These are the ones that have in the past usually been regarded as 'psychosomatic' disorders. As examples we will consider bronchial asthma and eating disorders.

Asthma

Bronchial asthma is characterized by paroxysmal attacks of difficulty in breathing. The smaller air passages in the lungs become constricted due to contraction of the muscles in their walls; secretions accumulate and the walls of the passages swell. The subject has difficulty coughing up the secretions. The lungs tend to get over-filled with air and the chest cavity is over-expanded.

The muscles of the air passages are supplied by nerves of the autonomic nervous system. This network of nerves, arising in the brain, transmits impulses which see to the correct ordering of various physiological functions – for example, heart rate, blood pressure and the diameter of the air passages in the lungs. It is not under conscious control. As well as responding to the needs which arise in activities such as exercise (during which increases are necessary in the blood supply to the muscles and the supply of oxygen to the blood by the lungs), the system is also sensitive to emotional changes. This is a primitive physiological process, deriving from the need the startled or frightened animal has to be ready for 'fight or flight'. A quick physiological response to danger was important for our phylogenetic ancestors, even if it is not for some humans today.

Two further factors may affect the diameter of the air passages. One is infection; the other is allergy. 'Allergy' describes the adverse reaction of the body to a substance which is not harmful to most people. Pollen, dusts and many other substances may provoke such reactions, causing the air passage walls to swell and produce liquid secretions. Infections provoke similar reactions.

Only certain individuals are prone to asthma. In infancy and early childhood many of them have also suffered from infantile eczema, in which there is a widespread eruption with inflammation and irritation. Such constitutionally susceptible individuals are liable to react to some combination of infection, allergy and emotional tension by developing asthma attacks. A circular process involving mind and body operates. The asthma attack, perhaps precipitated by infection or allergy, may lead to increased anxiety in the child (which may be related also to parental anxiety). This in turn may increase the severity of the asthma and thus raise anxiety levels still higher ... and so on. Anxiety may be one of the factors which helped precipitate the attack in the first place; the infective element may become more significant as the attack continues and the patient is unable to cough up secretions as a healthy person does.

Asthma is thus the result of the interaction of three groups of factors in a biologically predisposed individual. The role of emotional factors varies from case to case, depending on the temperamental style

of the child, the personalities of all family members and the characteristics of the family system. Treatment should take all these into
account.

While the emotional aspects of a case of asthma should never be
overlooked, the place of psychiatry and psychotherapy depends on the
severity of emotional disturbance in the child and the family. Minuchin
et al. (1975) suggest that certain types of family organization favour the
development and maintenance of 'psychosomatic' symptoms, which in
turn may play major roles in maintaining the current homeostatic
balance of the family. They believe that this situation is liable to arise
when a physiologically vulnerable child is a member of a family
characterized by the following transactional patterns:

- enmeshment (see Chapter 2);
- overprotectiveness;
- rigidity;
- lack of conflict resolution.

In such families the sick child plays an important role in the family's
pattern of conflict avoidance. These enmeshed families, in which
everyone is deeply involved with and responsive to the emotional state
of everyone else, show a high degree of protectiveness between all
members. The rigidity is shown in reluctance to change in response
either to outside circumstances or to internal events, such as a child
reaching adolescence. The enmeshment, overprotectiveness and rigidity combined cause these families to have a low threshold for conflict.
Their conflicts are not resolved, however, each family having its own
way of avoiding conflict. These involve the continuation of the child's
symptoms.

This pattern is not universal in so-called 'psychosomatic' disorders
but it is often encountered. Using treatment based on this
formulation, Minuchin *et al.* (1975) report good results in asthma,
anorexia nervosa and 'superlabile diabetes'.

Other factors play their parts in the evolution and maintenance of
asthma – for example, the secondary gain a child may obtain as a result
of having attacks of sickness. These children may come to enjoy being
the centre of attention, getting special foods or other treats, receiving
indulgent handling by parents and others and being able to avoid
school by use of the symptoms. Sometimes other dynamic forces are
at work. A family member may have died of asthma; the parents may
be unable to agree on how to deal with the child who then exploits
their lack of unity; or there may be competition with a sibling who has
some other defect or disease.

Mrazek (1986) discusses what he calls 'two central questions for
child psychiatry' regarding asthma. One is whether asthmatic children

'suffer a greater incidence and prevalence of psychiatric disturbance'; the other asks what role 'emotional stressors' play, given genetic vulnerability, in causing asthma to appear. The second question, to which no precise answer can be given in the present state of our knowledge, is an important and reasonable one, though the answer must vary from case to case. The first, however, seems to make the assumption that mind and body are separate. Clearly they are not, despite the tendency for psychiatrists and specialists in respiratory medicine to practise separately. It also raises the issue of what is meant by 'psychiatric disturbance'. This may be defined on the basis of the number and severity of symptoms of anxiety, depression, disturbed conduct and so forth, displayed by the child. When these reach a certain level 'psychiatric disturbance' may be deemed to exist and a psychiatrist may be brought in on the case. But this is a practical management issue, an important one perhaps but not one bearing upon the fundamental nature of the condition.

Better questions might be, 'Are the emotions ever uninvolved when a child has attacks of asthma?' And, if and when they are involved, 'How do emotional factors interact with other factors that are operating in each particular case?'

A fundamental question raised, though not asked, by Mrasek (1986) is thus whether we are to regard psyche and soma, or mind and body, separately or as one. Can the psychiatric aspects of the cases of children with asthma (for example) be separated from the somatic ones in any meaningful way? Traditionally, medicine has tried to do this, perhaps not very successfully. It is interesting that Rossi (1986a), who has produced a scholarly treatise on mind-body relationships, is not a physician but a psychologist.

The important practical point may be that one should always bear in mind that emotional factors and family dynamics, as well as organic processes, may be involved in cases of asthma. Their importance will vary from case to case and sometimes it may be slight. But these factors should not be overlooked, whether or not the expert attentions of a psychiatrist are required

Eating disorders

DSM-III-R, unlike ICD-9, has a section for eating disorders. Included are anorexia nervosa, bulimia nervosa, pica and 'rumination disorder of infancy'. (The latter two categories are discussed in Chapter 14.) Anorexia nervosa and what may be considered its converse, obesity, are the principal eating disorders of older children and adolescents.

Bulimia is primarily a disorder of adult life but it also occurs in adolescence.

Anorexia nervosa

Anorexia nervosa is a good example of a disorder in which physical and psychological problems are interwoven in a seemingly inextricable way. Predominantly a disorder of adolescent girls, its essential feature is a profound aversion to food, leading to serious weight loss. Not only do anorexic subjects lose weight, but their body images are distorted and they deny being unduly thin, even though they appear cachectic to others.

The symptoms include excessive activity, for example running long distances and other forms of 'working out'; depression; amenorrhoea, which is always present in female adolescent and adult patients once the disorder is established; and preoccupation with food and an interest in preparing it for others, though not in consuming it. Anorectics usually have accurate knowledge of what foods are 'fattening' and carefully avoid them. Laxative abuse and induced vomiting are other means whereby they try to keep their weight down. In due course the physical effects of the self-starvation come to dominate the clinical picture; the patient becomes weak and lethargic, with slow pulse, low blood pressure, constipation, hirsutism and blue and cold extremities. In severe cases death may occur from heart failure. The blood levels of luteinizing hormone, follicle stimulating hormone and oestrogens are all very low.

Although adolescent girls make up the bulk of new cases, the disorder also occurs in boys and in prepubertal children. Fossen *et al.* (1987) report 48 children with early onset anorexia nervosa, 35 girls and 13 boys; of these 23 were prepubertal (7 boys and 16 girls), 20 pubescent (6 boys and 14 girls), and 5, all girls, postpubertal. The age of onset ranged from 7.7 to 13.7 years, mean 11.7. Youngest children, who comprised 44 per cent of the study population, were over-represented compared to census figures (15 per cent); there was a bias towards the higher socioeconomic classes, as other studies have found. Depression was present in 56 per cent, also a finding similar to those of other studies.

Jacobs and Isaacs (1986) reviewed 20 prepubertal cases, 6 of whom were boys, and compared their characteristics with those of control groups of postpubertal anorectics and prepubertal neurotics. Sexual anxiety (see below) was equally prevalent in the pre- and postpubertal anorectics but significantly less so in the neurotics.

Prevalence depends on the population studied. Crisp *et al.* (1976)

studied the girls in 7 'independent' (that is fee-paying) schools in England and found a prevalence of about one severe case in every 200 girls; in girls over 16 years of age the rate was one in every 100. They also studied two large 'comprehensive' state-run (non-fee-paying) schools and found only one case (aged over 16) among 2786 girls, a discrepancy to which various factors probably contributed. Higher prevalence figures have been reported in certain populations – for example fashion students (3.5 per cent) and professional ballet students (7.6 per cent) (Garner and Garfinkel, 1980). A study in Munro County, New York, revealed an annual incidence of new cases of 0.64 per 100,000 population (Jones *et al.*, 1980). Boys seem to make up a larger proportion of prepubertal cases than of postpubertal ones. The disease is rare in impoverished populations and underdeveloped countries.

Mind-body relationships in anorexia nervosa

According to Russell (1985) 'there remains deep uncertainty about the fundamental causes of this illness', despite the many explanatory theories that have been put forward. Whatever the 'fundamental causes' may be, however, disorders of mind and body are clearly present.

Certain psychological features have long been recognized in anorexia nervosa. These include the fear of growing up and assuming the adult role; and sexual anxiety, manifested in fear of puberty, menstruation and sexual maturity generally, anxiety about motherhood or fatherhood, and loss of interest in any boyfriend or girlfriend the young person may have had. The unconsciously intended purpose of the refusal to eat seems to be to remain in, or go back to, a prepubertal state. As Crisp (1977) put it, 'The search for security and self-esteem has proved incompatible with growth, which has therefore come to be stifled and avoided'.

In some cases other psychopathology is present and in many social pressures seem important. A study of the measurement data of the centrefold girls in *Playboy* magazine for the years 1969 to 1978, revealed that the percentage of average weight for height decreased significantly. Bust measurements decreased, waists got larger and hips smaller (Garfinkel and Garner, 1982). Similar changes occurred in the Miss America contestants, especially the winners, between 1959 and 1978 (Garner *et al.*, 1980). Moreover, the nude women painted by many old masters would nowadays be considered seriously over-weight. A slim figure has, for whatever reasons, become desirable in western cultures (though not in many others, which may have something to do with the infrequency of the disorder in non-western countries). The high prevalence of the disorder in fashion models and ballet students fits in with these ideas, since those in such occupations must be under pressure to have 'perfect' figures. Alternatively, these occupations might differentially attract those prone to anorexia.

There is evidence that family factors play their part in the genesis of anorexia. The features of 'psychosomatic families', mentioned above in the discussion of asthma – enmeshment, overprotectiveness, rigidity and lack of conflict resolution – are also said to characterize the families of many anorectics (Liebman *et al.*, 1974; Minuchin *et al.*, 1978). Generational boundaries appear weak, the parents are divided and ineffective, individuals are given little autonomy or privacy, and these families have trouble solving problems and dealing effectively with stressful, frustrating situations.

Fosson *et al.* (1987) conceptualize anorexia nervosa as 'a distorted and overly focused struggle for self-control and autonomy'. They postulate that the likelihood of parents adopting the role of adversary in the child's struggle for autonomy depends on the age, sex and ordinal position of the child. They continue: 'In our culture parents are more likely to be intrusively involved with and/or overly controlling of girls and youngest children than offspring in complementary categories. In some of these families parents will not withdraw in response to the child's emancipatory stirrings. Given this situation, some children will attempt to resolve the ensuing conflict by focusing the controversy on food and control of intake. This is an effective option only if food consumption is consistently at their discretion – that is, not subject to availability or threatened by the family's financial resources.' (Fossen *et al.*, 1987, page 117.)

This is an ingenious explanation which accounts for many of the features of anorexia nervosa. It also seems compatible with Minuchin's views.

The psychological features of this disorder are thus legion, complex and major and they involve family as well as child. There is also evidence that anorexia nervosa may have a genetic basis. Holland *et al.* (1984) studied 30 female twin pairs in which at least one twin was anorectic; 9 out 16 (56 per cent) monozygotic pairs, but only 1 out of the 14 dizygotic pairs (7 per cent), were concordant for the disorder. This suggests that there is a substantial genetic contribution.

The hormonal abnormalities have been mentioned above. They appear to be due to dysfunction of the hypothalamic centres which affect production of hormones by the anterior pituitary gland and gonads. The endocrine changes and the cessation of menstruation are in part explicable as secondary to the weight loss, but sometimes amenorrhoea is an early symptom, occurring before the onset of weight loss (Halmi, 1974). It has also been suggested that hypothalamic dysfunction may have a role in causing the loss of appetite and disordered temperature regulation. In any event there are profound bodily changes along with the failure to eat, as we have seen above. In prepubertal cases puberty is delayed and growth is retarded.

In the past there has been a tendency to look for either a physical or a psychiatric cause for anorexia nervosa, as for other conditions on the borderline of psychiatry and 'organic' medicine. Perhaps this is neither necessary nor helpful. We are dealing with one organism, not a mind and a body. Under normal circumstances all developmental processes, psychological and physical, proceed in step with each other at their appointed rates. Various combinations of biological (including genetic) and environmental factors may speed them up or slow them down. Sometimes there are differential effects on particular areas of development, as in the specific developmental disorders discussed in Chapter 7. There must, however, be some somatic correlate of any functional change. Thus loss of appetite must be associated with some change in brain functioning. Probably the hypothalamus is involved, but it may well be that other parts of the brain are also. But which comes first? Perhaps neither. Anorexia and the corresponding changes in the brain centres responsible for appetite might occur simultaneously. What stimulates these changes? Some as yet imperfectly understood perturbation of the organism.

The perturbations responsible may be psychosocial, including family ones such as we have discussed above, producing the syndrome of anorexia nervosa in a genetically susceptible individual. Whatever they are, however, the condition is a disorder of mind *and* body.

Treatment of anorexia nervosa

Because anorexia nervosa is a complex condition in which many psychological and physical functions are disturbed, treatment should be what Fundudis (1986) calls 'multimodal'. Illustrating this by reference to the case of an 11½-year-old anorexic girl, Fundudis suggests that a treatment strategy be devised to deal with each of the patient's problems, in an appropriate sequence. In the illustrative case, the treatments used included stimulus control, systematic desensitization, cognitive restructuring, relaxation training, family therapy, dyadic therapy, social reinforcement and 'vicarious modelling'. In practice the treatment programme will depend on the details of the case and the treating physician's views on the best way of tackling each of the problems. An interesting multimodal treatment regime is also described by Ney and Mulvihill (1985).

We will now briefly review some measures which are usually needed, at least in the more severe cases. While milder cases may be treated as outpatients, the more severe ones should be admitted to hospital. When there has been serious weight loss a major initial objective must be to restore the patient's weight to a safe level. This may be a difficult undertaking.

In treating anorectics and their families the establishment of rapport is particularly important. Without it treatment is likely to fail; even with it, it may not be easy. Young people with anorexia nervosa are usually skilled in manipulating those around them for their own devious ends – notably to maintain their symptoms. They may promise to eat if they do not have go into hospital, they plead for 'one more chance' (and then for another, and yet another . . . and so on), and they are experts in the application of 'divide and rule' strategies. As Fosson *et al.* (1987) observe, 'Children with anorexia seem to be particularly adept at creating conflict, not from planned behaviour or malice, but as a habitual way of relating, generalised from family interaction'.

A firm, accepting, non-punitive but unyielding approach is required. The adults concerned, that is the parents and the treatment staff, must be united and supportive of each other. This implies that the parents trust and have confidence in the treatment team, especially the physician who is ultimately responsible. It must be made clear to the child that she (or he) must eat. This is not negotiable and if necessary all privileges, including family visits, watching TV, listening to the radio, even getting up to go to the toilet, may have to be contingent on eating or, preferably, weight gain. The environment must be structured so that it is not possible for the child to dispose of food without eating it.

All this implies skilled nursing care, close teamwork and frequent contact with and support for the parents. Perhaps in no other branch of the profession are psychiatric nursing skills so crucial; nurses with expertise and experience in relating to and treating these patients are priceless assets.

Being firm with their daughter and not yielding to her threats, pleadings and guilt-provoking statements (like 'You hate me', 'You've never loved me', 'I hate you' or 'You just want me to die in this hospital'), is exceedingly hard for parents accustomed to surrendering to such emotional blackmail. Thus the parents, too, require skilled management.

A high calorie intake is necessary to ensure weight gain and catch-up growth. Close cooperation between psychiatrist and paediatrician pays dividends. Both must agree on the treatment plan. The paediatrician may monitor the child's physical state, electrolyte balance and diet, prescribe the necessary dietary intake, and advise on the weight gain needed before it is 'safe' for the child to have certain privileges; while the psychiatrist coordinates the psychological care and treatment of child and family. It must always be clear who is ultimately responsible for the treatment; usually it is the psychiatrist when the child is in the psychiatric unit and the paediatrician when she or he is in the paediatric one. Given skilled management by an experienced team, tube feeding should rarely be needed, though it may occasionally be necessary to define a minimum weight at which it will be initiated.

It is helpful to have target minimum and maximum weights. These patients have a great fear of becoming fat and it seems to reassure them to say not only that they must reach a certain weight (for example, before they can leave hospital), but also that you will not allow their weight to go above a certain figure.

Once the predetermined weight has been attained, family therapy may commence. It is not appropriate, or practical, to start it while the young person is still seriously underweight and is subject to an intensive, behaviourally structured programme as described above. The therapy needed for the family will depend on the particular dysfunctional interaction patterns that are identified. By the time it starts the parents may already have learned quite a lot, having observed their formerly controlling and manipulative child's response to the measures used to get her to eat and gain weight. The child, too, may have learned from this experience. An excellent account of a structural approach to treating these families is to be found in *Psychosomatic Families: Anorexia Nervosa in Context* (Minuchin *et al.*, 1978).

Various drugs, for example chlorpromazine and insulin, have been suggested but they probably have little or no part to play, except in the treatment of co-existing diseases. If the patient is depressed, antidepressant medication may be indicated.

Hypnotherapy may be a useful adjunct (Gross, 1983; Baker and Nash, 1987). It may help promote the intrapsychic changes, including development of self-esteem, which are essential prerequisites to a successful outcome. But further study is needed to establish its role and value.

Outcome

Most anorectics gain weight in hospital if treated along the above lines but weight gain, while necessary, is not a sufficient objective. The associated problems, including the family ones, must be tackled also. If a comprehensive treatment plan, which may also involve individual therapy with the anorectic subject, is carried through most patients recover, though there are some who pursue a chronic course or become bulimic. The patients reported by Minuchin *et al.* (1978) did remarkably well but not all outcome studies have been so encouraging.

The outlook may be better for cases of younger onset than for those commencing in mid or late adolescence.

Bulimia

Bulimia, sometimes called bulimia nervosa, consists of episodic binge eating, usually followed by self-induced vomiting. The subject is aware that the eating pattern is abnormal, has a fear of being unable to stop eating voluntarily and entertains self-deprecating thoughts. Abuse of laxatives and/or diuretics, designed to promote weight loss, and episodic dieting, are other common features of the disorder. Diarrhoea and potassium deficiency may result from the laxative abuse. The condition may be preceded by anorexia nervosa which after some years gives way to bulimia. In other instances the bulimia arises *de novo*.

Bulimics share with anorectics a pathological fear of becoming fat but they are not necessarily underweight. Indeed some of them are obese. Their obesity may serve to intensify those symptoms designed to promote weight loss, while they feel unable to control their episodes of gorging themselves with food, usually of high calorie content. The onset of bulimia is usually in mid or late adolescence or early adult life. It may continue for many years.

Like anorexia nervosa, bulimia is a disorder of mind and body. The psychopathology also has much in common with that of anorexia nervosa, but it is a more inwardly-directed disorder. Bulimics often conceal their symptoms, even from their husbands who may live in the same household for years unaware of their wives' binge eating and vomiting. Comprehensive, multimodal treatment is required. In bulimic adolescents many of the same individual and family issues arise as are encountered in treating anorectics. Issues of control, autonomy, self-image and unresolved family conflict are usually central, though issues of genital sexuality are less evident. Substance abuse is common among bulimic subjects.

Obesity

It seems that childhood obesity may result from various combinations of genetic, biological and emotional factors (Grinker, 1981), though its etiology is not fully understood. Some individuals have a high count of adipose cells, which may be genetically determined, though there is evidence that it may be caused by over-feeding in the early months of life. Bruch (1974) described various family patterns which may lead to obesity in predisposed children.

Various psychosocial situations appear to contribute to childhood obesity. Thus the deprived, rejected child may eat excessively as a compensation for lack of affection. Or a parent who feels guilty, perhaps at an unconscious level, about harbouring rejecting attitudes towards a child may over-feed the child in an attempt at compensation. Over-feeding may also be motivated by a parent's desire to keep the child in a close and dependent relationship. While some children may rebel and even become anorexic in response to such handling, others accept it and remain obese and emotionally immature.

Obesity can also contribute to the development of emotional problems, whatever its cause. The fat child may be teased and so come to feel self-conscious. It can be hard to get children to keep to a reducing diet when one has been prescribed, and this can lead to tension or open strife between family members. In this way pre-existing family problems may be exacerbated. In some instances it is hard to know whether obesity is the cause or effect of the family problems, or whether it has simply become the focus of a problem which would have been centred around something else if the child had not been obese.

Other disorders

Complex interactions of mind and body characterize many other disorders. Conditions in which such interactions may be especially important include migraine; the periodic syndrome (attacks of head-ache with photophobia, abdominal pain, vomiting and a miserable, whimpering appearance occurring in children in the first year of life); cyclical vomiting (a variant of the periodic syndrome); ulcerative colitis (an inflammatory condition of the large intestine); and peptic ulcer.

Chapter 14

The Psychiatry of Infants and Young Children

Although early experiences have long been thought to have important influences on human development, the psychiatry of infancy and early childhood has only recently received much attention. Previously, psychiatrists and their colleagues tended to follow the example of Sigmund Freud, who was content to formulate theories about psychological development in young children without actually studying the children. This is no longer so. Infants and preschool children, and their psychiatric and developmental disorders, have become the focus of much interest and study. Bowlby's (1951) challenging views on the effects on children of early maternal deprivation, and the work of Thomas and Chess (1977) on the temperaments of young children (discussed in Chapters 1 and 2) were among the stimuli which led to these developments. Although some of Bowlby's views proved incorrect, he directed our attention to the importance of early mother-child relationships.

There are certain difficulties inherent in the study of young children. Among these are the following.

(1) In infancy and early childhood we are dealing, to an even greater extent than in later childhood, with development and its disorders, rather than with identifiable psychiatric syndromes. While a developmental viewpoint is useful at any age, in older children it becomes increasingly possible to identify specific syndromes and disorders, with their characteristic signs and symptoms. This is less often possible in infancy, and the borderline between psychiatry and developmental psychology may be hard to distinguish.

(2) Neither of the currently used diagnostic schemes, ICD-9 and DSM-III-R is well adapted for use in this period of life. Indeed the old fashioned 'medical model' of disease entities may be only marginally relevant when we are dealing with the, largely interactive, psychiatric problems of early childhood. Although both diagnostic schemes have categories for developmental disorders, these are limited to rather specific areas of development. We do not have any comprehensive method of categorizing the ways in which the development of infants

and young children may go astray. Any that might be developed should take into account not only the young child, but the interactional processes occurring between child and parents or parent-substitutes. (3) Studying children in isolation from their social contexts makes little sense, so we must decide how much to focus our attention on the individual child, and how much on the interactions between child and environment, especially family. In infancy the question is particularly important because of the almost total dependence of infants on those caring for them. To some extent infant psychiatry is the psychiatry of infant-adult relationships; the question remains, though, to what extent?

(4) The assessment of infants and young children demands special skills and the use of techniques different from those needed in assessing older children. Children who have not developed speech, and those whose speech and language development is at an early stage, cannot give us the sort of information we rely on when dealing with older patients. They cannot tell how they feel, nor what they are thinking or subjectively experiencing. We must become skilled in interpreting non-verbal behaviour, the natural means whereby infants communicate.

(5) The intimate involvement of child and family in this age period means that the child is particularly susceptible to tensions and other problems in the family group. It may not be easy to determine whether the problem is primarily the child's or the family's, or both.

Despite the above problems, infant psychiatry is now well established, as evidenced by the appearance of books on the subject (Osofsky, 1979; Howells, 1979; Call *et al.*, 1983; 1985), and the publication of increasing numbers of journal articles.

Disorders of infants and young children

Despite points 1 and 2 above, there are some recognized and reasonably well defined disorders occurring in this age range. Infantile autism and severe developmental delay are discussed in Chapters 7 and 16 respectively. Disorders of speech, language and motor development (Chapter 10), enuresis and encopresis (Chapter 11) and hyperactivity and attention deficit disorders (Chapter 9), all of which may become evident in the preschool period, are also discussed elsewhere.

Many other management and behaviour problems, including sleeping and feeding difficulties, occur in young children. These are discussed in this chapter. Psychiatrists are also interested in the processes of bonding and attachment occurring between parents and young children, and the relationship of problems in this area to the physical and emotional abuse of children.

Prevalence

A survey of 3-year-old children in a North London borough revealed that 7 per cent had moderate or severe behaviour problems and a further 15 per cent had mild problems (Richman *et al.*, 1975). There were no significant sex differences in overall prevalence rates but overactivity and wetting and soiling problems were more frequent in boys, and fearfulness in girls. Behaviour and management problems were the subject of most of the complaints voiced by the parents. Children with delayed language development are not included in these figures, nor are immigrant families, but later studies of the children of West Indian-born parents, both at age 3 and at follow-up 12 to 18 months later, showed prevalence rates that were not significantly different (Earls & Richman, 1980a; 1980b). A study in a rural USA community, using the same methods, also yielded similar results, 24 per cent of the children showing problems (Earls, 1980).

A study of 135 children attending a preschool day treatment centre showed that 30 per cent had severe management problems, 15 per cent were retarded, 13 per cent were autistic, 11 per cent had speech and language problems and 10 per cent showed severe separation anxiety, the remainder being there for such reasons as failure to thrive, feeding problems and risk of non-accidental injury (Bentovim and Boston, 1973). This list does not tell us what the prevalence is of these problems in the community, but it gives us an idea of the distribution of problems that may come to psychiatric attention.

Assessment of infants and young children

The principles and general approach to assessment set out in Chapter 3 apply to preschool children as they do to older ones. In the assessment of neonates and infants in their first year or two, however, the procedures require some modification. Moreover, there is but a small body of information on the psychiatric assessment of infants. Emde (1985) points out that the expression of emotion is particularly important in infancy. Infants do not talk; instead they cry, smile, make cooing noises and in various non-verbal ways which the perceptive parent soon learns, communicate fear, anger, sadness, joy, contentment and so on. The psychiatrist must evaluate such communications, striving particularly to understand the communication occurring between the infant and the parents and other adults.

Cognitive development may be assessed using either Piaget's approach or psychological tests such as those mentioned in Chapter 3. Although the results of testing in infancy generally correlate poorly with those of tests carried out later, the main purpose of assessment is to reveal the present state of affairs.

Emde (1985, page 327) points out the importance of 'times of developmental transition, or biobehavioural shifts'. The first of these occurs at 2 months, when there is a shift 'from a predominance of endogenous control to more exogenous control'. The baby comes to be awake more than asleep, with the wakefulnees mostly during the day. Exploratory and manipulative behaviour and the 'social smile' appear, and there is more eye-to-eye contact. This is the start of the 'awakening of sociability' (Emde, 1984).

At 7 to 9 months there is another shift, as signs of anxiety and displeasure arise when strangers approach and there is separation anxiety, or 'protest', when mother or father leaves. This behaviour peaks in the middle of the second year and then declines. The infant is giving the parents the message 'no-one else will do' (Emde, 1983).

Further major transitions occur when the child starts to walk, at about one year, and at 15 to 18 months, when representational intelligence emerges, problem-solving skills develop and the child begins to show a sense of success or failure in activities, and of right and wrong in relation to the parents' expectations. Above all this is a time when the sense of self seems to become consolidated (Emde, 1985).

Emde (1985) also suggests that our assessments of infants may be particularly coloured by our social values; he points out that early characteristics do not necessarily persist into later life, and that assessment is increasingly an interdisciplinary undertaking.

It is important to observe infants directly as well as to obtain information about them from their parents or other adults. Gaensbauer and Harmon (1981) describe a systematic assessment procedure for use in the age range 9 to 21 months:

(1) A free play period with mother and infant, during which the infant can play either with toys or with the mother.
(2) Approaches to the infant by a stranger and by the mother. This is designed to discover the extent to which the mother is used as a source of security.
(3) Developmental testing using the Bayley Scales of Infant Development.

(4)   A separation and reunion sequence involving the mother's departure and return three minutes later.

The authors report differences in the responses to all four experiences when a group of 'abused/neglected' children was compared to a group of normal controls.

Questionnaires for administration to the parents of young children, and to those caring for them in group settings, have been devised. The Behavioural Screening Questionnaire (Richman and Graham, 1971) has been found useful in large scale epidemiological studies, and has been further validated by Earls *et al.* (1982). It contains 12 items dealing, respectively, with eating, sleeping, soiling, activity level, concentration, attention-seeking/dependence, moods, 'several worries', 'many fears', relationship with siblings/peers, temper tantrums, and 'difficult to manage' behaviour. Each is scored 0 (absence of the behaviour), 1 (mild) or 2 (severe), according to the perceived severity of the behaviour.

The Preschool Behaviour Checklist (McGuire and Richman, 1986) has 22 items and is designed for use by the staff in group settings where preschool children receive care. It is intended as a screening instrument and has satisfactory inter-rater reliability, internal consistency and validity. It is not intended to be used for the assessment of individual children, but it may have value in directing the attention of staff to problems displayed by particular children, especially those who are isolated, nervous or withdrawn. Inconsistencies between the ratings of staff members may also draw attention to the differential effects of different management methods.

Common problems of young children

Temper tantrums

Temper tantrums are normal in toddlers but may represent a problem if they are severe and persistent and fail to respond to the parents' attempts to deal with them. This may happen if they are reinforced by attention and gratification. Whether tantrums continue or escalate depends on how they are handled. Firm but kind limit-setting in an emotionally warm and accepting context usually leads to rapid improvement. Tantrums should be ignored as far as possible. Children having tantrums because they want something, or are not allowed to engage in a particular behaviour, should not be given their wishes. Physical restraint is only necessary when children are doing things dangerous to themselves or others, or are physically damaging or destroying property. Persisting tantrum behaviour is especially likely in unstable and chaotic families in which the parents handle their children inconsistently.

The outcome, with this and many other problem behaviours, depends partly on how secure the child's relationship with the parents is. The greater the degree of security, the easier it usually is to deal with behavioural difficulties. Nevertheless, some children seem constitutionally more prone to tantrum behaviour than others, and the ease with which this behaviour can be extinguished varies from child to child. The 'goodness of fit' (see Chapter 2) between the parents' and the child's personalities is another relevant factor.

Sleep problems

When young children fail to sleep as and when the parents expect, it may simply be that the parents' expectations are unrealistic, or the parents may lack knowledge of the amount of sleep needed by a child of the age in question. Children's need for sleep also varies; and at about the age of 2 months infants undergo a shift 'from a predominance of endogenous control to more exogenous control' (Emde, 1985). They are now awake more than they are asleep, and they use the waking hours for more exploratory and manipulative behaviour. This transition may take the parents by surprise.

Failure to conform to a regular sleeping pattern may occur in chaotic and disorganized homes in which there are no regular bedtimes or bedtime routines, so that children do not have the opportunity to learn a set pattern of sleeping and waking behaviour. Failure to sleep, with crying, is common in babies, but normally settles after a few months at most, if the feeding and general care of the infant are satisfactory. Persistence of the trouble into the toddler years is nevertheless quite common. There seems to be an association between waking at night and other behavioural and temperamental difficulties, particularly lack of malleability and rhythmicity (Richman, 1981a).

Many young children with sleep problems are in other ways mentally and physically healthy, and the trouble is a transient developmental problem which clears up after a few weeks or months.

Night terrors may be alarming to parents who have not encountered them before, but are common in normal, healthy toddlers. The child wakes up in a frightened, even terrified, state and is inaccessible, not responding when spoken to nor appearing to see objects or people. Instead he or she appears to be visually or auditorily hallucinated, talking to and looking at people and things not actually present. The child may be difficult to comfort, and the period of disturbed behaviour and altered consciousness may last up to 15 minutes, occasionally longer. Eventually the behavioural manifestations subside, with or without comfort from an adult, and the child goes back to sleep, awakening in the morning usually with no recollection of the incident.

Night terrors occur on waking from 'stage 4' (deep) sleep. They persist into later childhood in 1 per cent to 3 per cent of children (Keith, 1975).

Nightmares are unpleasant or frightening dreams. The child does not wake up, nor necessarily become overtly disturbed while having the nightmare, and if woken up reacts normally. There is no period of altered consciousness or inaccessibility such as occurs in night terrors. Nightmares occur during REM ('rapid eye movement' or light) sleep.

Sleepwalking, or somnambulism, like 'sleep terror disorder', has been elevated to the status of a disorder ('sleepwalking disorder') by DSM-III-R but it is doubtful if it should be regarded as a specific psychiatric disorder. It is commoner in school-aged children but is described here for convenience. It may accompany night terrors or nightmares and it may also occur without there being evidence of either. Apparently the content of a dream is acted out in a state of sleep or altered consciousness. The child has a blank, staring facial expression, does not respond much when people try to communicate with him or her and can only be awakened with difficulty. Sleepwalking occurs in deep sleep (stages 3 and 4). Episodes may last from a few minutes to half an hour.

Any of the above forms of sleep disorder may be exacerbated by physical or emotional disorder. Nightmares and restless sleep are common in acute febrile illnesses. The possibility of sleep disturbance being due to nocturnal epilepsy must also be considered; some epileptic children only have seizures at night.

In many instances no evidence is found of any other abnormality or disorder and the sleep problem is appropriately regarded as a transient developmental disturbance. The parents and child can then be reassured. Any associated emotional problems should be treated as described elsewhere in this book.

Sleep apnoea may occur at any age but is mentioned here for convenience. Its occurrence in children is described by Guilleminault *et al.* (1976). It consists of frequent waking at night, associated with periods of reduced breathing or complete apnoea. Other features are loud snoring when asleep and excessive sleepiness during the day. The syndrome's main psychiatric significance is that symptoms include intellectual deterioration; depression, sometimes with suicidal thoughts; personality changes; sudden outbursts of irrational behaviour; and suspiciousness. Morning headaches and hynogogic hallucinations, that is hallucinations occurring as the person is falling asleep, have also been reported. The condition can be fatal and it is therefore important not to mistake it for a psychiatric disorder. Martin and Lefebvre (1981) provide a review of the disorder's characteristics and describe the successful surgical treatment of a 13-year-old boy.

The treatment of sleep disorders

Any associated emotional or behavioural problems are usually best dealt with first. Once they are resolved the sleep problem may no longer exist. When the problem is sleeplessness unassociated with any other disorder, the best approach is probably a behavioural one. Richman *et al.* (1985) describe the results of such an approach designed to help the child stay in bed quietly without disturbing the parents, and to settle down to sleep without parental attention. Alteration of the parents' responses to the children's night-time behaviour seemed often to lead to rapid resolution of the problem, suggesting that 'parental responses were important in maintaining waking behaviour'. The treatment programme was an individual one in each case, based upon a behavioural analysis (see Chapter 19). Complete or marked improvement occurred in 27 of 35 cases treated, but 5 did not complete treatment, so that the improvement rate in those that did was 90 per cent. At 4-month follow-up it was 80 per cent.

Drug treatment has little part to play in treating the sleep problems of young children. A double-blind trial of the drug trimeprazine tartrate (Richman, 1985) confirmed clinical impressions that the benefits are limited, though there was a significantly better response in the drug-treated than in the placebo-treated children.

Night terrors occurring in the absence of other disorders may need no treatment beyond reassuring the parents that they occur in many normal young children. If they are severe and troublesome they may respond to the drug diazepam (Keith, 1975).

A useful review of the sleep problems of young children is that of Richman (1981b).

Feeding problems

Appetite and eating disturbances in young children may be symptoms of various physical disorders but in many cases emotional factors and, especially, dysfunctional family relationships are prominent. Children may eat, or be thought by their parents to eat, too little or too much; they may be excessively fussy about what they will eat; or they may eat items not normally regarded as edible ('pica').

Food refusal may become the focus of a battle of wills between parent(s) and child, rather as soiling may be. It sometimes accompanies psychogenic soiling (see Chapter 11). The parents wish to control the child, perhaps in a rigid and obsessive way, and the child reacts by refusing to eat what the parents consider necessary. The parents may have exaggerated ideas about the importance of particular dietary regimes and unrealistic fears about what will happen if their child does not eat a certain diet. The child, consciously or unconsiously aware of this, chooses to strike a blow for independence by declining to eat what the parents wish. There may be numerous food fads, the child resolutely refusing certain specific foods. Such children are usually well nourished, indicating that they have been receiving adequate diets, though it is not always easy to persuade the parents of this.

The management of these cases resembles that of negativistic soiling. A general assessment of child and family, especially the nature of the parent-child relationships, should precede treatment. Some education of the family about children's nutritional requirements may be needed. If there are no other serious problems, treatment should address the parent-child relationship issues. An ordinary menu, made up of foods which provide a nutritionally balanced diet, should be offered on a 'take-it-or-leave-it' basis. If this is done children usually select an adequate diet, perhaps after some initial testing out of the situation. Unless there are severely disturbed parental attitudes or the family system is very dysfunctional, the outlook is generally good. (This approach does not apply in anorexia nervosa, a disorder of older children and especially adolescents – see Chapter 13.)

Mild food fads are common and are probably in part a means whereby children instinctively select a balanced diet suited to their current nutritional needs.

Pica is the eating of items not usually regarded as edible, for example paper, soil, paint, wood and cloth. Many other materials may be eaten also. The symptom has many causes, including adverse environmental circumstances and emotional distress. The children often have relationship difficulties. Pica is often associated with distorted developmental patterns, brain damage and mental retardation, but it also occurs in children of normal intelligence. Iron deficiency anaemia, due to a generally poor diet, may be present. Another possible cause of anaemia is lead poisoning, which may result from the ingestion of old lead-containing paint. Lead poisoning can also cause severe brain damage (see Chapter 8).

Associated sleep and behaviour problems are common and the families of children with pica tend to be disorganized and poor. In severe cases admission to hospital and intensive work with the family are usually needed. *Pica: A Childhood Symptom* (Bicknell, 1975) is a good source of further information.

Rumination disorder of infancy, as defined in DSM-III-R, consists of repeated regurgitation of food in the absence of other gastrointestinal symptoms, with failure to gain weight or loss of weight. Onset is between 3 and 12 months of age. In many cases this is probably a manifestation of a disturbed relationship between mother (or mother-substitute) and child.

Breath-holding spells

These are common in preschool children. They usually start before age 2 but seldom before 6 months. Livingstone (1972) reported a mean age of onset of 12 months and a peak frequency between ages 2 and 3. The spells usually cease by age 5 or 6.

Breath-holding spells are usually precipitated by some minor upset or frustration. This is followed by crying which increases in intensity until the child reaches a state of rage. Breathing then stops, usually in expiration, and cyanosis becomes manifest in blueness of the face, especially aroung the lips. Occasionally the spell leads to a major epileptic seizure, but in most instances the child starts to breathe again in half a minute or so and recovery quickly occurs. The three distinguishing features are a precipitating factor, violent crying and cyanosis. The spells seem to be used by some children to alarm, or express anger towards, their parents. The parents may then reinforce the symptom by a show of concern or by indulgence. The attacks are better treated calmly and with a minimum of fuss; it is important to ensure that the behaviour is not reinforced by any reward. The prognosis is good if there is no associated serious disorder.

Thumbsucking and Nailbiting

Both these behaviours are common in young children, though nailbiting is also frequently observed in older ones. In a population study it was found to reach a peak at 9 years in boys and 11 years in girls (Shepherd *et al.*, 1971). Thumb and fingersucking are normal behaviours in babies and gradually lessen during the second and subsequent years. Persistent thumbsucking has little psychiatric significance on its own, but it may be a feature of regressive behaviour in a child who is anxious or under stress. It often requires no treatment but if necessary it can usually be stopped by simple reminders, rewards or even sanctions. Occasionally it becomes a severe, compulsive behaviour associated with rocking or masturbation. Severe thumb-sucking can cause dental malocclusion in older children and may merit treatment for this reason. If treatment of the symptom itself is necessary a behaviour therapy programme (see Chapter 19) should be developed.

Nailbiting, like thumbsucking, seems often to be a tension-reducing habit occurring in anxious, tense children. The symptom itself rarely needs to be treated, but the underlying anxiety state or other disorder may.

Separation anxiety and disorders of attachment

Parent-child relationships and interactions are central issues in infant psychiatry. The emotional attachments of infants and young children to the adults in their lives have therefore been extensively studied. Ainsworth *et al.* (1978) studied the effects of brief separations and reunions of infants and their mothers. They identified three groups of infants, on the basis of their responses to the procedure:

- Securely attached infants, who seek contact with their mothers when under stress, are calmed by this and explore actively in the presence of their mothers.
- Anxiously attached infants, who seem ambivalent towards their mothers, seeking contact but apparently failing to be comforted by it. The anxiously attached infant is chronically anxious in relation to the mother and is unable to use her as a secure base from which to explore an unfamiliar situation. These mothers are less responsive to crying and other communications than the mothers of the securely attached infants.
- Anxious-avoidant infants, who show avoidant behaviour when reunited with their mothers after a period of separation. They do not seek close contact with their mothers, even in high-stress situations, and seem undisturbed when separated from their mothers. The mothers are rejecting and angry, rebuffing or roughly treating their infants when the latter seek physical proximity. The infants thus learn to avoid seeking proximity. In other situations and with other adults, however, these infants can respond positively to close physical contact.

For optimal attachment to develop, it seems that sensitive maternal care, which should be neither too highly involved with the child, nor too uninvolved, is best. The former may tend to produce 'avoidant' infants, and the latter 'anxiously attached' ones. An intermediate degree of involvement may be the one most likely to lead to secure attachment (Belsky *et al.*, 1984).

Much remains to be learned about attachment processes and the consequences of different patterns of attachment. It is believed, however, that secure attachments to specific people in infancy, as opposed to the more general attachments of institutionally reared children, may lead to high levels of self-esteem and autonomous functioning, and generally healthy personality development. The insecurely attached child may cope with stress less well and have impaired feelings of autonomy. The precise role of attachment experiences as opposed to other factors in personality development, however, remains to be established. There may also be a relationship between the nature of the parent-child attachment and the risk of child abuse.

Heard (1981; 1987) provides helpful summaries of the findings of research in this field.

The treatment of young children

Direct or indirect treatment methods may be used (Minde and Minde, 1981). Only a few psychoanalysts and psychodynamically oriented therapists have reported treating infants and it is not clear whether such therapies have a place in this age range. Behavioural approaches have been used and seem to offer more promise; parents and other involved adults may be trained to act as therapists.

Indirect treatment methods include the counselling of parents and others caring for infants and young children and the provision of 'early intervention' programmes for children at risk. These may be provided in day-care, preschool or home settings. Attention to the family system of which the child is a part may reveal problems likely to be responsive to family therapy.

The optimal care of small children who must spend long periods in hospital is likely to pay dividends. Minde *et al.* (1980) reported a study in which parents of very small premature infants were randomly allocated to self-help groups or to control conditions, that is no group meetings. They found that the parents in the self-help groups and their infants appeared to benefit.

Outcome

Many feeding, sleeping and behavioural problems are transient and resolve without any special treatment. They may be little more than minor upsets in the processes whereby parents and their children learn to adjust to each other and meet each others' needs. The stability of the family unit, the 'goodness of fit' between the temperaments of those concerned, and the parents' maturity and experience of children are all factors which influence the outcome.

Nevertheless, behaviour problems appearing in the preschool years may presage later problems. Stevenson *et al.* (1985) followed up 535 children from age 3 to age 8, and found that behaviour problems at age 3 were strongly related to behavioural deviance at age 8, especially in boys. Poor language development at age 3 was also correlated with deviant behaviour at age 8. A smaller scale study, rather differently designed, yielded similar results (Lerner *et al.*, 1985). It seems that aggressive children, withdrawn children, hyperactive children and speech- and language-disordered children in the age range 3 to 5 are specially at risk of developing later psychiatric disorders.

Chapter 15

Special Problems in Adolescence

Some special points about examining adolescents were made in Chapter 3. Adolescents are prone to feel threatened when they meet a psychiatrist, so that the establishment of rapport is particularly important. Interest in and acceptance of their points of view, and a respectful, non-judgmental approach are essential. The limits of confidentiality should also be made clear. Many adolescents want to know if you will tell their parents what they tell you and who you will report to on your assessment. These are reasonable questions which must be dealt with openly and honestly.

The developmental tasks of adolescence were reviewed in Chapter 1. In essence they comprise the gradual adoption of the adult role in the social, vocational and sexual spheres of life. This process occurs more easily in some young people than in others but many experience doubts, fears and feelings of inadequacy as it proceeds. This may lead to anxiety which is not always openly expressed; instead the young person may become aggressive and defiant, or moody and unpredictable. Adolescents often make a show of rejecting adult standards and of having interests and pursuits of which their parents disapprove.

The prevalence of adolescent psychiatric disorders

The prevalence of psychiatric disorders in adolescence differs from that observed in childhood. Studies of adolescent populations have yielded prevalence rates varying from 8 per cent to 21 per cent, depending on the criteria used, the population studied and the sex of the subjects. Most studies have found higher rates in adolescence than in childhood, but even more striking is the change in the sex ratio. In prepubertal children, disturbed boys outnumber disturbed girls by roughly a 2 to 1 margin, but as puberty arrives and adolescence proceeds the ratio becomes equal, and it is reversed in adult life. Urban rates are substantially higher than rural ones, though this applies also in childhood. Prevalence studies are reviewed by Graham and Rutter (1985) and by Rutter (1980b) in the book *Changing Youth in a Changing*

Society. This book contains much other useful information about the psychiatric problems of this age period. Offord *et al.* (1987), in their Ontario study, found the prevalence of disturbance in boys aged 4 to 11 (19.5 per cent) to be similar to that in boys aged 12 to 16 (18.8 per cent), but the rate in girls in the younger age group was 13.5 per cent, while that in girls aged 12 to 16 was 21.8 per cent.

The pattern of psychiatric disorders changes as childhood gives way to adolescence. Schizophrenia, rare before puberty, becomes commoner. Major affective disorders, particularly depression, are also encountered more frequently, while encopresis, enuresis and some developmental disorders become less common. Much of the change in the sex ratio is due to the increased prevalence of affective disorders, principally depression, in girls; in addition some of the developmental disorders and encopresis, which affect boys more than girls, have resolved by this time. Suicide, very rare before puberty, becomes more frequent; and mania, also rare before puberty, increases in prevalence, though it is still rare in early and middle adolescence. Alcohol and drug abuse and anorexia nervosa are other conditions which are uncommon before puberty and may make their appearance in adolescence. (An exception is solvent and petrol (gasoline) sniffing which often starts before puberty.)

It is convenient to consider adolescent disorders under three headings, though the subdivisions are somewhat artificial, especially that between categories 2 and 3:

(1)   unresolved childhood disorders;
(2)   disturbances related to puberty and adolescence;
(3)   early-developing adult-type disorders.

Unresolved childhood disorders

Conduct disorders

Conduct disorders are often exacerbated with the onset of puberty; the tendency to rebel and reject adult standards which is often encountered in adolescence may accentuate pre-existing antisocial feelings. In one study the children who were most aggressive at age 8 to 10 were found to be particularly at risk of becoming violent delinquents (Farrington, 1978). Adolescents who do not have secure relationships with their parents and lack internal controls based upon identification with them, are especially at risk of becoming involved in antisocial behaviour.

Anxiety/neurotic disorders

Neurotic disorders, which generally have good prognoses, sometimes improve around the time of puberty, as the biological drives towards independence develop. The support of the peer group, as it becomes more influential, may also help. In the United Kingdom the change from primary to secondary school usually occurs at about the time of puberty; if the child can face and meet the challenge of an often larger school, requiring more responsibility and independence of decision on the part of its pupils, this may be a useful experience. In North America a similar change from elementary to junior high schools usually occurs at about age 12 but by the time children reach high school, at about 15, adolescence is well under way. Their changed peer group circumstances may assist emotionally immature children who have been overdependent on their parents to become more self-reliant.

Sometimes these aids to emotional growth are insufficient. Faced with the challenges of adolescence, some neurotic children lack the emotional resources to cope. Such drives towards independence as exist are not enough, and the young person seeks to fall back into the security and comfort of the family. Such children, realising unconsciously if not consciously their incapacity to fill age-appropriate roles, may become even more anxious, with a worsening of their condition.

School refusal in adolescence may represent a continuation or exacerbation of a problem which existed before puberty, or it may be a symptom appearing for the first time. Even if the onset is during adolescence, however, its origins can often be traced to earlier years. The onset of school refusal is usually more gradual in adolescence than it is in middle childhood, with increasing withdrawal and isolation from peers. Symptoms of separation anxiety are less prominent and difficulties in school more so. The 'problems' there, which often concern relationships with peer group or teachers, are such as would not usually be problems to children whose emotional development had been normal and whose family relationships were secure.

School refusing adolescents tend to have difficulty expressing aggression and asserting independence in normal ways, difficulties they often share with their parents. The adolescent's desire, conscious or unconscious, to be independent, and awareness of the parental protectiveness which prevents this, can cause a build-up of intensely aggressive feelings. These may be expressed by violently angry outbursts under stress in a young person who at other times behaves in passive and dependent fashion. In such cases treatment of the whole family group is often the best approach. If the family is not prepared to participate, admission to a residential setting may be indicated. School refusal in adolescence tends to be associated with more serious pathology in child and family than it often is in earlier childhood. Depressive or conduct disorder symptoms may also be present (Hersov, 1985b).

Affective disorders

Depression is commoner in adolescents than in younger children. This applies also to suicide and attempted suicide. Mania, and bipolar affective disorders, from being exceedingly rare in childhood, become less so in adolescence. These conditions are discussed more fully in Chapter 6.

Autism

The handicaps of autistic children persist in adolescence and epilepsy is sometimes added to them. Hyperactivity may lessen and autistic adolescents are often underactive. They lack initiative and drive, and their inappropriate social responses and behaviour and their lack of empathy for others isolate them from their non-autistic peers; consequently they tend to remain in closer contact with their families than normal adolescents. But perhaps because of the hormonal changes of puberty and their increase in size and physical strength, these children may become more assertive and difficult for the parents to manage. This may lead to their placement in institutions.

Developmental disorders

Developmental disorders are less evident in adolescence, children often having overcome their speech, language and motor problems by puberty. Reading difficulties frequently persist, however, and may be associated with conduct disorders.

Hyperactivity

Hyperactivity usually lessens in adolescence. So also do the symptoms associated with it (distractibility, impulsivity and aggression) but they remain more prevalent than in the general population. Low self-esteem, poor school performance and poor peer relationships characterize these adolescents; some exhibit antisocial behaviour, though different studies have yielded widely varying estimates of how many (Weiss and Hechtman, 1986, Chapter 4).

Disorders related to puberty and adolescence

The emotional, social, psychological and physical changes of adolescence provide the context for some of the disorders occurring at this time. The following are issues which may be relevant:

(a) *The dependence-independence conflict.* Adolescents are neither dependent children nor independent adults. They feel, in varying degrees, the urge to be independent and they are subject also to social pressures which foster this. But they are as yet uncertain about how far they can act independently. The evident desire to fall back on the family for support may alternate with shows of independent, but sometimes ill-judged, decision making. Help and support given by parents may be accepted in off-handed and ungracious ways. Handling this behaviour requires patience, tolerance and understanding in the parents.

(b) *Uncertainties about sexual role and sexual adequacy.* The main physical and emotional changes of puberty may occur as early as 10 or as late as 17, though on average puberty comes earlier and is completed more quickly in girls than in boys. Consequently some young people feel out of step with their peers, especially if puberty comes late to them. Fears of sexual inadequacy are common during this period.

The upsurge of sexual feelings and activity and the development of sometimes intense relationships with the opposite sex, may provoke feelings of anxiety and confusion. The young person may wish to enter into relationships, while feeling shy and lacking the necessary confidence. On the other hand some adolescents become involved in sexual activity early; this may lead to unwanted pregnancies which, whether carried to term or aborted, are stressful experiences.

(c) *Peer group influences.* During adolescence the peer group assumes increasing importance in the individual's life. Adolescent groups are sometimes all of one sex or they may be mixed. They give support to their members in meeting the social and emotional challenges of adolescence. With the support of the group, young people who still lack self-confidence are able to do things they would shy away from if on their own. Adolescent groups may be as small as 2 or 3 but membership may run to as many as 10, 20 or even more. Some remain quite constant, but most change as members leave to join other groups, and others join. One young person may belong to several groups of differing type and size.

The influence of adolescent groups is not always beneficial. Delinquent gangs may have seriously adverse effects on their members. Some young people feel 'different' from other group members, and some are treated differently because of appearance, race or religion. Adolescent groups usually demand a fair amount of conformity to their standards and unwritten rules. Inability to meet the group's standards may cause individual members anxiety, or even lead to their rejection from the group.

(d) *Discrepancies between individual development and the demands of society.* A recent newspaper cartoon pictured a couple at the box office of a theatre over which there was a sign saying 'Children under 16 must be accompanied by a parent'. The stylishly dressed couple are explaining to the person selling tickets that, 'We're under 16 but we're parents'. This sums up a dilemma faced by many young people in modern day society. Puberty is occurring earlier (in western countries the average age of the menarche is now about one year earlier than it was 50 years ago), yet many of society's institutions take no cognizance of this. For many young people formal education and financial dependency are increasingly prolonged, and those who choose not to remain in formal education beyond their mid-teens are unable to find satisfactory work and places in the adult world. This can lead to feelings of defeat and low self-esteem, as well as anger directed at the adult world in general.

(e) *Family development problems.* Accepting the arrival of adolescence in the children, and making the necessary adjustments in the family system, proves difficult for some families. Attitudes and methods of control which have been appropriate, and have worked well previously, may no longer do so. A process that should be a gradual, sensitively monitored handing over of responsibility from parents to child may become instead a battle of wills; or the opposite may happen, the parents relinquishing control before the young person is ready to shoulder the responsibilities the parents are giving up.

Adolescent conduct disorders and delinquency

Conduct disorders are described in Chapter 4. They are at least as common in adolescence as in middle childhood, and the numbers of antisocial activities engaged in by conduct disordered adolescents are probably greater (Shapland, 1978). Legally defined delinquency is only possible once the age of criminal responsibility is reached, and it reaches its peak in the mid-teenage years. Truancy, running away, stealing, and disruptive behaviour are common in early adolescence, but violent crime is more prevalent in late adolescence. The abuse of alcohol and other drugs often accompanies antisocial behaviour and is discussed below.

Some adolescent conduct disorders are continuations of behaviour patterns established in middle childhood, but others have their onset in adolescence. These latter cases lack the association with reading problems found in cases of earlier onset, and their symptoms and the associated family problems are generally less severe and chronic. They are sometimes no more than exaggerated reactions to some combination of the five circumstances affecting adolescents listed above. The soundness of the parent-child relationship before puberty, and the way the parents react to rebellious behaviour on the part of their child, also affect the severity and persistence of disorders. Sometimes rebellious and antisocial behaviour seems to have the unconscious aim of stimulating the parents to take control of the behaviour of a child who is insecure and afraid of his or her own aggressiveness. In other instances the behaviour is a protest against over-strict demands made by the parents. In yet others it is associated with feelings of rootlessness and aimlessness in children who have been deprived of love and emotional security. There may be a background of physical or sexual abuse. Children, especially girls, who have been sexually abused are especially prone to act out sexually.

Some conduct disorders develop in the context of seriously deviant personality development. The poor quality of the young person's past relationships may have led to defective conscience formation; the conflicting pressures and anxieties of adolescence then upset the delicate and uncertain balance upon which reasonably conforming behaviour has been based.

Although some adolescent conduct disorders are associated with serious personality pathology, many seem worse than they really are. The reported severity of the behavioural disturbance is on its own an inadequate criterion. Many adolescents emerge as mentally healthy individuals, adjusting satisfactorily in society, after going through a period of difficult behaviour. The prevalence of antisocial behaviour is considerably lower in young adulthood than it is in adolescence, suggesting that it is often a transient phenomenon. Factors to be considered in deciding how serious the problem is include the child's adjustment before puberty, family stability and parental attitudes, and the young person's adjustment in circumstances where the parents are not directly involved. These include school, peer group and the interview situation with the physician or other professional.

Running away from home is a common problem in adolescents, and it occurs also in younger children. The term is applied to leaving or staying away from home, with the intention of staying away for a period of time, in circumstances in which the individual will be missed by those remaining at home. In the USA about 10 per cent of adolescent boys and 8.7 per cent of girls report having run away at least once (Russell, 1981); 733,000 adolescents are said to have run away from home in 1975 (Opinion Research Corporation, 1976). The homes of runaways are characterized by high rates of parent-child conflict, parental death and divorce, and physical and sexual abuse. Physical abuse was reported by 78 per cent of 199 youths admitted to a runaway shelter (Farber *et al.*, 1984). Running away may be seen by the child as an attempt to escape from conflicts in the family, or as a means of avoiding defeat in the battle for independence from the parents.

Alcohol and drug abuse

Adolescent drug abuse has become a serious problem in the last few decades. In this section the term 'drug' is used to include alcohol, except where the context indicates otherwise. Alcohol is a powerful mind-altering drug and its use often leads to abuse and dependence.

Prevalence rates vary from place to place and from time to time. Different drugs come in and out of fashion, and availability and cost are factors influencing their use. Jalali *et al.* (1981) surveyed 2131 adolescents in five New Jersey schools. Their ages ranged from 12 to 18, with most in the 15 to 17 age bracket. Over 80 per cent of the subjects reported alcohol use from an early age, 34 per cent from age 8 or younger. Most of the children were introduced to alcohol in the family setting, whereas other drugs were first obtained from peers, usually at school. Of the other drugs used the most frequently reported, as in other studies, was marijuana. Only 49 per cent of the subjects said they had never used this drug. Amphetamines (26.3 per cent), barbiturates (25.3 per cent), hallucinogens (21.1 per cent), cocaine (13.6 per cent), inhalants (13.2 per cent), and opiates (9.3 per cent) had also been used. The onset of drug use was most often in the age range 13 to 15, but earlier in the case of marijuana. Alcohol use among adolescents is closely associated with its use, and especially its abuse, by the parents.

Table 15.1   Prevalence of drug use (Ontario Child Health Study).

	Boys	Girls
Tobacco		
Occasional use	31.1	45.6
Regular use	15.8	23.4
Alcohol		
Occasional use	42.5	48.8
Regular use	10.6	15.9
Marijuana	13.3	17.6
'Hard' drugs	5.3	7.5
Inhalants	3.8	4.5

In 1983, in the course of the Ontario Child Health Study, drug use was investigated in a representative sample of 1302 adolescents, of whom 1265 (97 per cent of those eligible) participated (Boyle and Offord,

1986). The age range studied was 12 to 16. The percentage prevalence figures found in the 14 to 16 age range were as shown in Table 15.1.

'Hard' drugs included amphetamines, stimulants, barbiturates, sedatives, tranquillisers, hallucinogens, psychedelics, heroin or opiates. The prevalence rates for all categories of drug except inhalants were much lower in the 12 to 14 age bracket. Inhalants, however, were used by 8.3 per cent of the boys and 9.6 per cent of the girls in the younger group. It seems that girls may be more prone to drug use than boys, though only in the case of cigarette smoking was the difference statistically significant. There is a clear progression with age and the mid-teens are a common time for drug use to commence. The findings of a study conducted in New York suggest that the major risk period for initiation into the use of cigarettes, alcohol and marijuana is completed by age 21, and that for illicit drugs other than cocaine by age 21 (Kandel and Logan, 1984).

Daily cigarette use has been found to occur in 15 to 25 per cent of most adolescent populations studied. There is a strong correlation between parental smoking and smoking in adolescents; the chances of becoming a teenage smoker are about five times greater in smoking than in non-smoking households.

There is a stepwise progression in drug use. This starts with the use of beer or wine, going on to, successively, tobacco and hard liquor, marijuana, and then other illegal drugs such as LSD, tranquillisers, heroin and cocaine. Fortunately only a few of those who start out on this sequence complete it (Yamaguchi and Kandel, 1984a; 1984b).

Kovach and Glickman (1986) suggest that a period of drug use has become a normal feature of adolescence in western society, and that the onset of use is around age 14. They studied the characteristics of users, defined as those who had used marijuana or alcohol at least once a week for 3 months, or had used any 'high-risk' drug (tranquillizers, barbiturates, sedatives, hallucinogens, phencyclidine or amphetamines) in the past year. Comparing users with those who had used no drugs in the past year, they found that the users were:

- more often male;
- more often Caucasian;
- older;
- children who had repeated school grades 8 times more often than non-users;
- more involved with family crises and conflict with parents;
- more likely to be arrested, incarcerated, and convicted of property, drug and weapons offences;
- experiencing less enjoyment and satisfaction in school, and more dislike of and fights with teachers;

- more argumentative and disruptive in class.

Table 15.2 Some drugs of abuse.

Drug	How used	Main characteristics
Tobacco	Smoked Chewed	Powerfully addictive, but widely advertised and readily available to young people
Alcohol	Drunk as beer, wine and distilled spirits	Causes physical and psychological dependence; widely abused; introduced to children in families
Cannabis products – marijuana, hashish, 'hash oil'	Smoked in cigarettes ('joints') and pipes	Intoxicant and euphoric; causes psychological dependence; relatively cheap; readily available, circulates in schools
Stimulants – amphetamines, 'speed', methylphenidate	Orally Intravenous (I.V.)	Euphoric, cause feelings of well-being; increased energy; may cause psychoses, dependence common, mainly psychological
Hallucinogens – LSD ('acid'), mescaline, phencyclidine (PCP, 'angel dust')	Orally	Altered consciousness, hallucinations, unusual subjective states, psychological dependence
Barbiturates	Orally I.V.	Sedative effect; may be used to counter effects of stimulants; can cause serious dependency
Tranquillisers – especially benzodiazepines ('Valium', 'Halcion', 'Librium')	Orally Rarely I.V.	Lightheadedness, relief of tension; used for 'coming down' after using cocaine, amphetamines and other stimulants; psychological dependence
Narcotics – heroin, morphine, methadone, codeine and related compounds	I.V. Orally	Feelings of wellbeing, pleasant drowsiness, contentment. Major physical dependence may occur
Cocaine	Inhaled as powder, smoked ('freebasing'), I.V.	A stimulant, producing great euphoria briefly, and stimulation of heart and other organs. May cause psychotic state and severe psychological dependence
Inhalants – solvents in glue etc., gasoline/petrol	Inhaled, often from plastic bag	Brief euphoria and confusion. Psychological dependence may occur; may cause brain damage

The users associated with, and claimed as friends, more drug users than the non-users did, and the prevalence of other behavioural and psychiatric problems was higher. The regular drug users stood out as having more personality and family problems. Vicary and Lerner (1986) report the results of an extensive longitudinal study. They found that early parental conflict over child-rearing, and harsh and restrictive parenting, were associated with drug use in the teen years.

Table 15.2 lists the principal drugs which adolescents have been reported to use and some characteristics of each. The list is not exhaustive. Various other psychoactive preparations, cough syrups containing codeine, and compound tablets containing mixtures of analgesics, sedatives, antihistamines, caffeine and other drugs are abused. Drug use among young people is seldom confined to one drug. Any opportunity to get 'high' that presents itself may be taken. If only one drug is used it is likely to be either alcohol, marijuana or tobacco.

Drug users may be divided into experimental, situational (or recreational) and compulsive groups. Most adolescents experiment, at least with alcohol, cigarettes or marijuana, at some stage. A smaller number use drugs at parties and in particular social situations, while an even smaller number become dependent on a drug or, more commonly, drugs. The factors which determine whether a person becomes dependent are not completely understood. Social class does not seem to be a major factor, though economic factors may play their part. Social pressures can lead to drug use but probably do not determine who becomes dependent. That may be a more a matter of the emotional stability and personality characteristics of the individual. There is a small subgroup of drug users who have serious personality problems or psychiatric conditions such as recurrent depression (Amini *et al.*, 1976). They may have a history of early deprivation or other adverse rearing experiences. It is among this minority that serious drug abuse, leading to addiction, is most likely to occur.

There is a correlation between drug abuse and both delinquency and school failure, though it is not clear what the causal relationships are. It may be that common factors lead to all three sets of problems. Other factors which have been found to be associated with drug use are social isolation, low self-esteem, poor relationships with parents, depression, and unconventional beliefs and values concerning drug use. Individuals may seek to have their felt needs for affiliation, satisfaction of curiosity, altered states of consciousness, recreation, anxiety reduction, and general drive reduction met by the use of drugs in the company of other users.

Other disorders related to adolescence

Anxiety/neurotic disorders may arise during adolescence and in the etiology of some of these the stresses of adolescence play a part. Clear-cut obsessive-compulsive, conversion, and dissociative disorders become commoner in adolescence; so also do social phobias and agoraphobia. The manifestations of these conditions are reviewed in Chapter 5; the form of the disorders is little different from that seen, albeit rarely, before puberty. Neurotic depression/dysthymic disorder may arise in the context of difficulties in adolescent adjustment.

Anorexia nervosa is predominantly a disorder arising in adolescence. Many of its features seem to be associated with difficulties in making the adjustments necessary at this stage of development. It is described in Chapter 13.

Adult-type disorders arising in adolescence

Any of the major psychiatric disorders of adult life may arise during adolescence. Both schizophrenia and the major affective disorders (depression, mania and bipolar disorders) become commoner as adolescence proceeds.

The onset of schizophrenia may be insidious. Its early symptoms can be hard to distinguish from the shyness, diffidence and vagueness of expression common in anxious adolescents who are feeling unsure of themselves but are not developing schizophrenia. It is important not to make the diagnosis of schizophrenia lightly, since the implications of wrongly labelling a disorder in this way can be serious. The criteria set out in Chapter 8 should be the basis on which the diagnosis is made, though in some cases it is necessary to await developments, while bearing the possibility of schizophrenia in mind. Sometimes a period of observation in hospital, away from the family and the peer group, may serve to clarify the diagnosis.

Apart from conduct disorders, depression is the commonest form of major psychiatric disorder occurring in this age period. Its features are described in Chapter 6.

Suicidal behaviour in adolescence

We have seen that suicide is very rare before puberty, following which its incidence increases. Around, and shortly after puberty it is still relatively uncommon, but as the teenage years progress it becomes less so. In the USA in 1978, 151 children between the ages of 10 and

14, 117 boys and 34 girls, committed suicide; this represents an age-specific rate of 0.81 per 100,000. Most were over 12. In the age range 15 to 19 there were 1686 suicides, 1367 being boys and 319 girls; this is 7.64 per 100,000 (Shaffer and Fisher, 1981). The incidence of adolescent suicide seems to be increasing in most western countries.

The incidence of suicidal attempts, otherwise known as parasuicide, is much higher though difficult to estimate accurately. 'Attempts' may be as mild as a few superficial scratches on the wrist, or as serious as the taking of massive overdoses of drugs which would have been fatal had not prompt and intensive medical treatment been available. What is clear is that the sex ratio among suicide attempters is the reverse of that found in completed suicides, girls being much more prone to parasuicide (Hawton *et al.*, 1982).

Self-poisonings, wrist-slashings and other self-mutilations do not necessarily represent suicidal attempts. Nor does the declared wish of the young person to die or to commit suicide necessarily mean that the wish or intention actually exists. Such acts or statements are sometimes expressions of distress or attempts to stimulate concern, solicitude or attention, or to achieve other changes in the environment. Despite this they may have unintended fatal outcomes. They should always be taken seriously because they indicate that a serious problem exists, even though the risk of suicide may be slight. On the other hand adolescent suicide can come out of the blue, either because pre-existing depression has not been recognized or because it is an impulsive act, rather than a planned one or the result of a period of increasing distress.

The psychiatric assessment of an adolescent should always include an evaluation of suicidal risk. At some point during the interview, preferably after rapport has been well established, you should ask questions such as, 'Have you ever felt life isn't worth living any more?' or 'Have you ever wished you were dead?' If such questions are answered in the affirmative you should explore when, and under what circumstances, the young person has entertained these thoughts. How severe and frequent have they been? When was the last time they were present? Was the subject facing a lot of stress at the time? If so, is that stress continuing or has it been resolved?

The next set of questions should address suicidal intent, for example, 'Have you ever thought of harming yourself physically in some way?', and 'Have you actually thought seriously about killing yourself?' If the answers are yes, you should ask, 'Have you thought how you would kill yourself?' If the answer is again yes, you should explore what the young person's suicidal plans are, how carefully they have been laid and how effective they would be if carried out.

Finally you should ask about previous attempts at suicide, and explore the precipitating circumstances, the actual events and the consequences that followed. Was the young person taken to hospital? If so, what treatment was provided? Was he or she admitted? If so, for how long? What was the reaction of the parents and other family members?

The risk of suicide is greater when the subject has been getting steadily more depressed over a period of time. It varies with the severity of the depression. Suicide is more likely the less communication there is with others. The isolated depressed person is very much at risk, especially when communication channels have recently broken down. If there have been previous suicide attempts, especially serious ones, the risk may be greater. A long history of self-destructive behaviour is particularly serious. Also important are the extent to which parasuicidal behaviour has been intended as a means of communication and whether the communication has been heeded by those to whom it has been directed. If there has been little impact on the environment, the risk of recurrence is greater. Most serious of all are attempts at suicide in isolation, especially when accompanied by a strong desire to die.

The treatment of adolescents

The treatment of the main psychiatric disorders from which adolescents may suffer has been outlined in the chapters dealing with those conditions. Many disturbed adolescents, especially those with conduct disorders, tend to resent those in authority. Adolescents' negative attitudes towards their parents are sometimes displaced and directed towards the therapist. The establishment of rapport and a good working relationship, and the clarification of treatment goals, are therefore especially important. If treatment is embarked upon on the basis of the parents' goals, or those of the young person's social worker or probation officer, or the family court judge, success is unlikely. Similarly we must temper our own enthusiasm for making the changes we believe are desirable, rather than those the adolescent is seeking. Time spent discussing, clarifying and agreeing goals is always well spent.

Sometimes the picture given by adolescents of their family situation or of themselves is quite different from that supplied by their parents. They may even deny the existence of any problems, while the parents, and perhaps their teachers, have a long list of complaints. In such situations family therapy may be the best approach. The points of view of all concerned can be stated with everyone present, and the differences of opinion, or the disputed facts, can be examined. This is often an essential first step in therapy. Haley (1980) discusses therapy with the families of adolescents and suggests various approaches which can be productive.

Some severely disturbed adolescents, especially those from highly dysfunctional families, are best admitted to residential treatment. While this is no panacea, well structured programmes using behaviour modification methods may be of benefit (Romig, 1978; Shamsie, 1981). Involvement of the family is sometimes better postponed until some work has been done with the adolescent (Burquest, 1979).

Particularly difficult to treat are adolescents who have suffered prolonged and severe deprivation, especially if this has been combined with physical or sexual abuse. Many of them have great difficulty establishing trusting and intimate relationships with people and their willingness to get involved in a psychotherapeutic relationship is similarly limited. Initially, involvement instead in a living situation in which opportunities are available to learn interpersonal skills may be more helpful. An excellent account of the treatment of an adolescent girl with such difficulties has been provided by Rossman (1985).

Medication has a well established, if limited place in the treatment of adolescent psychiatric disorders. Antidepressants are usually indicated for major depressive disorders; and antipsychotics, either phenothiazine compounds or haloperidol, for schizophrenia. Lithium carbonate may be effective in the treatment of bipolar affective disorders, and it may have a part to play in the treatment of some behaviour problems of adolescence. It does seem to be more effective in controlling disturbed behaviour than either placebo or haloperidol (Campbell *et al.*, 1984), and causes less drowsiness and depression of cognitive function (Platt *et al.*, 1984). How far drugs should be used to control aggressive and antisocial behaviour is a moot point. Such treatment is only symptomatic; therapy designed to improve the young person's relationships, self-concept or other more basic problems is generally to be preferred.

Adolescent drug abuse is hard to treat. Most teenage drug abusers deny that their use of drugs presents a problem. Kicking a drug habit can be difficult for the person whose motivation is strong; those whose motivation is minimal or absent, as is the case with many adolescents, are unlikely to stop unless they undergo some experience (for example the death of a friend from an overdose) that makes them see drug use in a different light. Suffering the psychological craving for drugs and/ or their physical withdrawal effects is simply not worthwhile for young people whose drug use has not as yet caused major problems – or problems they are prepared to acknowledge. Since many of these young people are members of disturbed families, a family approach often offers the best chance of success. There is extensive, if inconclusive, literature about the families of drug addicts (Kaufman and Kaufman, 1979; Stanton and Todd, 1982; Reilly, 1984; Friedman *et al.*, 1987).

It is possible to stop adolescents taking drugs by placing them, willingly or protesting, in treatment centres where drugs are unavailable but unless they can be 'hooked' into therapy while there, the effects do not usually last long after discharge. Self-help organizations like Alcoholics Anonymous and Narcotics Anonymous, while helpful to many adult addicts, may be less useful to adolescents. They are based upon acceptance by the addict that he or she *is* an alcoholic or an addict and has an unmanageable life. This usually involves first reaching a psychological 'bottom' which many young people entering the world of drug abuse have not yet done.

In the management of suicidal adolescents any associated depression or other psychiatric disorder should receive appropriate treatment. In addition it is usually important to open up communication between these patients and their families, as well as exploring their communication, relationship and other problems psychotherapeutically. Some combination of individual and family therapy may be the best way of achieving this. Inpatient admission is usually indicated when the suicide risk is judged to be high but some families are able to provide a good degree of supervision at home; in such circumstances it may be possible to manage the patient as an outpatient or a daypatient even though there is some risk of suicide.

Many of the treatments that have been advocated for a wide range of adolescent problems are summarized and reviewed in *Therapies for Adolescents* (Stein and Davis, 1982).

Outcome

There is a strong association between antisocial behaviour in adolescence and similar behaviour in adult life. But while most antisocial adults have shown antisocial behaviour as adolescents, most antisocial young people do not become antisocial adults (Robins, 1978). Many delinquent youths abandon their antisocial behaviour between the ages of 17 and 20; this seems in part a maturational process, associated with changes in attitudes towards drug use, consciously formulated changes in priorities, and support from girlfriends, boyfriends, siblings or others (Mulvey and LaRosa, 1986).

The outlook in anxiety/neurotic disorders seems to be better than that for antisocial behaviours; most do not presage adult problems of the same type. On the other hand the risk of recurrence of major affective disorders, including bipolar ones, is high. Schizophrenia has a relatively poor prognosis, though with continuing treatment the symptoms may be kept under control.

Hyperactive adolescents are mostly found to be functioning within normal limits in adult life. One-third to a half become indistinguishable from the normal population, but there are higher prevalences of the use of alcohol and cannabis products, and of antisocial personality disorder when these adults are compared with normal controls (Weiss and Hechtman, 1986).

Autism and other pervasive developmental disorders usually persist into adult life. Many autistic individuals remain severely handicapped and up to half are eventually admitted to institutions. Others survive in the community with varying degrees of support from family members or others; only a small minority find places in the labour force.

Helpful sources of further information about the problems of adolescents and their treatment are *The Clinical Psychiatry of Adolescence* (Steinberg, 1983) and *Basic Adolescent Psychiatry* (Steinberg, 1987).

Chapter 16

Psychiatric Disorders in Mentally Retarded Children

Mental retardation is usually defined in terms of both social and intellectual functioning. To use either criterion alone can lead to unfortunate results. If social functioning were taken as the sole criterion, those with intelligence in or near the average range might be treated as retarded if their social skills were impaired for other reasons. If assessed intelligence is the only criterion, some of those whose intelligence is well below average, but who nevertheless function satisfactorily in society, may be stigmatized, admitted to institutions or otherwise deprived of opportunities they could use.

It is helpful to take children's levels of intellectual and social functioning into account in planning their education and vocational training. But for the purposes of providing them with psychiatric services, dividing them into those who are mentally retarded and those who are not has disadvantages. It is better to consider the psychiatry of all children, whatever their level of functioning, as part of the mainstream of clinical child psychiatry. In the past the psychiatric care of intellectually retarded children has often been provided in hospitals and institutions for the retarded, sometimes far from their homes and families and administered separately from other child psychiatry services. Moves to reverse this trend have fortunately been under way for some years now (Kushlick, 1972).

The prevalence of psychiatric disorders in the mentally retarded

The Isle of Wight study of 9- to 11-year-old children (Rutter, Tizard and Whitmore, 1970) indicated that 'intellectually retarded' children (those whose IQs on the Wechsler Intelligence Scale for Children – see Chapter 3 – were two or more standard deviations below the mean for 'control' children) had psychiatric disorders 3 to 4 times more frequently than children in the general population. Among severely retarded children not attending school, psychiatric disorder was found in 50 per cent, compared with 6.6 per cent in the general population. In this group psychoses and the hyperkinetic syndrome were proportionately commoner than in children of higher intelligence (Rutter, Graham and Yule, 1970).

Not only are specific psychiatric disorders more common in children of lower intelligence, but so also are a variety of forms of deviant behaviour. Table 16.1 illustrates this point using data culled from the Isle of Wight findings.

Table 16.1   Symptoms reported in 10- and 11-year-old girls (Isle of Wight survey).

	IQ 120 or more	*IQ 79 or less*
Poor concentration		
Parents' report	2.6%	26.4%
Teachers' report	9.1%	62.3%
Fighting		
Parents' report	1.3%	9.9%
Teachers' report	2.6%	11.0%

Corbett (1979), in a study in South-East London, found that there were 140 children aged under 15 with IQs below 50, in a population of about 175,000. Of these 43 per cent showed evidence of behavioural disturbance. Common problems among this group were psychoses (17 per cent), stereotypies and pica (10 per cent), and adjustment disorders (6 per cent). Conduct, emotional and hyperkinetic disorders were each found in 4 per cent of these children.

Clinical associations and causes of mental retardation

Some of the causes of mental retardation have been mentioned in Chapters 2, 7 and 8. Genetic factors, physical disease of the brain, brain injury and environmental factors may all contribute. The high prevalence of psychiatric problems in individuals of very low intelligence is probably due chiefly to the brain damage which is usually present in these cases. The relationship is not, however, a simple one and many other factors may play their parts. The following points are relevant:

(1) There is a relationship between IQ and deviant behaviour in children of normal intelligence as well as in intellectually duller children, brighter children showing less deviant behaviour. This may be in part because greater intellectual capacity makes social adaptation easier.

(2) Organic brain disease is commoner in children of lower intelligence

than in those with IQs in the average range, and it is virtually universal in those with IQs below 50. Epilepsy is present in many children with brain damage and is associated with an increased incidence of psychiatric disorder. Behaviour often improves following hemispherectomy, an operation sometimes performed to remove half the cerebral cortex when this is badly damaged in children with infantile hemiplegia; similar improvement may occur following the surgical removal of an epileptogenic focus from the brain, especially from the temporal lobe. All these points suggest that brain damage can contribute to behaviour problems.

(3) Social factors such as depriving, hostile and rejecting parental attitudes may adversely affect both intellectual development and emotional stability. Instability has been found to be commoner in the families of retarded children that in other families. Retarded children may also be subject to rejecting attitudes on the part of other children which may adversely affect their development and mental health.

(4) The developmental immaturity of retarded children means that their language and other social skills compare unfavourably with those of their peers. These differences, and their delay in achieving motor and toilet training skills, are additional handicaps which may predispose to psychiatric disorder.

(5) Educational failure is associated with psychiatric disorder (a finding of the Isle of Wight study). As a group, children of lower intelligence progress more slowly than other children. Sometimes longstanding failure at school is a factor contributing to psychiatric disorder.

(6) Institutionalization can adversely affect both intellectual development and emotional growth. The adverse effects of the environment in some children's institutions was well demonstrated by the sociological studies reported by King *et al.* (1971).

(7) There is little evidence that emotional disorders cause poor intellectual functioning, though they may impair children's cooperation in intelligence testing. High anxiety levels can also result in underachievement in school, even though intellectual capacity is unimpaired.

Specific forms of mental retardation

Down's syndrome

Down's syndrome, also known as trisomy-21, is the commonest specific clinical entity associated with mental retardation. It occurs in about 1 in 700 births. In this condition there are usually three of the chromosome 21s, though sometimes the additional material is attached to another chromosome. Older parents are at greater risk of having children with this condition; Down's syndrome afflicts about one in every 100 children born to women over 40 (Mikkelsen, 1981).

Down's syndrome children are usually recognizable at birth. They have marked epicanthic folds, inwardly slanting eyes, small heads, short necks, small and low-set ears and protruding tongues. There is usually only a single palmar crease and the fifth finger typically curves inwards. Moderate to severe mental retardation is present in nearly all cases, though chromosomal mosaics (individuals in whom some cells contain normal chromosomes and others show trisomy-21) may have near-normal intelligence. About 40 per cent have congenital cardiac abnormalities and there is a high incidence of other congenital defects.

It used to be thought that there was a particular personality type associated with Down's syndrome, but this does not seem to be the case. Formerly many Down's children were admitted to institutions early in life, but nowadays they are usually cared for in the community while being provided with specialized schooling. This helps promote normal development and it seems that many of the behavioural abnormalities seen in the past were due to institutional life and experiences.

The verbal skills of these children are more impaired than their non-verbal ones and few achieve reading skills better than those of an average 8-year-old. They exhibit behavioural problems more often than children of normal intelligence, but apparently less often than other retarded children of comparable levels of intellectual functioning. Hyperkinetic behaviour, short attention span and aimless activity are common features (Gath, 1985).

Phenylketonuria

The genetics of this condition were mentioned in Chapter 2. Phenylketonuria is quite rare, occurring in fewer than 1 in 10,000 children. Untreated children are usually, though not invariably, retarded and may be hyperkinetic and show other behavioural abnormalities. They tend to have light coloured skin and hair, often have eczema and also a characteristic urinary smell. Early detection can be achieved through the screening of newborns by means of a simple urine test. Treatment is by means of a diet low in phenylalanine during the child's early years. This usually leads to normal or near-normal development.

The fragile X syndrome and autism

These conditions have been mentioned in Chapters 2 and 7. The fragile X syndrome was originally believed to affect only boys, who were mildly or moderately mentally retarded and had large testes, jaws and ears. It is now clear that girls with this chromosome abnormality may be retarded, though usually only mildly. The fragile X condition also appears to be associated with infantile autism, though it is present only in a minority of autistic children.

Infantile autism, whether associated with the fragile X chromosome or not, is associated with mental retardation in at least 75 per cent of cases.

The Lesch-Nyhan syndrome

This rare sex-linked inborn error of purine metabolism is character-ized by severe mental retardation, self-mutilation, aggressive beha-viour, increased muscle tone, other neurological abnormalities and renal failure. Symptoms appear during the first year of life. The self-mutilation, consisting of biting the lips, fingers or other parts of the body, usually commences during the first few years of life.

The Prader-Willi syndrome

This is another form of mental retardation in which chromosome abnormalities are sometimes, but not invariably, present. Obesity, underdevelopment of the gonads and behavioural problems are other features. These children often seem to have insatiable appetites, gorging themselves, stealing food and displaying the symptoms of pica (see Chapter 14).

Cerebral palsy and related neurological disorders

Some children with cerebral palsy and other syndromes associated with brain damage are mentally retarded, though many are of normal intelligence. The combination of a serious physical handicap with limited intellectual skills provides a particular challenge to those caring for, treating and educating such children. This applies, sometimes with even greater force, to deaf and blind retarded children.

Many other, mostly rare, disorders are associated with moderate or severe mental retardation. Some are mentioned in Chapter 8, since they may present with a psychotic picture. Further information is available in textbooks on mental retardation.

Sociocultural retardation

While severely retarded children are usually suffering from specific clinical syndromes or disorders, many of the mildly retarded show no other medical or neurological abnormality. Their retarded development is probably due to some combination of sociocultural deprivation and polygenic inheritance. The innate, genetically determined intellectual potential of some children falls at the lower end of the normal range; if such children also lack cognitive stimulation and suffer general sociocultural deprivation, a mild degree of retardation may result. This frequently becomes apparent only when the child goes to school; in their home environments these children are often considered to be functioning normally.

Clinical management and treatment

There are two populations of retarded individuals. The larger one comprises those who are mildly retarded and do not suffer from any specific clinical syndrome or medical problems. A smaller group consists of more seriously handicapped people who either suffer from specific syndromes, such as those we have mentioned here or in Chapter 8, or who have major brain damage. The boundary between the former group and the normal population is not a distinct one. Whether the mildly retarded are identified as having problems depends on such factors as their personality characteristics, social supports and the educational and vocational opportunities available to them.

Also important is the nature of the society into which retarded children are born. Such children have more difficulty adapting to the needs of technologically sophisticated societies and those which have a high level of literacy, than children of normal intelligence. The industrial revolution led to the setting up of many institutions for the mentally retarded, for whom no place could be found in the industrial workforce. Formerly these people had been able to find appropriate niches in the rural, village societies in which they lived. Even today most mildly retarded individuals usually function well in 'third world' societies. The tasks which fall to many young people in these societies, such as minding cattle, sheep or goats, or carrying water from the river to the homestead, are well within their capabilities. If, however, they needed to acquire reading or mathematical skills to function in society, they would have great difficulty.

Nowadays, in many parts of the developed world, the potential of the mildly retarded to become integrated into the mainstream of society is better understood. Educational programmes, either in special classes or special schools, are provided for children who cannot benefit from the regular school programme. Families are given support and sometimes financial assistance to enable them to retain their retarded children, rather than have them placed in institutions. Employment opportunities still exist for those with practical, rather than academic, skills and sheltered workshops and factories provide work for some who cannot survive in the regular workplace.

The assessment of the skills and potentials of retarded children is usually carried out by educational psychologists. Educationalists also play a major part in the management of these children, who require skilled and specialized teaching. These children and their families often have social problems, so that the services of social workers may be required as well. Family physicians, paediatricians, neurologists and speech therapists all have contributions to make in the management of retarded children, especially in the assessment and treatment of the more severely retarded. Psychiatric skills are required primarily in the management of the emotional and behavioural problems which are often present. Ideally the management of retarded children should be a multidisciplinary undertaking, to which all the above professional groups contribute.

As with other disorders, a comprehensive assessment should first be made of the child in the context of his or her family, school and neighbourhood. The medical and biological aspects of each case must be considered along with such factors as the stability of the family and its capacity to provide needed cognitive stimulation and to promote the child's self-esteem; the educational situation; and any emotional and behavioural disorders which the child presents. In many developed countries centres have been established for the early detection, assessment and remediation of developmental delays and problems. These are usually staffed by teams made up of professionals from the disciplines mentioned above. A careful appraisal of each child's developmental and learning problems, perceptual deficits, emotional status and social background leads to a plan of action by one or more members of the team.

Treatment methods

The treatment of emotional and behavioural problems in mentally retarded children follows the same general lines as the treatment of these disorders in children of higher intelligence, though some special considerations apply. The following approaches may all be used with retarded children:

(a) Behaviour therapy

This is widely used in the treatment of the behavioural problems of retarded children (Yule and Carr, 1980). The laws of learning theory apply as much to retarded children as to others, though they tend to learn more slowly and more behavioural trials may be needed to achieve the same results. Suitable programmes can promote toilet training, the extinction of such behaviours as temper tantrums, rocking or head banging, the acquisition of motor and language skills and other therapeutic aims.

(b) Other forms of individual psychotherapy

Action-orientated therapy methods are particularly suitable for use with retarded children. These include role playing, from which retarded young people can often learn more than they can from the verbal discussion and explanation of things; the prescription of tasks and rituals, which may have metaphorical significance (van der Hart, 1983; Barker, 1985); and play therapy in its various forms. In using any of these methods the level of cognitive functioning of the child must be taken into account.

(c) Family therapy

Many of the problems of retarded children or adolescents are intimately grounded in their family systems. Family therapy approaches are as applicable to families containing retarded members as they are to those in which there are normally developing children. Retarded family members of any age often participate enthusiastically in the various action and other special techniques available for use in family sessions (Barker, 1986, Chapter 11).

(d) Medication

The indications for the use of drugs in retarded children are similar to those that apply in the treatment of other disturbed children. Epilepsy, if present, should be controlled by the use of anticonvulsants. Hyperactivity may respond to methylphenidate or amphetamines; if these prove ineffective, haloperidol or phenothiazine drugs may be helpful. The use of medication to control aggressive and disruptive behaviour should be avoided if possible. Suitable behavioural management, the provision of appropriate general care and schooling, and proper treatment of speech and physical and perceptual problems are much to be preferred. These children's problems are long-term ones and the prolonged use of drugs can lead to unwanted side-effects; adequate control of disturbed behaviour with drugs often involves a degree of sedation which impairs learning, already a problem for these children.

(e) Residential care
Institutional care is necessary for some children, including most of the very severely retarded. Whether it is needed depends on the degree of intellectual retardation, the presence and severity of any associated physical handicaps or psychiatric disorders, and the capacity of the child's family to provide the care needed. When residential care is necessary, it should be in small, well staffed units as near as possible to the child's family. Only a minority of the most severely retarded require the full facilities of a hospital. Most do better in small hostels or group homes, which are also less expensive to run.

Other points

In dealing with intellectually handicapped children a middle course has to be steered between asking too much of them and asking too little. Facing such children with tasks, for example in school, which are beyond them can be emotionally damaging and lead to anxiety, or even despair, and a needlessly poor self-image. On the other hand, asking too little, as may happen to the inmate of a large hospital ward, may mean that the child's potential is not realized.

The assessment of developmentally retarded children should be a continuing process. Their progress, including their responses to the education, treatment or other help they may be receiving, should be monitored regularly. New management plans invariably need to be made from time to time.

Continuity of care is also important. Retarded children often find change difficult and the care of these individuals should be looked upon as a long-term commitment. The needs of the family must always be borne in mind. It is possible for the special attention given to a handicapped child to have adverse effects on the care given to other children in the family. For the parents, the presence of a seriously retarded child, especially one who also has behavioural or emotional problems, can prove a severe emotional strain and may affect the stability of their marriage.

Outcome

Clinical experience suggests that retarded children can respond to treatment in much the same ways as other children. It is important that the symptoms and behaviours due to superimposed psychiatric disorders are not confused with those due to the underlying delays in cognitive development. Retarded children may be depressed or anxious, they can suffer from adjustment disorders or psychotic ones or from any of the other problems discussed elsewhere in this book. While their limited cognitive skills mean that non-verbal rather than verbal treatment approaches are usually more appropriate, treatment should not be withheld because they are retarded.

While we have no effective treatments for many of the conditions responsible for severe retardation (phenylketonuria being a notable exception), the adverse sociocultural circumstances many more mildly retarded children face can often be ameliorated through the provision of appropriate educational, social and recreational programmes. Much of the help given should be directed to these children's families, since they are in the best position to stimulate their children's development.

The development and adjustment of retarded children, like that of all others, depends very much on the general care and the cognitive and other stimulation they receive. Given suitable care, stable family backgrounds and appropriate treatment of any added psychiatric problems, most mildly retarded children are able to make a satisfactory adjustment in society. Their intellectual limitations do, however, complicate management and place constraints on the ultimate out-comes that may be expected. Perhaps the biggest limiting factor, however, is that imposed by therapists, parents, other professionals and even the children themselves who so often take too gloomy a view of what these children can achieve.

Further reading

Useful sources of further information include *The Modern Management of Mental Handicap* (Simon, 1980) and *Mental Handicap* (Heaton-Ward and Wiley, 1984), a concise text on the subject. *Scientific Studies in Mental Retardation* (Dobbing *et al.*, 1984) contains reviews and discussions of research into various aspects of mental retardation.

Chapter 17

Child Psychiatry and the Law

Child psychiatrists' involvement with legal matters usually arises out of their work in assessing and treating children and families. Forensic psychiatry is a more specialized field which 'is not primarily concerned with medical or psychiatric treatment of the individual. It is an interface discipline in which psychiatric theories, concepts, and practices are applied to legal issues for the ends of the legal system' (Pollack, 1974). The psychiatrist's two roles – that of therapist to child and family, and that of expert who assists the court in its efforts to ensure that justice is done – are not always distinct. In this chapter we will consider primarily some legal issues with which clinical child psychiatrists may be confronted in the regular course of their practice:

(1) They may see children who have been abused or neglected. In many jurisdictions they are legally obliged to report such cases to the appropriate authorities.
(2) Child welfare (or child protection) agencies (in Britain, the children's departments of local authorities) may seek their advice concerning the management of children and families with whom they are dealing. Legal issues may be involved when the child has been or may be removed from the care of the parents against their wishes.
(3) Children appearing in court because of delinquent acts or for other reasons may be referred for psychiatric assessment.
(4) They may be asked for opinions by separated or divorced parents, or lawyers acting on their behalf, to assist in the resolution of disputes concerning the custody of or access to children of the marriage. In some jurisdictions lawyers are appointed by courts to act as advocates for children involved in divorce and these lawyers may ask for psychiatric opinions. Courts may also directly request psychiatric input.
(5) Their opinions may be sought by courts on other legal issues, for example whether a child or adolescent should be admitted involuntarily for residential treatment; the competency of children to act as witnesses; or whether a child placed for adoption should be returned when the natural mother requests this before the adoption is finalized.

The use of procedures such as artificial insemination and surrogate motherhood may result in requests that psychiatrists advise courts on what they believe to be in the best interests of the children concerned. (6) Psychiatrists may be involved in malpractice suits.

(1) The child psychiatrist and child abuse

It is hard to practise child psychiatry without becoming involved in issues of child abuse. Abuse occurs in many of the disturbed and dysfunctional families which come to psychiatric attention. Many abused children suffer from psychiatric disorders, and many disturbed children have been subject to physical, sexual or emotional abuse, or have been neglected in some way.

It may become apparent that a child referred for psychiatric assessment is being or has been abused. The abuse may be mentioned by the child, by the parents or by a sibling; or suspected abuse may be one of the problems mentioned by the referring person. In other cases, however, abuse comes to light later, often during psychotherapy with the abused child or with the abusing person. These situations present difficult dilemmas for therapists. One of the most difficult arises when abuse comes to light in the course of therapy with an abusing adult, as Guyer (1982, page 80) points out:

> 'In its most difficult form this dilemma arises when, during the course of psychotherapy, the therapist learns that a patient is engaging in child abuse. Such a revelation creates a clinical crisis and can place the therapist upon the horns of a dilemma. If the admission is reported, the therapist in effect becomes a witness against [the] patient and the therapeutic alliance may be destroyed, to the ultimate detriment of the child as well as the patient-parent. Alternatively, failure to report places the therapist squarely in opposition to the letter of the law and open ... to sanctions.'

Such situations can also arise when a child or a family group is engaged in therapy. Guyer (1982) discusses the options available to the therapist in situations of this sort. These are:

(1) To ignore the law's requirements 'in the service of a higher ethical imperative'.
(2) To inform patients at the start of treatment of the reporting obligation. If the need to report arises, patients may not then feel that the confidentiality of the therapeutic relationship has been betrayed.
(3) To use the reporting obligation to 'coerce' the patient to cease the abuse by threatening to report if this does not happen.

(4) Simply to comply with the law's requirements and deal .with the therapeutic consequences on an *ad hoc* basis.

My own practice is to explain to children, parents and families, when they first attend, the confidential nature of the interviews I will be having with them. I explain that a record of my interviews is made and assure them that information in it will not be communicated to anyone without their permission, though I report my findings and recommendations to referring physicians – something to which patients rarely object. If referral comes from someone other than a physician, for example a member of the staff of a school or social agency, I discuss what information should be sent to the referring person; if patients wish to limit this or to have no information passed on, I abide by their wishes. Older children and adolescents are assured that what they say will not be passed on to their parents without their consent, except for things so serious, such as suicidal plans, that the parents must know. Finally, I mention the law's reporting requirements, assuring them that I would inform them if I was going to make a report. This final piece of information thus comes as part of a package presented to all families. There is no implication that it applies to any particular family to which it is given.

It is important to be aware of the law in the jurisdiction in which you practise. Each of the 50 United States and the 10 Canadian provinces has its own child welfare legislation; so also do England and Wales, Scotland, Ireland and other countries. Definitions of abuse vary and the circumstances in which suspected abuse must be reported are variously defined. In some jurisdictions the law is more rigid in its definitions than in others; phrases like 'reasonable grounds to suspect' often occur, leaving scope for interpretation of what is reasonable.

When I find myself in a position in which I must make a report to the child welfare authorities, I make clear my willingness to continue to be of service to the family. When appropriate, I also offer to act as the family's advocate. This applies especially when the family is actively involved in therapy. In such cases the child welfare authorities may be willing to allow treatment to continue uninterrupted, perhaps themselves adopting a watching brief. It is helpful to have close working relationships with your local child welfare or child protection staff. This facilitates joint efforts to help families and children.

In these, often difficult, situations it is important to keep families you are treating fully informed. While few like having their cases brought to the attention of child welfare authorities, many understand why this is necessary once it is explained. The role of child welfare workers in helping families overcome their problems, and their aim of keeping families together whenever possible, should also be emphasized.

(2) *The psychiatrist and child welfare agencies*

Some psychiatrists act as consultants to child welfare agencies; others see children referred for advice by or at the suggestion of the staffs of such agencies.

Child welfare agencies may use psychiatric consultation in several ways. They may seek psychiatric advice on the programmes and services they provide; they may request psychiatric input concerning the management or treatment of particular families or children; or they may request the help of psychiatrists in dealing with issues which come to court or threaten to do so. The first two of these activities are part of the psychiatrist's role in the community and do not necessarily involve legal issues. Any work with children in care or otherwise involved with child welfare authorities may, however, lead to requests for, or subpoenas requiring, the psychiatrist's appearance in court.

The extent to which courts and child welfare agencies seek psychiatric input when questions arise concerning the removal of children from parental care varies. Many of these children, and their families, have psychiatric problems requiring treatment. Input from psychiatrists can therefore assist courts and agencies in the decisions they make and in developing appropriate plans of management and treatment. The psychiatric report or evidence usually supplements reports by the agency's social worker and perhaps other professionals (teacher, psychologist or residential child care worker, for example).

(3) *The psychiatrist and delinquent children*

Although the psychiatric contribution to the treatment of delinquent children is limited, courts sometimes ask for psychiatric reports on children appearing before them. There are two main reasons for such requests:

(a) To ascertain whether the young person is fit to stand trial; and
(b) To gain understanding of the young person's mental state and delinquent behaviour and obtain guidance as to the best disposition of the case.

(a) Fitness to stand trial

Only a small minority of delinquent young people are suffering from a psychotic or other major psychiatric disorder such as might lead them to be unfit to be tried. Occasionally young people who are suffering from schizophrenia, a dementing process, severe mental retardation or some other major psychiatric disorder commit serious crimes for which they cannot, because of their mental state, be held responsible.

The criteria for fitness to stand trial differ from one jurisdiction to another. Generally, however, the two main points to be determined are whether the subject understood what he or she was doing when the crime was committed; and whether he or she was aware that it was wrong to do it. Thus the young man who commits murder on the basis of a firmly held delusional belief that God wished him to kill the victim because of the latter's sins, might be considered unaware that the act was wrong. Delinquent acts may also be committed in states of altered consciousness or confusion so that the person is unaware of what he or she is doing or has done. Difficult situations can arise when crimes are carried out while the person is under the influence of alcohol or drugs; the law applying to such cases also differs between jurisdictions.

(b) Guidance for the court

Many delinquents have long histories of behaviour difficulties, educational failure and emotional problems; their families are often disturbed and unstable and they may have been subject to abuse in one of the forms mentioned in Chapter 18. A psychiatric assessment may help clarify for the court how these circumstances have led to the current situation and what may be the best way of helping the young person overcome his or her problems.

(4) *The psychiatrist and divorce and custody proceedings*

With the rising marriage breakdown and divorce rates in most western countries, disputes over which divorced or separated parent should have custody of the child(ren) of the union are becoming more frequent. So, too, are issues of access to such children by non-custodial parents. While these issues usually arise in association with divorce proceedings, they may continue long after a divorce, perhaps as vicarious ways in which the parents maintain their relationship.

Some psychiatrists are reluctant to get involved in such cases since they can be time-consuming and they may not see them as the best use of scarce psychiatric time. Sometimes, however, custody and access issues arise in cases with which the psychiatrist is already dealing. When this happens involvement in the legal processes may be unavoidable.

In the past it has often happened that each party to a custody dispute has obtained the services of a psychiatrist or other mental health professional and has, almost inevitably, presented that person with a one-sided view of the situation. This usually led to a court hearing in which the psychiatric and other expert testimony was conflicting and the interests and points of view of the parents, rather than the best interests of the child, tended to be the focus of the proceedings.

A better plan is for the psychiatrist or other professional to be retained by both parties, each contributing to the fee (Chamberlain and Awad, 1979); or for them to be employed directly by the court or retained by a lawyer appointed to represent the child's interests. This should be followed by a process of 'family mediation' (Irving, 1981; Kaslow, 1984; see also *Basic Family Therapy* (Barker, 1986, Chapter 13)). This work is increasingly being done by 'family mediators' – specialized mental health professionals of various disciplines. They usually deal with all the outstanding issues between the parties, not just the custody of the children. Once an agreement is reached by this means, it is put into writing and used by the lawyers as a basis for a settlement to be confirmed by the court.

Ash and Guyer (1986) report on 200 court-ordered custody and visitation evaluations. The assessments were carried out in a specialized programme in a university teaching hospital. The result was that in only 11 per cent of cases did the judge have to make the decision. 'Highly adversarial' parents had reached agreement by the end of the evaluation in 18 per cent of cases, and the recommendations of the experts functioned 'as a bargaining chip which promoted resolution in 71 per cent of cases'. This approach is preferable to adversarial legal proceedings.

(5) Other issues

The 'other' issues mentioned above require a careful assessment of all the parties and issues involved. The child psychiatrist's primary concern must always be for the child patient(s) concerned and their welfare. The issue of children appearing as witnesses in court is a difficult one, especially when the proceedings concern sexual or other abuse of the child. If a parent is accused the child is in a very difficult, and usually highly conflictual, situation. Psychiatric help and support for the child, as well as advice to the court as to whether the child can act as a reliable witness or should be required to do so, may be needed. The handling of these cases is discussed by Nurcombe (1986) and Terr (1986).

(6) Malpractice issues

Malpractice suits are fortunately relatively uncommon in child psychiatric practice. Careful attention to the establishment of rapport, the maintenance of high professional ethical standards, the willingness to seek further opinions in difficult and doubtful cases, and the keeping of scrupulously accurate and up-to-date records are the best ways of reducing their likelihood.

Assessment in cases involving legal issues

If a child, a family or parents are being assessed primarily for legal as opposed to therapeutic purposes, it is essential to know precisely what questions are to be answered and what the relevant law is in the jurisdiction concerned. As Benedek (1983) points out, 'If the questions had to do with termination of parental rights, an evaluation which focuses on the mental status of the adolescent and his or her parent does not address the question of termination directly. It may be interesting reading but is not a useful document.' Thus the assessment of children and families in these cases, while using similar procedures to those described in Chapter 3, must pay special attention to the particular issues in dispute. In the case of termination of parental rights, for example, an excellent discussion of this difficult field is that of Schoettle (1984), who points out the many ethical issues and the role conflicts which these cases present for psychiatrists. Schoettle also provides an appendix in which he lists the 'basic aspects of the psychiatric evaluation' and the criteria which he believes should be considered when termination of parental rights is suggested.

There are some other special points about these assessments. The limits of confidentiality are quite different from those that apply in regular clinical practice. Reports must be sent to the lawyers concerned and they are usually seen by all parties to the dispute. They may also be produced as evidence in court and psychiatrists may be questioned under oath about any of the interviews they have had with the family members concerned. All this should be made clear to family members before the assessment is started.

In addition to the interviews recommended in Chapter 3, it may be appropriate to carry out individual assessments of the parents in cases in which the care or custody of the children are at issue. The parents' histories, mental states and personalities are often relevant factors in the matters which are in dispute.

The expert witness

Psychiatrists and their professional colleagues are usually used by the justice system as 'expert' witnesses. That is to say, the evidence they offer describes their professional opinion, as experts in their field, on the matters before the court. This stands in contrast to evidence of fact, when witnesses describe things they have seen or heard. Some factual evidence will be included in that provided by experts, for example behaviours they observed or bruises that were apparent when a child was interviewed. But giving an opinion on how those bruises might have been caused would constitute an expert opinion, provided on the basis of the witness' status as a physician.

In giving evidence and writing reports it is important to distinguish between what you have observed; your interpretation of your observations; what you have been told by those you have interviewed in the course of your assessment; and your professional opinion arising out of all the information available to you.

Writing reports for courts

The form and content of a court report will depend on the nature of the court proceedings, the purpose for which the psychiatric examination and report are intended, and local practice. Certain general principles are, however, widely applicable. These apply also to reports prepared for lawyers acting on behalf of clients; such reports may later be used in court or they may be factors which influence decisions on whether to go to court.

A report can never be better than the clinical assessment on which it is based. It is inadvisable to submit a definitive report with recommendations if the assessment has been incomplete or certain key figures have not been interviewed. It is usually important to obtain reports from the child's school and from any relevant social or other agencies. If it proves necessary to submit a report before assessment has been completed this should be emphasized in the report.

General points

(1) Write in plain, readily understandable language, avoiding the use of jargon. Remember that lawyers, magistrates and judges may not understand medical or psychological terms.

(2) Bear in mind that your report may be read out in court. It will probably be shown to all those involved with the case, including the young person whom it concerns. If the report contains essential information which should not be disclosed in court (which is not, for example, the best place for children to learn that they were born illegitimately or were adopted), this information should be plainly marked 'confidential'. It may be helpful to add a note explaining why the information should not be disclosed.

(3) Avoid referring to questions of guilt or innocence. These are for the court to decide.

(4) Do not quote information given by the child, the family or others as if it were fact. It is better to use phrases like 'She said that ...' or 'They described ...'

(5) Do not repeat information given in other reports which will be available to the court, unless you have a special reason for emphasizing certain points in those reports.

(6) Ensure that your meaning is expressed plainly and unambiguously, avoiding terms like 'immature' or 'borderline intelligence' unless you explain clearly what you mean by them. Rather than using phrases like 'He is immature' say, 'In his relationship with his parents and other family members he behaves more like a child four years younger than his true age'. Do not quote IQ figures; rather explain your view of the child's level of intellectual function and its significance in the case.

The precise form of the report is less important than ensuring that all relevant information is included. I have found the following scheme useful as a guide to setting out reports. Each numbered paragraph in this scheme can be the subject of a paragraph or, in a long report, a section with its own subheading.

(1) State the sources of information you have used, including any reports from schools, social agencies etc., you have read, as well as when, where and who you interviewed.

(2) Draw the court's attention to what you consider to be the important points in the history you obtained and that presented in other reports.

(3) Describe the results of your examination of the child, avoiding technical terms and explaining in language a lay person will

understand the nature and implications of any disorder which
you found to be present.
(4)   Present a formulation of the case in lay terms; include in this your
understanding of how the events which led to the child's
appearance in court have arisen. The formulation should take
into account all relevant emotional, biological, social, educational
and other factors.
(5)   Conclude with any recommendations for treatment or management you may have and make any other suggestions you believe
may be helpful to the court in deciding how to deal with the case.

This scheme may require modification when applied to some types
of court proceedings. For example, if the issue is whether the child
should be placed or retained in the care of the child welfare authorities,
the emphasis will probably be on the functioning of the family, the
parents' skills at parenting and the prospects of improving the care the
child gets in the family, rather than on the child's mental state.
Some other guidelines:

• Word your report in moderate terms.
• Avoid apportioning blame.
• Remember that you are giving guidance to the court, not telling it
  what to do.
• Use short words and sentences as far as possible.

Most children assessed for juvenile and family courts prove not to
have a major psychiatric condition such as a psychotic illness. The
psychiatrist's report, while useful to the court in ruling out such a
condition, may be of value mainly in the understanding it provides of
the case as a whole and in the suggestions it makes as to how child and
family may best be helped to overcome their problems.

An example of a Court Report

Child Psychiatry Clinic
Endhampton Hospital
Farr Road
Endhampton

Special Psychiatric Report on Andrew Barry Charles,
born 1.1.74 [Address].

Charged with theft of bicycles and breaking and entering.

I saw this boy on December 31 1986. He was accompanied to the clinic by his parents,
his brother Luke (born 7.7.72) and Miss Harris, the social worker concerned with his
case. I first interviewed the whole family, then saw Andrew on his own, following

which I met with the parents on their own. I then had a discussion with Miss Harris. I have also read Miss Harris' social report dated 26 December, 1986; the report prepared by Mr James, the principal of Andrew's school, dated 18 December, 1986; and that of the educational psychologist, Dr Keen, dated 15 December, 1986.

History

Miss Harris' report covers the main features of Andrew's development and the family situation. I think that the following aspects of the history are particularly relevant.

(1)   Andrew was born with a harelip and cleft palate which caused feeding difficulties and repeated admissions to hospital during his first two years of life. Although these deformities were in due course surgically repaired, the Court will notice that there is still some slight disfigurement.

(2)   Andrew's relationship to his mother seems never to have been a close one. The parents attribute this to his frequent admissions to hospital early in life and they say he was never a 'cuddly' baby like their other son, Luke.

(3)   Andrew had difficulty adjusting when he first went to school and he was late learning to read. His educational progress has always been poor and I note that the educational psychologist finds his reading skills to be about 2½ years behind the average for his age, though his intelligence is assessed as being in the average range.

(4)   Andrew's adjustment in the secondary school he entered at the start of this academic year has been particularly poor. Andrew is said to have played truant repeatedly and the offences with which he is charged are alleged to have been committed while he was missing from school in company with another child.

(5)   Andrew has been a lifelong bedwetter.

(6)   There have been difficulties in the relationship between the parents. Mr Charles left Mrs Charles 18 months ago to live with another woman but returned home 6 months later. The parents say that the relationship between them has now improved but they also indicated that tensions between them persist.

(7)   Miss Harris reports that the neighbourhood in which the family lives is one with a high level of delinquency.

Examination

My interviews with the whole family and with the parents lead me to believe there are considerable problems in the relationships between family members. The parents are far from being a united couple. Luke is a better looking and academically more successful boy than Andrew and seems to be favoured by both parents. During the family interview he repeatedly sided with the parents in criticizing Andrew. Neither parent had much that was positive to say about Andrew; yet they repeatedly expressed disagreement about how he should be handled and it seems they have been quite inconsistent in their dealings with him. The marital tensions were also evident and, during my interview with the parents alone, Mrs Charles expressed considerable resentment about having been 'deserted for 6 months', as she put it.

When I saw Andrew on his own I found him to be a friendly, cooperative and pleasant boy. He was well dressed and seemed well cared for. I noted the scar and slight facial deformity mentioned above.

Andrew spoke freely and answered questions readily. He gave me a full and apparently frank account of his family life and his situation at school. I detected no abnormality in his thought processes, nor did I find evidence of delusions, hallucinations or other abnormal mental processes. His mood was appropriate to the situation and the subjects under discussion.

Andrew tells me he has never liked school. He particularly dislikes his present school which is 'too big' and where he feels bullied and teased. He says he finds most school subjects difficult but he enjoys woodwork and games. According to Andrew another boy he met on the way to school suggested they skip school and steal the bicycles which are the subject of one of the charges. Andrew proved willing to talk freely about the events leading to his appearance in court. He expressed regret about what happened but I did not detect any deep feelings of guilt.

Andrew also spoke about the tensions in the home. He said he feels his parents favour his brother who has been more successful in school and has never been in trouble with the police. He is also sensitive about his bedwetting, a problem his brother does not have. He spoke about the period when his parents were separated during which, it seems from his account, his mother was quite depressed. I think he is concerned that his parents might again separate.

I found no abnormality on physical examination, apart from the facial abnormality mentioned above.

Opinion

In my opinion Andrew is not suffering from a major psychiatric disorder but there are emotional, educational and family factors which have contributed to his current difficulties. He seems to have a poor self-image, is not secure in his family relationships and is not getting much satisfaction in school. There also appear to be family relationship problems. Andrew seems to be very much the odd person out in this family and he is clearly the less favoured of the two children. His parents see him as a less attractive child, less well behaved and less successful at school than his brother with whom they openly compare him unfavourably. His congenital deformity, the consequent periods in hospital, the difficulty in feeding him and his bedwetting may all have militated against the development of a warm relationship between Andrew and his parents.

A further problem is the marital tension. This is probably a factor contributing to the inconsistent way Andrew is handled by the parents; his behavioural and school problems may also serve to divert attention from the marital problems. Lacking fulfilment at home and at school, Andrew seems to have become involved with other children who are prone to delinquent activities and among whom he can achieve more acceptance and status than he gets elsewhere.

On the positive side, Andrew has an engaging, friendly personality and relates well in the interview situation. He is of average intelligence and is seeking satisfying relationships. He would like to achieve his parents' approval, though he despairs of doing so. The parents acknowledge the difficulties in their relationship and expressed interest in receiving family therapy when I raised this possibility with them.

Recommendations

I believe that if Andrew's problems are to be resolved several issues must be addressed;

(1) The family difficulties need attention. Family therapy may be of help and the marital tensions might be the first of the issues to be tackled in treatment.

(2) Andrew's poor self-esteem and feelings of rejection and disapproval by his family are central issues. Any treatment plan must take these into account.

(3) Andrew needs help with his reading. I hope a plan to provide him with this can be worked out by Mr Keen in conjunction with the school staff. If Andrew's reading skills can be improved he should find school an easier place in which to achieve success.

(4) The bedwetting has not been properly investigated or treated. A physical cause is unlikely but should be excluded by appropriate investigations. These could be arranged by his family doctor. Treatment with an enuresis alarm might then be instituted and would have a good chance of clearing up this problem.

The successful implementation of the suggestions in paragraphs 1, 3 and 4 is likely to lead to improvement in Andrew's self-esteem; later some individual therapy with him may also be helpful. It may be possible to arrange for family therapy by a therapist at this clinic and I also suggested to Miss Harris another agency which might be able to help. Miss Harris is willing to set in motion suggestions 3 and 4 above.

I believe that Andrew's problems should be dealt with in the context of his home, family and neighbourhood school. It would not be helpful for him to be removed from home at present but a supervision order would enable Miss Harris to monitor progress and support the family in becoming and remaining involved in therapy.

Andrew will remain 'at risk' of getting into further trouble for some months after treatment starts, but I believe that if the measures I have suggested are implemented the chances of longterm improvement are good.

[Name, qualifications, appointment(s), signature and date]

Chapter 18

Child Abuse and Neglect

Children may be abused in various ways, and the last few decades have seen increasing awareness of these. Child abuse is not a new phenomenon, however. Lynch (1985) points out that it is alluded to in literature as far back as the second century AD. The London Society for the Prevention of Cruelty to Children dealt with 762 cases in the three years following its foundation in 1884. These comprised assaults (333), starvations (81), dangerous neglect (130), desertions (30), cruel exposure to excite sympathy (70), other wrongs (116), and deaths (25). 132 cases, many 'almost incredible' were taken to court; there were 120 convictions (Lynch, 1985). Charles Dickens, in his novels, described graphically the plight of many children in Victorian days.

In 1946 Caffey, a radiologist, described cases of multiple fractures of the long bones in association with subdural haematomas in children. He suggested that the fractures were due to inflicted trauma, and it has since been established that physically abused children often show X-ray evidence of old fractures. Kempe *et al.* (1962) coined the term 'battered child syndrome'. This seemed to capture the imagination of the medical profession and led to increased interest in and recognition of what has also been called 'child abuse' or 'non-accidental injury in children' (Scott, 1977).

In addition to abuse causing identifiable physical injury, other forms are recognized. These include neglect, which seems to have existed from time immemorial, and sexual and emotional abuse.

Child abuse is important to psychiatrists because of its role in the development of psychiatric problems in abused children. It is frequently associated with other family problems; and other members of the·families often suffer from serious psychiatric, including personality, disorders.

The incidence of child abuse

Incidence figures depend on the definition of child abuse used, the population studied, the age range of the children and the sources from which information is gathered. Studies of severe abuse, especially fatal cases, are more likely to provide results that reflect the true incidence of such abuse; many milder cases go undetected or unreported so that it is hard to obtain accurate data on their incidence. Sexual abuse is often hidden within families; it may not be revealed until the victim speaks of it in later life. This may happen during psychotherapy or in the course of the investigation of another problem. Emotional abuse is less easy to detect than physical injury. It is also harder to define.

Baldwin and Oliver (1975) studied severe child abuse involving children under 5 in north-east Wiltshire, England, over a 7-year period. The last $1\frac{1}{2}$ years were studied prospectively, the others retrospectively. Strict criteria for abuse were used. In the prospective study a rate of abuse of nearly 1 per thousand was found for the first 3 years of life; this was 2.6 times the rate found in the retrospective study. There were 4 deaths in the retrospective study and 2 in the prospective. 225 separate incidences of abuse were recorded in 38 children, a mean of 5.9 per child, with a range of 1 to 23. Both studies probably underestimated the true incidence because they aimed to cover only severe cases. In Britain, increasing numbers of physically injured children are being reported to the National Society for the Prevention of Cruelty to Children. In 1979 the rate was 0.43 per thousand children and by 1982 it had risen to 0.63 per thousand (Creighton, 1985). The increase in reported cases does not necessarily mean that the true incidence is rising; it may be due to increasing awareness of the problem by professionals concerned with children and more complete reporting. All reported figures are likely to be underestimates, since inevitably some cases go undetected and/or unreported.

In the USA the National Centre for Child Abuse and Neglect (1981) estimated, on the basis of a study of a representative sample of the US population, that 1,151,600 cases of abuse and neglect were suspected by professionals in the period May 1979 to April 1980. Of these, 652,000 met their strict criteria of abuse and neglect.

It is particularly difficult to discover the frequency with which the sexual abuse, neglect and emotional abuse of children occur. One British study reported that 10 per cent of a nationally representative sample of men and women reported that they had been sexually abused before the age of 16. For women the rate was 12 per cent, for men 8 per cent. Some studies have yielded much higher rates but the criteria used have generally been looser. Neglect is certainly widespread but its prevalence depends on the definition used; moreover, the socially accepted norms for the care of children vary in different cultures.

Child abuse is not confined to the western world, although

statistical data on its incidence elsewhere are scarce. Cultural standards vary greatly; practices such as the severe physical punishment of
children are acceptable in some societies, whereas in others they would
be considered abusive.

The causes of child abuse

The etiology of child abuse is complex. As Schmidt and Eldridge (1986,
page 269) put it:

> 'Child maltreatment is a multiply-determined phenomenon that
> does not lend itself to definitive explanations. The parent, the child,
> the circumstances, and the environment all contribute to the
> occurrence of maltreatment.'

Parental factors

Many adults who abuse children have themselves been abused during
childhood. Their unconscious model of parenthood is a violent one and
they instinctively see physical punishment as the preferred way of
dealing with undesired behaviour in children. On the other hand
abuse is not inevitably transmitted from one generation to the next;
many factors may diminish the likelihood of this happening (Kaufman
and Zigler, 1987).

Abusing adults, not all of whom are parents, sometimes have
serious personality disorders. They may lack adequate impulse control
and have difficulty showing children love in affectionate, caring ways.
The abuse may occur when the abuser is under the influence of alcohol
or other drugs, which may further impair impulse control.

Neglectful and abusive parents often have problems in other areas
of their lives. Their social and vocational skills may be poor, their
intelligence may be low and they may have difficulty with the
instrumental tasks of everyday living. Nevertheless abuse also occurs
in families with good incomes and middle class respectability, though
it is probably less frequent in families that function well in instrumental ways.

Child factors

We have seen that children vary in their temperaments. Some are
easier to rear than others and sometimes there is a serious clash of
temperaments between child and parents – or other adults. Some

children find they only get parental attention when they behave in provocative ways, so that they learn patterns of behaviour which stimulate their abusively prone parents to acts of violence, emotional abuse or incest. Abused children often seem to have poor self-images; they may consider themselves worthy of nothing more than the treatment they receive, though this may be a consequence of abuse as well as a contributory factor. Children with handicaps or disabilities of various sorts may be at increased risk of abuse; in individual cases this sometimes seems to be the case, but how far it is generally true is unclear (White *et al.*, 1987).

Interactional, family and social factors

Child maltreatment seems often to have its origins in the early relationship between parent and child, that is the period during which attachment is normally developed and consolidated. Disorders of attachment, as discussed in Chapter 14, may increase the chances of abuse occurring (Schmidt and Eldridge, 1986). Various other family problems may be found in association with child abuse. An extreme example is the extended family network described by Oliver and Buchanan (1979). Starting with a mentally retarded young woman and the six men she successively lived with, these authors studied her children and their descendents. In all, 40 members of the family, and their spouses or partners, were investigated. There was revealed a tragic saga, transmitted from generation to generation, of physical neglect, assaults on the children with hammers or knives, incest, prostitution (sometimes taught to the children by the parents), burns causing persisting poker marks, bites, beatings and hair pullings. While families as severely dysfunctional as this one are relatively uncommon, they do exist and there are many others with problems that differ only in degree. Tonge *et al.* (1975), in their controlled study of 33 problem families, found that neglect and poor care of the children was much commoner in these families than in the comparison families they studied.

Child abuse is not confined to families and children living at home. It may occur at the institutional level, as in day care centres, schools, courts, child care agencies, welfare departments and correctional and other residential settings. Gil (1975) suggests that it may also occur at a third level, that of society at large, which allows 'millions of children in our society' to live in poverty and to be denied adequate nutrition, health care, education, housing and neighbourhood conditions generally. These latter problems are perhaps sociological ones, rather than those of individuals or family groups.

Clinical considerations

Only rarely do families come asking for help because they are abusing their children. Physically abused children are often brought to hospital emergency departments, perhaps with a story that they have fallen downstairs, out of bed or against an item of furniture or household appliance. The tales told by parents can be detailed and imaginative, but they are usually inconsistent and nearly always incompatible with the nature of the child's injuries. Moreover, a full and careful examination of the child usually reveals evidence of previous injury.

Suspected child abuse is sometimes reported to child welfare agencies by neighbours or relatives, who may have heard the child screaming in pain or have observed injuries. Other cases come to notice at school, in day care centres or during routine physical examinations. The injuries may consist of bruising of any degree of severity, fractures, injury to internal organs, perhaps with internal bleeding, intracranial haemorrhage with consequent damage to the brain, or loss of vision due to eye injuries. Death has been reported in various surveys as occurring in from 1 per cent to 23 per cent of cases (Scott, 1977).

Physical abuse may be associated with neglect or emotional abuse. Abused children may be malnourished and ill-cared for. Medical attention may not be sought when it is needed. Both physical and psychological development may be adversely affected. Some physically abused children seem well cared for in other ways; satisfactory general physical care may be interrupted by episodes of parental rage, during which the child is injured. Some abusing parents adopt an offhand, uncaring attitude and show a lack of concern about the child's condition. They may be reluctant to accept admission to hospital or investigation for their child, and may have been to many different hospitals. Evidence may emerge of such other family problems as marital conflict or the abuse of alcohol or other drugs.

Abused children tend to have difficulty enjoying themselves, behaviour problems, withdrawal, oppositional behaviour, hypervigilance, compulsive behaviour, a pseudo-adult manner and learning problems at school (Martin and Beezley, 1977). Low self-esteem seems to characterize both the children and their mothers (Oates *et al.*, 1985; Oates and Forrest, 1986). In infants language development may be delayed (Allen and Wasserman, 1985). Abused children may appear fearful towards their parents, perhaps getting upset when they hear father returning home; and they may show 'reversed caring' by anxiously looking out for their parents' needs, offering mother one of her cigarettes and so on. In severe cases the child may appear obviously ill-cared for, dirty, undernourished or dehydrated.

Sexual abuse may occur in the absence of other forms of abuse or neglect and can continue for long periods undetected. It often happens within the family. The sexual abuse of girls occurs more frequently than that of boys; it may consist of anything from fondling of the child's breasts or genitals to vaginal or anal intercourse. Another form of sexual abuse is the sexual exploitation of children in pornographic movies, videotapes and photographs. The abuser is often someone known to the child, frequently a family member. Parents, stepparents and foster parents are responsible in many instances. The incest taboo which operates in many natural families seems often to be less strong in reconstituted families, a situation which may lead to stepfather-daughter incest. Sexual abuse by someone outside the family or the family's intimate circle of friends is likely to be reported sooner and thus to come to attention more quickly.

Apart from physical signs of damage in the genital area and evidence of sexually acquired disease, sexual abuse may be suspected if the child shows seductive behaviour, sexual knowledge inappropriate for his or her age, severe psychosomatic or acting-out behaviour (especially non-epileptic seizures or running away) or sexually precocious behaviour. Self-destructive behaviour in the absence of other stress, or pregnancy in a young teenager, especially if the father is not named, are other ways in which sexual abuse may present.

Ghent *et al.* (1985) provide useful guidelines in detecting physical and sexual abuse.

Emotional abuse

Many children's emotional and other psychological needs are not adequately met in their families. How severe the family's failure to meet its children's needs must be to justify use of the term 'emotional abuse' is an arbitrary judgment, although extreme cases are easily identified. The term could be applied to many children with psychiatric disorders.

Many jurisdictions in the western world have enacted laws defining emotional abuse. The aim is to have a legal basis for intervention in cases in which there is no obvious physical abuse or neglect but there is gross failure to meet children's psychological needs. An example of such legislation is contained in the Child Welfare Act of the Canadian province of Alberta (Government of Alberta, 1984), which uses the term emotional 'injury' rather than 'abuse'. It states that a child is emotionally injured

(i)   if there is substantial and observable impairment of the child's mental or emotional functioning that is evidenced by a mental or behavioural disorder, including anxiety, depression, withdrawal, aggression or delayed development, and

(ii)   there are reasonable and probable grounds to believe that the emotional injury is the result of
   (a)   rejection,
   (b)   deprivation of affection or cognitive stimulation,
   (c)   exposure to domestic violence or severe domestic dishar-mony, or
   (d)   inappropriate criticism, threats, humiliation, accusations or expectations of or towards the child, or
   (e)   the mental or emotional condition of the guardian of the child or chronic alcohol or drug abuse by anyone living in the same residence as the child.

Garbarino *et al.* (1986) use the term 'psychologically battered child'. They define five forms of 'psychically destructive' behaviour:

- Rejecting: the adult refuses to acknowledge the child's worth and the legitimacy of the child's needs.
- Isolating: the child is cut off by the adult from normal social experiences, prevented from forming friendships and made to believe he or she is alone in the world.
- Terrorizing: the child is verbally assaulted by the adult who creates a climate of fear, bullies and frightens the child, and leads the child to believe the world is capricious and hostile.
- Ignoring: the adult deprives the child of needed stimulation and fails to respond in suitable ways, stifling emotional growth and intellectual development.
- Corrupting: the child is 'mis-socialized', being stimulated to engage in destructive antisocial behaviour and reinforced in such deviant behaviour.

Garbarino and his co-authors (1986) provide examples of how each of the above types of behaviour by adults may affect children at different stages of development. In extreme cases the syndrome of 'non-organic failure to thrive' (Bullard *et al.*, 1967) may result. 'Deprivation dwarfism' (Silver and Finkelstein, 1967; Powell *et al.*, 1967) is another term that has been used for growth failure related to adverse rearing experiences. In most instances, however, the child's growth and physical condition are within normal limits but there are problems of psychological development and adjustment. These may be poor self-esteem, unresolved anger or almost any of the psychiatric syndromes described elsewhere in this book, the main exceptions being those of predominantly organic origin. Conduct disorders, chronic anxiety disorders and academic failure are common consequences; and as the children grow older some come to meet the criteria for personality disorders.

Many parents who fail to meet their children's emotional needs have themselves experienced poor parenting as children. Covitz (1986) refers to emotional child abuse as 'the family curse', handed down from generation to generation. He points out that it is what the parents are and do, rather than what they tell their children, that are most important. He describes three 'abusive styles of parenting', labelling these 'the inadequate parent', 'the devouring parent' and 'the tyrannical parent'. Later in his book he suggests various approaches to breaking the intergenerational cycle of emotional abuse. Many children's behavioural, emotional or physical symptoms may be seen as danger signals – signs that their needs are not being met and opportunities for intervention.

Assessment and treatment

Children who have been abused, and their families, should be assessed and treated using the principles and approaches set out elsewhere in this book. There are, however, certain special points to be borne in mind in dealing with these families. Mature clinical judgment and a patient, painstaking and empathic approach are essential. These families tend to be especially defensive. They are often aware that they may face criminal charges and risk having their children removed from their care against their wishes.

A physical examination should be carried out when physical or sexual abuse is suspected. It should include examination of the genitals, and X-rays and other special investigations as indicated.

In most jurisdictions the law requires that established or suspected child abuse be reported to the appropriate authorities. It is usually better to deal with the responsible child welfare agency, the staff of which make the necessary liaison with the police.

Once abuse has come to light, the child welfare agency staff are responsible for the immediate welfare of the child; they must decide whether to remove the child from the care of the parents or guardians. Admission to hospital and medical or surgical treatment may be necessary. Meanwhile investigation of the family is carried out, usually by a social worker from the child welfare agency. At this stage psychiatric help may be sought, either for the whole family or for one or more members.

Evidence of abuse, or reason to suspect it, may emerge during the psychiatric assessment of a child or family. In many jurisdictions the person discovering or suspecting the abuse then has a legal obligation to report the facts or suspicions to the appropriate statutory agency. In that case, the family should be told that the report is being made. In such situations I explain to the family members my legal obligations and assure them of my willingness to continue to offer them help. If the family chooses to remain under my psychiatric care it is often possible for me to act as its advocate in dealings with the child welfare agency.

In working with abusive families it is important to adopt an empathic, non-punitive attitude, however distressing you may find the situation. It can be hard to remain objective and non-judgmental when one is faced with parents who have gravely physically injured or sexually abused a child. Nevertheless, it is unhelpful to express the anger or outrage we may feel when confronted with such situations; to do so militates against forming therapeutic relationships. It is important also not to get emotionally over-involved. Many child abusers are plausible, attractive, even charming people. We may come to feel sorry for them because of the hard and deprived lives they have led, or because they have themselves been subject to abuse as children. They need skilled treatment rather than sympathy, however. They may be expert at manipulating social agencies and authority figures, for example by suggesting that their behaviour and attitudes are changing, thus flattering the therapist, when there has been no real change. The naive therapist can easily be deceived.

It is not necessarily helpful to extract a confession from parents or other relatives who have abused children. Sometimes it may be enough to tell them that the child's injuries are not compatible with the story given. Investigation and treatment can then proceed on the basis of an unspoken understanding of the parents' (or other relatives') part in the problem.

The situation is different when a child has been abused by someone outside the family. In such cases the family is usually united in condemnation of the perpetrator and cooperates actively in the investigation and treatment of the case. There can nevertheless be great emotional repercussions in the family; there may be guilt feelings, perhaps denied, on the part of the parents for allowing their child to be in a position to be abused. Sometimes pre-existing family problems are brought to light by an episode of abuse by an outsider.

Many sexually abused children are quite young. Mian *et al.* (1986) report that one-third of such children presenting to an acute care hospital were aged 6 or less. In investigating sexual abuse, especially in young children, the use of 'sexually anatomically correct' dolls has been found helpful. The child is interviewed in a playroom containing, among other items, a series of dolls representing adults and children of both sexes. During the course of the interview the child is given the opportunity to play with the dolls and talk about them. The procedure has not been standardized and more information is needed on the responses of normal children than is currently available, but White *et al.* (1986) have described a procedure for the use of these dolls. It consists of five parts:

- Identification of the dolls by sex and name.
- Assessment of the child's knowledge of the body parts, sexual and non-sexual, by name and function.
- 'Private part knowledge'.
- 'Abuse evaluation', consisting of asking the child about being touched, hurt, having secrets, receiving threats and other items which might indicate sexual abuse.
- 'Abuse elaboration', in which any 'positive answers' to the questions in the previous stage are followed up.

The treatment needed by abused children and their families depends on the type and duration of the abuse, and whether the abuse is intrafamilial or is committed by a stranger. Therapy for the whole family may be needed when the abuse is intrafamilial; in such cases there often prove to be serious family system problems. Individual psychotherapy may be needed by children who have been abused, epecially when there has been a longstanding incestuous relationship with a parent. Jones (1986) provides a helpful discussion of the use of individual psychotherapy in the treatment of sexually abused children.

Sometimes group therapy, in which children are treated along with others who have been similarly abused, proves more helpful than individual therapy. Abusive parents are also frequently in need of psychiatric help; not only may they have established personality disorders, but they may be suffering from depression, anxiety disorders, alcoholism or the effects of drug abuse, all of which may respond to treatment.

When the abuser is someone outside the family circle the main need may be for individual or group psychotherapy with the child. The parents may need guidance in how to deal with the child and help in dealing with their own feelings.

The treatment of abusive families should be a multidisciplinary process. Close cooperation between whoever is providing therapy for the family members and the child welfare authorities, especially the social worker dealing with the family, greatly improves the chances of success. The police and the courts may also be involved, and sometimes the possibility of legal action against abusive parents or other relatives is retained with the objective of increasing the family members' motivation for treatment. This may be achieved by postponing court proceedings, or sentence, while the effects of therapy, and the family's or the parents' involvement, are monitored. Alternatively an abusing adult may be placed on probation with a condition that he or she undergoes treatment. A preferable situation is that in which the family voluntarily and willingly enters therapy; unfortunately many families do not do this.

Sometimes it is necessary to remove abused children from their homes. This can be temporary while treatment is instituted or, if treatment is refused or fails, it may be permanent. In cases of parent-child (it is most often father-daughter or father-stepdaughter) incest it may be more appropriate to arrange for the parent's removal to another setting, perhaps a treatment one. Separation of child and parents may not be harmful if it is managed properly and is part of a long-term plan of treatment and rehabilitation for the whole family. Frequent episodes of removal of abused or neglected children, with their periodic return, which occurs too frequently in many jurisdictions, should be avoided. The treatment of children who have been victims of incest in discussed by Boatman *et al.* (1981).

In cases of emotional abuse treatment should be addressed to rectifying the underlying family problems. The disorders in the children themselves should be treated as set out in the respective chapters of this book. The approach of Kirschner and Kirschner (1986) is often productive in these cases.

Treatment of abused children and their families is often a long and difficult process, requiring skilled personnel, close cooperation between therapists and agencies and careful long-term planning. Prevention is much to be preferred and there is reason to believe that a preventive health service for young children and their families, with frequent visits by nurses or other workers is helpful (Wynn, 1974).

Outcome

The physical consequences that may result from child abuse include permanent mental retardation, blindness, cerebral palsy and other forms of physical damage or deformity. The psychological consequences are harder to define but include poor self-image, personality and behaviour problems, and delayed development in various areas of functioning. In many cases it is difficult to separate the effects of physical or sexual abuse from those of other adverse circumstances. Children are rarely abused in healthy, well-functioning families and factors other than the abuse *per se* probably contribute to the poor outcomes reported in many studies (Lynch, 1978; Hensey *et al.*, 1983; Oates, 1984). Elmer (1986) found, in a comparative study of three groups of infants, two of them abused, that the effects of socioeconomic status were more marked than those of abuse. Oates (1984) compared the personality development of abused children with controls matched for age, sex, ethnic group and social class. On follow-up several years later the abused children were found to have fewer friends, lower self-esteem and more behavioural disturbance, and to be less ambitious than the controls.

Sexual abuse can lead to problems of psychosexual adjustment later in life; it seems to be associated with runaway behaviour, anxiety and suicidal behaviour in adolescents (McCormack *et al.*, 1986).

Chapter 19

The Treatment of Child Psychiatric Disorders

The formulation of each particular case (see also Chapter 3) should be the basis of the treatment plan. The formulation should be kept under review and modified as new information comes to light and the response to the treatments used is observed. Any of the following treatments may be useful:

- Individual psychotherapy.
- Therapy or counselling for the parents.
- Family therapy.
- Group therapy for children or parents.
- Behaviour therapy.
- Hypnotherapy.
- Pharmacotherapy.
- Daypatient treatment.
- Inpatient treatment.
- Alternative families.
- Educational measures.
- Speech therapy.
- Other measures, including removal from parental care.

Because child psychiatric disorders usually have multiple causes, it is often necessary to use more than one treatment.

Setting treatment goals

We considered how to define the goals of treatment in Chapter 3. The goals should be reviewed again before therapy starts. Therapist and patient(s) should be agreed on how things will be when the problems which treatment is to address are resolved. With children, especially younger ones, it will usually be the parents who are mainly involved in this process; but with older children, and especially adolescents, the patients themselves should also agree on the desired outcome. All the points in the section on 'defining the desired outcome' in Chapter 3 should be carefully reconsidered at this stage.

Individual psychotherapy

The essence of individual psychotherapy is the development of a relationship between therapist and patient (or client), in the context of which change in some aspect(s) of the patient's mental state is promoted. Every contact between child and therapist is of emotional significance and may be either therapeutic or antitherapeutic. Although there are many schools of psychotherapy, and great differences between some of them, certain principles apply. These are important even when psychotherapy is not the specific treatment being employed:

(1) Do not criticise the child. Children coming for psychiatric treatment must be accepted as they are. If a child's symptoms are expressions of repressed anxiety or hostility, disapproving attitudes in the therapist are likely to cause the anxiety or hostility to worsen. Acceptance of children does not imply the approval of all they do; child and therapist will often be able to agree on aspects of the child's behaviour, feelings or attitudes that need to change.

(2) Remember that most children do not come for treatment of their own accord. They are brought by others who are worried or concerned, or perhaps angry with them. They may arrive with the expectation that they will meet someone who is going to have similar feelings for them. Some parents even tell their children to expect 'a good talking to'; in such cases the therapist may have to work hard to gain the child's confidence, a process which may take several interviews.

(3) Do not plunge straight into a discussion of the symptoms, unless these are brought up by the child.

(4) Try to understand the child's feelings and point of view. It is only when there is such understanding between child and therapist that free communication, which is a prerequisite to successful treatment, becomes possible. The child should come to see the therapist as someone who is concerned about him or her. This will not prevent the expression of angry or other negative feelings, in fact when the child has a need to express such feelings it will help facilitate this. The experience of giving vent to negative feelings, or revealing 'bad' things about oneself and not being rejected, lectured or criticized as a result, can be therapeutic.

(5) Remember that, while the free expression of feelings is to be encouraged, limits have to be set in a psychotherapeutic interview, as in other situations. For example, physically hurting the therapist, dangerous activities like playing with live electrical

fittings, or damaging the fabric of the room and its furnishings and equipment cannot be allowed. It is a good plan to outline the limits of what is permissible during therapy in the first session. Limits should be imposed on the basis of 'I can't allow you to do that', and with an explanation why. The child's desire to carry out the activity should be acknowledged and accepted, however.

The techniques and application of psychotherapy can only be learned by working with children under supervision, though reading texts on the subject can be a useful adjunct. Before embarking on psychotherapy it is necessary to have a plan and to be clear what the therapy is aiming to achieve. These aims should have been set out in the diagnostic formulation.

There are many different types of psychotherapy, with varying aims, procedures and theoretical bases. 'Supportive therapy' aims at helping the patient to cope better with the current situation. It may be applicable when a child faces an acute or severe stress which is likely to subside in the course of time, for example the illness or admission to hospital of a parent or the grief reaction following a bereavement. It may also be needed when the stress is a continuing one which cannot easily be removed, though ideally treatment enables the child to live with the stressful situation without the need for therapy.

Quite different, and in some respects at the opposite end of the therapeutic spectrum, is psychoanalysis. This aims to bring about a radical change in the patient's emotional state and reactions. It is a highly specialized treatment for which long and rigorous training is necessary. It can involve hour-long treatment sessions up to five days a week over a period of many months or even years, so that even when trained psychoanalysts are available the number of patients they can treat is limited. The objective of the therapy is to explore fully the subject's unconscious life and fantasies, dealing with any problems found in the context of the relationship between patient and therapist. Child analysis is a specialized field in which Anna Freud (1966; 1972) and Melanie Klein (1932) were pioneers.

Between supportive psychotherapy and psychoanalysis there is a range of psychotherapies designed to achieve more limited goals than analysis or to deal with particular aspects of the subject's life. Psychoanalysis has helped us understand emotional disorders and mental processes but it is of limited value as a practical treatment for child psychiatric disorders. Its concepts have, however, contributed to the practice of psychotherapy generally.

Techniques of psychotherapy vary widely, depending on the theoretical orientation of the therapist, the treatment goals and the patient's age. Some therapists make extensive use of verbal interpretation of the child's statements and play, while others make little or no use of interpretation. Some therapists take more active roles than others. As a general rule, the younger the child the more contact has to be through the medium of play, though some children as young as three or four talk freely. How freely they communicate depends on their level of cognitive, especially language, development and their emotional state.

Common to all forms of psychotherapy with children are:

- The development of a working relationship with the child.
- An appraisal of the feelings and ideas the child expresses in the context of the relationship.
- The use of the relationship to help resolve the child's problems.

How does the treatment help the child? The first level of help is simply the process of accepting the child's feelings. We often feel better after we have spoken to an accepting and understanding person about things that are worrying us or which are sources of anger or shame for us. This applies equally to disturbed children. It accounts for the considerable improvement that sometimes follows a single interview, even one intended primarily as diagnostic. For some children it is a new experience to be listened to and given the full attention of an accepting adult. When such children find that their revelations do not shock, worry or provoke expressions of outrage in the therapist, this can be a considerable relief to them.

In many cases it is not sufficient for children simply to express their feelings and have them accepted by the therapist. There has also to be emotional interchange with the child over a period of time. In these emotional transactions children often manifest behaviour and attitudes similar to those they show towards their parents or other key figures in their lives. The feelings and behaviours which emerge can be worked through in the context of the therapist/child relationship. This, too, enables some children to overcome their problems.

At the next level, interpretation is added to the interchange between therapist and child. This aims to put the problems and conflicts into words, so helping the child to understand them. Interpretations are usually withheld until the meaning of a child's play or talk is clear. It is inadvisable to offer speculative interpretations, though incorrect ones may be ignored or rejected.

All the above therapy methods are based on the psychodynamic view of psychiatric disorders. With the possible exception of supportive therapy, they all aim to use the therapist/child relationship to resolve the postulated repressed conflicts which are held to be responsible for the child's symptoms. This is the essence of the methods of such therapists as Allen (1942), Maclay (1970) and Adams

(1982). Therapy may also be based on other theoretical ideas. These include family systems theory, learning theory and the principles of 'state-dependent learning, memory and behaviour' (Rossi 1986a; 1986b).

'Strategic' methods may also be used in individual therapy. These are essentially pragmatic (Cade, 1980), though they are based on the general belief that the problems of individuals are related to the operation of repetitive behavioural sequences between them and others. Intervening to change these repetitive behaviours is the essence of much strategic therapy. Strategic methods include 'reframing', changing the sequences of behaviours, giving paradoxical directives and offering therapeutic metaphors.

The term 'reframing' refers to the giving of a different meaning to something; this may be a symptom, a repetitive behaviour pattern or a belief system. A clinically useful form of reframing is 'positive connotation', which redefines the intent behind a behaviour. For example, the behaviour of a parent who physically abuses a child might be reframed as comprising a well-intentioned attempt to discipline the child and eliminate antisocial behaviours. The actual behaviour is not commended or approved of but the intent behind it is. Therapy then becomes a matter of finding better, socially acceptable ways of achieving the same ends.

Frankl (1960) pioneered the use of what he called 'paradoxical intention' for problems which worsened as the patient struggled to resist or counter the symptoms. He encouraged his patients to bring on or increase their symptoms, but in a humorous context and always in a way which enabled them to distance themselves from the symptoms. Rapid change and relief from symptoms can occur by this means (Barker, 1981; Weeks and L'Abate, 1982).

Therapeutic metaphors are stories related in some way to the patient's situation. They may serve various therapeutic objectives, for example reframing problem behaviours, helping patients find within themselves resources they have not been using, and suggesting solutions to challenges the patients may face. They are especially suited for use with children who are generally receptive to fairy tales and other types of story. Several books are available on metaphorical approaches to therapy (Barker, 1985; Wallas, 1985: Mills and Crowley, 1986).

Psychotherapy can only be learned through supervised clinical experience, though background reading can be helpful. In addition to the references mentioned above, *Play Therapy* (Landreth, 1982), which contains contributions by 31 authors, and *Psychotherapy with Adolescent Girls* (Lamb, 1986) are good sources of information. The latter contains a selective annotated bibliography. Rossman (1985) describes well what therapy with a severely disturbed adolescent may involve.

Therapy or counselling for parents

It is seldom sufficient to provide psychotherapy, or any other treatment, for the child and leave the parents uninvolved. Either counselling concerning their child's disorder and its treatment – often referred to as 'casework' – or psychotherapy for the parents themselves may be needed.

In parent counselling or casework 'the emphasis is clearly and constantly on the child as patient' (Kraemer, 1987). The aim is to enable the parents to understand the child's problems, the factors that have led to them and those that are contributing to their continuation. This will include the parts the parents have played. It is important to keep the parents interested and involved; there is always a danger, especially when the treatment extends over a long period, of their contracting out of the therapy process. They may then leave it to the therapist to 'fix' the child who, they expect, will in due course be returned to them, rather like a car that has been repaired in a garage.

Kraemer (1987) describes the caseworker as 'educator, adviser, supporter, manager and, sometimes, psychotherapist'. The child's relationship with the parents is the main focus of the work. The past history of the child and family relationships generally, as well as the current situation in the home, at school and in the treatment setting are all subjects that may be discussed. Casework may also include the promotion of environmental change, for example by mobilizing community resources (play groups, daycare centres, youth groups and the like) and community workers (youth leaders, school counsellors, credit counsellors and so forth) when a family is in need of help from them.

The borderline between casework and psychotherapy is ill-defined but it is crossed when therapy starts to focus on the parent and his or her emotional problems and mental state. The parents of many children referred for psychiatric assessment and treatment suffer from psychiatric problems of their own; for some of these individual psychotherapy may be needed. The relevance of the parents' psychiatric problems to the child's disorder will vary; in many cases the psychiatric problems of the parent(s) have been significant factors in the genesis and/or maintenance of the child's problems. In any event resolution or alleviation of parental problems is likely to be of benefit to the family as a whole, as well as to all the children in it. The skills required for casework/counselling are different from those required for individual therapy, so that sometimes referral to a different therapist will be necessary when the focus of treatment changes.

Occasionally the main focus of treatment will be on the parent(s) and the child will be involved in therapy very little or not at all. These cases are those in which, although the child's symptoms are presented as the main problem, investigation reveals that these are secondary to the parents' psychiatric problems. For example, to the depressed parent a child's behaviour may seem intolerably bad, although objectively it may not seem so and the parent could handle it without outside help if not depressed.

Kraemer (1987) provides an overview of the respective places of casework and psychotherapy in working with the parents of disturbed children, and reviews the relevant literature.

Family therapy

The focus of the family therapist is the family system. Family therapy may be the best treatment when a child's symptoms are features of a dysfunctional family system. Many children's psychiatric problems are best understood in this way, though determining which ones is an inexact science; in practice the philosophy and beliefs of the therapist are also major factors influencing the treatment recommendations that are made in particular cases. The indications for family therapy, and the various possible approaches to the treatment of families, are discussed more fully in *Basic Family Therapy* (Barker, 1986).

While the focus of family therapy is the family group rather than any of the individual members, this does not necessarily mean that all members of the family are seen at each therapy session. In many instances they will be, but changes in family systems can often be brought about by seeing family subsystems, for example the parents, the children or even single members, separately. The essential point is that it is the *functioning of the system* – that is, the way the family members interrelate and communicate – that is primarily being addressed, not the mental states of individual family members. The expectation is that changes in the family system will lead to the resolution or amelioration of the presenting problems.

In family therapy the therapist first joins the family – that is, enters into communication and establishes rapport with its members. This is usually done in the course of one or more meetings with the whole family group. This leads to an assessment of the way the family functions and to hypotheses about how the therapist may help promote change. Useful models of family functioning are the structural model of Minuchin (1974; Minuchin and Fishman, 1981), the

McMaster Model of Family Functioning (Epstein *et al.*, 1978) and the closely related Process Model (Steinhauer, *et al.*, 1984). Several other models are discussed in *Basic Family Therapy* (Barker, 1986). Interventions are then offered to the family, based on an understanding of how it functions and what may promote the desired changes.

The types of intervention used differ, depending upon therapists' theoretical models and philosphies. They may be classified into direct and indirect, or 'strategic', ones. The extent to which they are systemic, that is addressed to the system as a whole rather than to a part or parts of it, also varies. To be family therapy interventions at all, however, they must be in some degree systemic.

Direct interventions consist of offering the family alternative ways of functioning, usually by means of straightforward injunctions to do things differently or in different sequences. In some families this can be effective and adequate treatment but in many it is insufficient and a strategy has to be employed to promote change in a more subtle and, usually, indirect way. Strategic methods of therapy, which as we have seen may be used with individuals as well as with family groups, include reframing and positive connotation; metaphorical communication; giving paradoxical directives; prescribing rituals and tasks; declaring therapeutic impotence; prescribing interminable therapy; employing humour; using a consultation group as a 'Greek chorus'; offering split opinions as to the best course of action; and staging a debate about the family in front of it. Both direct and strategic approaches are considered in more depth in *Basic Family Therapy* (Barker, 1986). To learn to use them supervised experience is essential.

Group therapy

Children or the parents of disturbed children may be treated in groups (Ginott, 1961; Yalom; 1975). Various approaches to group therapy are possible but the essence of the process is to enable group members to help each other through their interaction and the modelling they can provide for each other. The active, outgoing child can act as a model for the quiet, inhibited one and *vice versa*. Group therapy may be particularly valuable for children who have difficulty with peer relationships.

Group therapy with younger children usually involves much use of play, while with adolescents discussion predominates, with the problems of individual members often being addressed quite directly. In all forms of group therapy the therapist or therapists (with larger groups especially it can be helpful to have two therapists) have important roles in facilitating constructive and helpful interchange between the group members.

Parent groups can sometimes achieve many of the aims of individual casework, but more effectively and economically. The focus of the group is usually on children's problem behaviours and their management. The emphasis is on finding solutions rather than on apportioning blame or elucidating causes; social learning theory principles and behaviour therapy techniques can be useful in this process (Philipp, 1979). Input may be provided by the group leader but an important part of the process is the interaction between the parents as they engage in problem-solving discussions as a group. Each brings his or her experience of dealing with various problems, successfully or unsuccessfully, and compares this with the experience of other group members. Such groups also provide mutual support for their members. It can be helpful for parents to know that they are not alone in their difficulties and that others have problems coping with their children's behaviours. They may also acquire a new perspective on their own children's problems.

Behaviour therapy

Behaviour therapy is based upon learning theory. It aims to achieve precise therapeutic goals, either the elimination of symptoms or the development of behaviour considered desirable. Behaviour therapists do not interpret the meaning of problem behaviours, nor promote insight into their psychodynamics. They believe that problem behaviours, like most other behaviours, are learned and can be eliminated or replaced by desired behaviours through the provision of new learning experiences. Behaviour therapy techniques now have an assured place in child psychiatry. The treatment is often located in the child's environment – home, school or treatment centre – rather than in the clinic or therapist's office.

The 'conditioning' processes which are the basis of behaviour therapy may alter either the circumstances leading up to an event – 'respondent' or 'classical' conditioning – or those following one – 'operant' conditioning. These procedures may be applied to individuals or groups.

A good example of respondent conditioning is 'systematic desensitization'. This is often an effective treatment for phobias. A necessary preliminary to behaviour therapy is a careful study, or 'behavioural analysis', of the patient; in the case of a phobic patient this would involve assessing the circumstances in which the fear is present and ordering these in a hierarchy according to the severity of the fear in each situation.

As the first step in the treatment proper, the patient is taught relaxation – that is, the reduction of muscle tension throughout the body. Once this has been achieved the phobic object is presented in mild form, perhaps as a small uncoloured picture or even by asking the child to imagine it. There is then a gradual, planned increase in the intensity of the stimulus, based on the hierarchy previously determined. A small, monochrome picture might lead to a larger one, then a coloured one, then a movie of the object, then viewing the object itself from a distance and so forth. The rate of increase in the intensity of the stimulus is such as to enable the patient to maintain a state of relaxation. The therapist does not proceed to the next stage of the hierarchy until the patient is perfectly at ease in the current one.

In the treatment of phobias of specific objects, for example water, snakes, dogs or other animals, systematic desensitization is usually effective. It may also be used for phobias of specific situations, for example heights, closed spaces, open spaces, or travelling on buses or aeroplanes.

Operant conditioning is the planned modification of behaviour through manipulation of the consequences which are seen to control the behaviour. If every time a boy touches something hot he receives a painful burn he will soon stop touching that particular object. If whenever he helps his mother with a household chore he gets a smile and a hug from his mother this will increase the likelihood of his helping – assuming that smiles and hugs are reinforcing for him. If every time we pass a door we try it and find it locked we will soon stop trying the door; in behaviourists' terms the behaviour has been extinguished by non-reinforcement.

Operant methods include the planned positive reinforcement of desired behaviour, negative reinforcement of undesired behaviour and extinction of behaviour by taking steps to ensure that there is no response to it. Positive reinforcers may be material items like candies but social ones, for example smiles, attention, or words of praise or thanks are often better. In some situations token economy systems have been found useful; the children acquire tokens for certain specific behaviours and in some systems they lose them for others; the tokens are later redeemable for rewards such as money, toys, privileges or status. Such programmes are used in some residential and day treatment centres. They have also been successfully used in schools, group homes and other institutional settings. They are also applicable to home and family situations. They lend themselves well to the treatment of groups of children (Wagner and Breitmeyer, 1975; Hoefler and Bornstein, 1975).

Behaviour therapy, usually using operant methods, has been used to treat many problems including temper tantrums, aggressive behaviour, delinquent behaviour, obsessive-compulsive symptoms, anorexia nervosa, tics, language disorders and enuresis. It has also been used to promote attendance at school and the development of social skills.

In treating obsessive-compulsive rituals 'response prevention', the active restriction of the rituals, has been found of value. It seems that if the rituals are consistently prevented, the urge to carry them out eventually disappears (Stanley, 1980). The use of the various forms of enuresis alarm is another example of conditioning, though there is some dispute as to how the apparatus works.

Patterson (1976; 1982) has been a pioneer in the development of learning theory-based treatments for children with severe behaviour problems. He has observed high levels of 'coercive behaviour' in these families, everyone trying to get everyone else to do as they wish by the use of aggression in some form. One person would make a coercive attack on another who would then retaliate with aversive behaviour designed to terminate the attack. Whenever coercive (that is, aggressive) behaviour succeeds in terminating another's coercive attack that behaviour is reinforced, so that over time the severity of each behaviour increases. Patterson's research has demonstrated that careful behavioural analysis, followed by appropriate interventions can reverse such processes.

The programmed texts *Living with Families* (Patterson and Gullion, 1968) and *Families* (Patterson, 1971) offer parents and others dealing with such children guidance on how to apply behavioural methods in dealing with their children. These techniques, when applied in family settings are more properly termed 'behavioural family therapy', the principles of which are summarized in *Basic Family Therapy* (Barker, 1986).

Hypnosis and hypnotherapy

Recent years have seen increasing interest in the use of hypnosis as an adjunct to other treatment methods in child psychiatry. Hypnosis may be defined as a state in which the subject's attention is focused upon inner ideas, realities and feelings. Hypnosis is best induced in the context of an intense rapport between therapist and patient. Self-hypnosis is a similar state which the subject enters without the presence of a therapist; it is usually first taught to the patient by a therapist. As attention becomes increasingly focused various 'hypnotic phenomena' may appear; these include the release of inhibitions, reduced capacity for volitional activity, heightened susceptibility to suggestion, arm levitation, catalepsy, ideomotor activity (involuntary movements and actions), dissociation, time distortion, age regression, 'positive' and 'negative' hallucinations ('negative' ones being the inability to see things which are actually there), amnesia and hypermnesia. Many of these appear only in states of moderate to deep trance.

The state of trance, which is the essence of hypnosis, is a commonplace one. All of us focus our attention on particular things from time to time – a daydream or a story we become deeply involved in. As we do so we are often in a state of light trance, a state not fundamentally different from that induced by the clinical hypnotherapist. In trance our awareness of certain things is heightened and that of others is decreased; those on which our attention is not focused are ignored even though we may be distantly aware of them. Many of us have had the experience of driving somewhere and having no memory of the journey on arrival at our destination. This is an example of an everday trance experience.

Children are generally good hypnotic subjects, at least once they have reached middle childhood. Brown and Fromm (1986) point out that they live naturally for much of the time in a world of imagery. The hypnotherapist may use this characteristic to advantage in the treatment of many of their disorders. The following are among the uses which hypnosis may have in our field:

(1) It may help children gain access to emotional or other mental states which are more conducive to adaptive behaviour. States which they have experienced in the past can often be recalled and put to use in the hypnotic state.
(2) It may promote access to material which is not currently available at the conscious level. Such 'repressed' or 'state dependent' material may be responsible for anxiety, phobic or other symptoms. Hypnosis may help make it available so that it can be dealt with in psychotherapy.
(3) It may enable patients to obtain access to resources of which they are consciously unaware. We have seen how important self-esteem is to the developing child. Most children (and adults too) are consciously unaware of many of their capabilities and have forgotten or repressed past achievements. In trance they can become aware of these things, so that their views of themselves are modified.
(4) It facilitates mind-body communication (Rossi, 1986a). Thus it helps promote physiological changes, for example to blood pressure, body temperature, bleeding (Swirsky-Sachetti and Margolis, 1986), healing of wounds and burns, enuresis (Edwards and van der Spuy, 1985) and nausea.

(5) It can assist in the control of anxiety, often through some of the processes mentioned in paragraphs 1, 2 and 3 above.

(6) It can assist in pain control.

(7) It can help diminish or remove abnormal repetitive behaviours.

(8) It may be a helpful adjunct in the treatment of various other disorders, for example 'learning difficulties; behaviour disorders; temper tantrums, hair pulling, nail biting, prolonged thumb sucking; phobic reactions, including school phobias, needle phobias and animal phobias; shyness; nightmares and sleepwalking; anorexia nervosa; stuttering; and drug abuse, (Brown and Fromm, 1986). The strength of the scientific evidence for the effectiveness of hypnosis in the treatment of these disorders varies; much depends on the skill of the therapist and the specific approach used.

In none of these conditions is hypnotherapy a panacea. Inducing trance in itself has little therapeutic value beyond facilitating a state of relaxation. Moreover, it is seldom sufficient simply to offer suggestions that the symptoms will improve. More important is the making of new associations and helping patients gain access to the psychological resources they need.

Hypnosis does not provide a means of 'mind control' but rather a heightened state of responsiveness and trust between patient and therapist. The hypnotherapist then leads the patient to become involved in a past experience or previous learning that may be of benefit in the present situation. For example, a child oncology patient receiving chemotherapy may be enabled to re-experience in trance, during the procedure, a previous enjoyable trip to a farm. This may lead to reduced nausea and enhanced feelings of well-being.

The major difficulty with hypnotherapy is that the susceptibility of individuals to hypnosis varies. Some achieve trance, especially its deeper forms, more easily than others. Nevertheless it can be successfully applied in a large proportion of the population, especially once a high level of trust and rapport exists between therapist and patient.

Hypnosis and Hypnotherapy with Children (Gardner and Olness, 1981) describes in detail how to use hypnosis with children and discusses its application in various conditions. Other useful books are those by Pratt *et al.* (1984), Crasilneck and Hall (1985) and Brown and Fromm (1986).

Pharmacotherapy

Psychoactive drugs can be of value in the treatment of hyperactivity, depression, severe tics and the Gilles de la Tourette syndrome, and major psychoses, notably schizophrenia. They may be of occasional value in the treatment of neurotic children. Anticonvulsant drugs play a major role in the control of epileptic seizures.

Drugs for hyperactive children

Stimulant drugs have an established place in the treatment of hyperactive children. Although these drugs act as psychic stimulants in adults, they have the paradoxical effect of reducing motor activity and improving attention and concentration in children.

Methylphenidate, the stimulant most used in North America, has a half-life (the time taken for the concentration of the drug in the blood to be reduced by half) of only 2 to 3 hours (Gualtieri *et al.*, 1982). This means that the drug has to be given every 3 to 4 hours to maintain an adequate blood level. It also means the value of the treatment can be assessed by comparing ratings of a child's activity level and behaviour on days when the drug is being given with those on days when it is not. Ideally, on the latter days 'placebo' medication, identical in appearance, should be given and the ratings made by observers who are unaware whether the child is on active or placebo medication. Various rating scales are available; a widely used one is that of Conners (1969). When the drug is used with children whose hyperactivity is causing problems in school, doses given half an hour before starting school and again at about midday usually constitute a satisfactory regime. The drug need not be given on non-school days unless the hyperactivity is causing problems at home or in other situations.

Amphetamine compounds and pemoline are other stimulant drugs which may be effective in children who do not respond to methylphenidate, but their longer action means that their effectiveness cannot be assessed by comparing successive days on and off them. Tranquillisers such as the phenothiazine drugs and haloperidol can be used to control hyperactive behaviour, but often at the cost of sedation which may impair cognitive function. These drugs also have other undesirable side-effects, especially when used long-term. Tricyclic antidepressants such as imipramine also diminish hyperactive behaviour and may improve performance on tests of attention, but their drawbacks may outweigh their advantages (Taylor, 1986b). Recent reports suggest that clonidine, an unrelated drug, may be of value (Hunt *et al.*, 1985).

Table 19.1 includes the principal drugs that may be useful in hyperactive children, with their doses and their most important adverse effects. A fuller discussion of the drug treatment of these children, and its problems, is provided by Taylor (1986b).

Table 19.1.   Drug doses and adverse effects.

Drug	Dose	Principal adverse effects
Stimulants (for hyperactive children)		
		Excitement
		Sleeplessness
Methylphenidate	0.25–1.0 mg/kg/24 hr	Loss of appetite
		Growth failure
Dexamphetamine	0.2–0.5 mg/kg/24 hr	Palpitations
		Headache
Pemoline	0.5–2.0 mg/kg/24 hr	Abdominal cramps
		Drug dependence (rare in hyperactive children)
Phenothiazine drugs		
		Drowsiness
		Tremor
Chlorpromazine	1–3 mg/kf/24 hr	Muscle rigidity and spasms
	(night sedative dose up	Precipitation of epilepsy
Thioridazine	to 3 mg/kg	Jaundice
		Blood dyscrasias
Fluphenazine	0.05–0.25 mg/kg/24 hr	Urinary retention and incontinence
Perphenazine	0.15–0.3 mg/kg/24 hr	Skin rashes (chlorpromazine may cause photosensitive skin reactions)
		Painful muscle spasms
Haloperidol	0.025–0.3 mg/kg/24 hr	Muscle rigidity and tremor
		Drowsiness
		Depression
Benzodiazepines (for over-fives)		
Diazepam	2–5 mg 2 or 3 times daily	Drowsiness
		Skin rashes
Chlordiazepoxide	5–10 mg 2 or 3 times daily	Muscle tenderness or weakness

Notes: (1) The above doses are guides only. Dosage should be individualized according to response.

(2) Long-term administration of phenothiazines or haloperidol may cause 'tardive dyskinesia' (see Glossary).

(3) Muscle spasms and tremor caused by phenothiazines or haloperidol may be countered by 'anti-Parkinsonian' drugs such as benzhexol (1–5 mg twice daily).

Drug treatment of affective disorders

Antidepressant drugs may be useful in the treatment of depression in children and, especially, in adolescents. Tricyclic drugs such as imipramine, amitriptyline and nortriptyline are used extensively in the treatment of major depressive disorders in adults; they seem to be of value also in some younger patients with depressive disorders. Well designed trials of these compounds in children have been few, however, and the results have not been clear-cut. The absorption and metabolism of the tricyclic drugs in children is highly variable, so that widely differing blood levels may be achieved with standard weight-related doses. Monitoring of blood levels is advisable (Puig-Antich, 1980; 1981).

The use in children of the other main group of antidepressant drugs, the monoamine oxidase inhibitors (examples are isocarboxazid and phenelzine), has been little studied. These drugs may have a place in the treatment of depressed adolescents who do not respond to tricyclic drugs.

Mania in young people is treated along the same lines as in adults. In the acute phase the administration of an antipsychotic drug – usually haloperidol or a phenothiazine such as chlorpromazine or thioridazine (see Table 19.1) – may be required to control the manic behaviour. These drugs are usually given orally but if oral medication is refused or acts too slowly intramuscular injection may be indicated.

Table 19.2. Doses and adverse effects of tricyclic drugs and lithium.

Drug	Dose	Principal adverse effects
Imipramine Amitriptyline	1.5–5 mg/kg/ 24	Arrhythmias, blood pressure changes and other cardiac disorders Dry mouth Difficulty with visual accommodation Tremor
Imipramine (for enuresis)	10–50 mg at bedtime	Precipitation of epileptic seizures Jaundice and blood disorders (both rare) Psychosis Drowsiness (amitriptyline)
Lithium carbonate	600–1200 mg per day (depending on blood levels)	Tremor Anorexia, nausea Abdominal discomfort Thirst, polyuria Goitre Fatigue, weakness

Note: The absorption and metabolism of tricyclic antidepressants by children is very variable. If possible blood levels should be checked regularly.

Lithium carbonate is often effective in the treatment of bipolar affective disorders and may be used in adolescents with such disorders. Given in doses which maintain a blood level of 0.8 to 1.2 milliequivalents/litre, it leads to a reduction or cessation of attacks of mania and depression in perhaps 80 per cent of cases (Hassanyeh and Davidson, 1980; Youngerman and Canino, 1978). A dose of 600 to 1200 mg per day is usually needed, but the blood level should be estimated regularly and maintained in the therapeutic range. Table 19.2 provides further information about the tricyclics and lithium.

Anxiety/neurotic disorders

Drugs have little place in the treatment of neurotic disorders. Individual or family therapy, casework with the parents and other measures to lessen any stresses the child is facing are usually the main needs. Hypnotherapy and behavioural approaches may also be of value. Occasionally the very short-term use of a benzodiazepine tranquillizer such as diazepam or chlordiazepoxide may be indicated. This may tide the child over for a few days, while other measures are instituted or take effect.

In adult patients with obsessive-compulsive disorders the antidepressant clomipramine is widely used and is believed by many to be an effective treatment. Its use in childhood has not been much studied, but it may have a place in the treatment of some childhood obsessive-compulsive disorders. Dosage is similar to that of imipramine.

Table 19.1 provides further information about the above drugs.

Schizophrenia

The phenothiazine drugs and haloperidol are widely used in the treatment of schizophrenia in adults, though they should never be more than one facet of a much wider management plan. Their use in juvenile schizophrenia has not been studied as extensively but they are often used to treat adolescents with schizophrenia and probably have a place in the treatment of some schizophrenic children (see Table 19.1).

Other conditions

Drugs have little place in the treatment of *behaviour disorders*, unless there is associated hyperactivity. Occasionally the major tranquillisers are used to control acutely disturbed behaviour, but physical restraint, along with other measures as described in Chapter 4, is generally to be preferred.

No drugs have been shown to affect the course of *pervasive developmental disorders* such as infantile autism. Associated problems such as persistent insomnia or severe hyperactivity may sometimes be ameliorated by the use of appropriate medication. The mainstays of treatment should be the measures outlined in Chapter 7.

Sleeplessness in young children is often a manifestation of disturbed parent/child relationships, rather than of problem in the children themselves. Although medication is sometimes given to children who do not sleep its effects are often disappointing. Some drugs which may be tried are listed in Table 19.3, but their use should be short-term, rarely extending for more than two weeks. Behavioural methods and counselling for the parents may yield better results (Richman *et al.*, 1985; Richman, 1985).

Table 19.3. Hypnotic drugs: doses and adverse effects.

Drug	Dose	Principal adverse effects
Chloral Dichloralphenazone Triclofos	20–50 mg/kg/24 hr Maximum dose 1 G per 24 hr	Nausea Vomiting
Promethazine	15–30 mg (in age range 5–12)	Dizziness Impaired concentration Blurring of vision Blood disorders (rare)

For *tics and Tourette's syndrome* haloperidol is probably the most effective treatment. Doses near or even above the upper end of the range suggested in Table 19.1 may be necessary.

Some general points about drug treatment

Caution should be exercised in the prescription of drugs for children. The suppression of symptoms, whether emotional or behavioural, may be possible but this involves at least two risks. One is that of masking underlying problems such as disturbed family relationships or difficulties in other areas of the child's life. The other lies in the message which the use of medication tends to carry, namely that the problem lies within the child and is a medical one. Sometimes there are elements of truth in this, for example in cases of schizophrenia, in some affective disorders and in Tourette's syndrome. But in many behavioural and anxiety/neurotic disorders this is not so and the use of medication may lead those concerned with the child's care to take an unrealistic view of the problems.

Many of these drugs have serious side-effects and can be lethal if taken in overdoses. This applies especially to the tricyclics, the phenothiazines and haloperidol, but all psychoactive drugs can be fatal if taken in sufficient doses. The families of children for whom drugs are prescribed should be warned of the dangers, and told that medication should always be kept in a secure place and the child's access to it controlled.

It seems that in practice the patterns of psychoactive medication use in children varies greatly. According to Taylor (1985) stimulant drugs are used 'very extensively in the United States and very seldom in Britain'. A study of the prescription of psychoactive drugs to children in the Canadian province of Saskatchewan also showed a pattern of use differing greatly from that suggested in this chapter, minor tranquillisers (mainly the benzodiazepines), sedatives and hypnotics being the most frequently prescribed. Stimulants were less used than might have been expected (Quinn, 1986).

Inpatient and residential treatment

'Inpatient treatment' refers to treatment in a hospital unit for disturbed children and 'residential treatment' to that provided in other specialized centres. The latter tend to be longer-term units than those in hospitals but there are many exceptions to this; some hospital units treat children for periods as long as a year, occasionally longer. Some non-hospital units offer short-term admission. Hospital and non-hospital treatment centres differ in other respects; hospitals are normally directed by psychiatrists and take a more medical approach, while other centres may be directed by psychologists, social workers or other mental health professionals. Nevertheless the two types of treatment facility share many features and treat similar types of children. Many specialize in certain age ranges or types of clinical problem.

Children may be admitted to units of either type primarily for assessment or for treatment. Admission for assessment may be necessary for one of three main reasons:

- Because the case is unusually complex and intensive observation and investigation beyond what is possible as an outpatient are needed. This applies especially when there is doubt about the roles of suspected organic neurological factors on the one hand, and psychological and family ones on the other. In such cases investigation in a hospital unit by a team of specialists may clarify the situation.
- Because there is doubt about how far the child's symptoms are being maintained by the current dynamics at home or, occasionally, in the wider social setting in which the child lives. Observing

whether symptoms persist, worsen or improve away from home may then be helpful.

- Because the child lives at a great distance from the centre, making repeated outpatient visits impractical. This is more commonly the case in North America, with its vast rural areas, than in more tightly populated European countries.

The main indications for admission for treatment are:

- Because the child's behaviour is so disturbed as to make treatment or even care elsewhere difficult or impossible. This applies to some children with very severe conduct disorders, especially those complicated by severe hyperactivity or extremely impulsive behaviour; also to some with schizophrenia and other psychoses.
- Because of danger to the child or others if the child remains at home. This applies to many suicidal young people, to a few who are a danger to others and to most severe cases of anorexia nervosa, that is those in whom there has been a dangerous degree of weight loss.
- Because the child's environmental circumstances are very unfavourable and efforts to ameliorate the situation have failed.

Adverse circumstances which might lead to admission include an unstable home with gross marital strife or other serious family systems problems, severe parental rejection of the child, or serious emotional deprivation or abuse. In such cases admission may be helpful if it seems likely, or at least possible, that more can be done to alter the adverse conditions in which the child has been living during the period of inpatient treatment. It is sometimes possible to do more to help the family, and promote improvement in parents' attitudes and handling of the children, while the latter are receiving treatment away from the family. The parents are relieved of the constant irritant of the child's disturbed behaviour and it may be possible, in due course, to return a less disturbed child to a better functioning family. Treatment can then be successfully pursued on an outpatient or daypatient basis.

Admission must always be considered carefully, in light of the family situation or the situation in the group home, foster home or other setting in which the child is living. Requests for admission are sometimes disguised attempts by parents or others to get rid of an unwanted child. Admission of the child for psychiatric treatment is not then usually the best response. Sometimes the request arises out of the 'scapegoating' of a child; in such cases the best response is often to offer family therapy, with the object of promoting changes in the family system such that the scapegoating will no longer be necessary.

Many inpatient units admit children for short periods of perhaps a few weeks during which intensive assessment and short-term treatment is carried out. This leads to the development of a long-term plan of treatment to be continued after discharge, usually on an outpatient basis, though transfer to daypatient treatment or, occasionally, to a longer-term residential unit may be recommended. As well as assessment procedures as set out in Chapter 3, and appropriate physical investigations and consultations with other specialists as indicated, an important part of the assessment is observing how the child responds to different management techniques and regimes. The best way to discover how a child will respond to a treatment is to try it and observe the result.

Most hospital units are staffed primarily by nurses and/or child care workers. These 'front line' staff are usually part of larger treatment teams consisting of psychiatrists, psychologists, social workers, occupational therapists, speech therapists, teachers and others. A central feature of the treatment is the general emotional environment or 'milieu' of the unit. An emotionally warm, relaxed atmosphere is much to be desired. However difficult and disturbed their behaviour may be, the children should be met with accepting, rather than rejecting or hostile attitudes and responses. These should be combined with firm, calmly applied limit-setting which is as necessary in residential settings as it is in other forms of therapy. The children's current clinical states and behaviours are accepted while work proceeds to bring about changes in each child's problem areas. The staff are working with, not against, each child to achieve this.

Residential treatment is invariably multimodal, a comprehensive plan being worked out to address the needs of each child and family. Keat (1979) presents a model of multimodal therapy which is based largely upon behavioural methods, and another is presented by Fundudis (1986). In addition to the therapeutic milieu of the unit specific treatments that may be needed by children include individual or group psychotherapy, behaviour therapy, occupational and recreational therapy, speech therapy, special educational help and pharmacotherapy. In most cases family therapy and/or counselling for the parents is also an important part of the treatment. Active involvement of the family is important; children who are left in residential units to be 'fixed', while their parents go about their business relieved of parental responsibilities seldom do well.

Ney and Mulvihill (1985) describe an interesting 12-week treatment concept. During the first 2 weeks the child and family are assessed comprehensively as outpatients. This is followed by a 5-week period of intensive, multimodal inpatient treatment, and then by a 5-week follow-up period. All children are admitted for 5 weeks, no more and no less, but they can be readmitted for a further 5 weeks at any time after the follow-up period. Ney and Mulvihill (1985) describe 44 treatment techniques designed to deal with a variety of symptoms. They also offer comprehensive treatment programmes for child abuse, anorexia, autism, depression, encopresis, firesetting, incest, school phobia, weight control and conversion reactions.

Residential treatment is discussed in *The Residential Psychiatric Treatment of Children* (Barker, 1974b), and by Barker (1982) and Hersov and Bentovim (1985). *Children in Residential Care: Critical Issues in Treatment* (Schaefer and Swanson, in press) provides an up to date review of many aspects of residential treatment. The drawbacks and potential dangers of residential treatment and means of lessening these are discussed by Barker (in press).

Day treatment

Treatment in a daypatient unit can provide many of the benefits of inpatient treatment without removing the child completely from home and family, and at less expense. Children treated in such units spend a substantial part of their waking hours in a therapeutic milieu and can receive comprehensive, multimodal therapy, much as in-patients do. Most day treatment units operate 5 days a week and the children attend from 8 or 9 a.m. until 4 or 5 p.m., though details vary. Treatment is usually organized round the school day, with active involvement also of the family. In some places there are half-day programmes for younger children and in some units the possibility of attendance less often than 5 days a week exists. More consistent staffing is usually possible in day units than in residential ones, because the shift changes and days off which inevitably characterize residential units are avoided.

Day treatment relieves parents and other family members of some of the strain which caring for a severely disturbed child may entail, yet child and family do not lose contact nor come to deny the existence of the problems – ever-present risks in residential treatment. The family are together every evening and weekend, so that the problems are kept in view and all concerned have ample opportunity to put into practice what they are learning in treatment. The risk of the child becoming dependent on the unit is much reduced and the treatment can be more cost effective than residential treatment.

Day treatment may be especially useful when a child's problems are selectively manifest at school and adjustment at home is satisfactory. Most day treatment units have teachers on their staffs, so that the educational needs of the children can be met during daypatient attendance. If the child has academic problems remedial measures can often be undertaken.

Day treatment may be contraindicated for:

- children who are dangerous to themselves or others;
- children whose cases can be adequately managed in an outpatient setting;
- children whose parents or other caretakers are themselves severely disturbed, dangerous and abusive;
- children with a physical illness or handicap which necessitates round-the-clock care.

Day treatment may be long- or short-term, extending from a week to several years, but periods of a few weeks or months are often sufficient, especially if treatment of the family is also undertaken. Many day treatment services are located in centres which also have inpatient and outpatient services. Day treatment may then be one phase in a programme of treatment which also includes outpatient and inpatient therapy.

Hersov and Bentovim (1985) and Zimet and Farley (1985) discuss day treatment and review the relevant literature. The latter authors also discuss the attempts that have been made to evaluate this form of treatment; it seems to be of value and should be one of the services available for disturbed children.

Alternative families

An alternative to residential treatment that has been used in various centres is the placement of children in alternative families where their psychiatric problems can be tackled. This may be helpful for children whose own families are so unstable or disturbed that treatment cannot be successfully carried out while they remain there. Examples include the 'parent-therapist' programme in Hamilton, Ontario (Levin *et al.*, 1976), the Alberta Parent Counsellors (Larson *et al.*, 1978) and the Kent Family Placement Project (Hazel, 1977).

In these programmes families are specially selected, trained and paid. They take into their homes disturbed children who need to be treated away from their own homes. They are provided with continuing professional help and consultation, often primarily by means of regular group meetings under the leadership of a professional worker. Meanwhile therapy is provided for the natural families, much as it would be during inpatient treatment. Contact between the 'alternative' families and the natural ones can also be beneficial as the natural parents observe how their child is handled and responds to the environment in the alternative home.

The 'family care programme' in Toronto was set up along similar lines. Alternative families were provided for children receiving inpatient treatment and who had no families able to provide them with suitable care (Barker *et al.*, 1978). The children were in the care of child welfare agencies, some of them on a permanent basis. As well as visiting their children in the treatment centre these 'foster care workers', as they were called, provided a weekend home for the children and, in many instances, a home for the child to live in upon discharge. This appeared to facilitate and shorten residential treatment in cases in which a child's family had broken up or rejected the child, and to help prevent subsequent relapse.

Educational measures

Many disturbed children have educational problems and we have seen that conduct disorders are frequently accompanied by reading problems. In such cases appropriate educational measures are an important part of treatment. These may include remedial teaching, a change of educational methods or transfer to a different class or school. Special educational approaches may be necessary.

In many jurisdictions special classes or schools are provided for children with psychiatric problems. Some are part of state-run school systems, others are private schools. The various British Education Acts have for long recognized 'maladjustment' as one of the categories of handicap for which children may require special education. Education authorities therefore have a legal obligation to provide such education. Some local education authorities run their own day classes or schools for such children, others use privately run schools, many do both. Many residential schools for maladjusted children also exist, some run by local education authorities but most by other organizations, the authorities paying fees for the children they place in those schools.

In North America arrangements for the education of disturbed children are more varied. There are some schools, mainly privately run, that specialize in the education of disturbed children. In addition many school boards have special, small classes for disturbed and disruptive children and those with learning problems.

The education of disturbed children requires small classes or groups, a high teacher/child ratio and skilled accepting care and teaching by specially trained teachers. Residential schools for maladjusted children are usually small (up to about 80 children, but usually nearer 40) and the treatment of the children's emotional and relationship difficulties is given as much attention as the remediation of their academic problems. While at school, the children are often able to develop relationships with the staff which are more satisfying and constructive than those they have with their parents. But they can maintain contact with the parents during school holidays and breaks and perhaps at weekends. Their adjustment at home often improves as they overcome their emotional and educational problems at school. Some of these schools have social workers on staff who work with the families while the child is at the school. The development of schools for maladjusted children, and their philosophies, were well reviewed by Bridgeland (1971).

While special schools and classes are valuable for some disturbed children, most are educated in ordinary schools and classes. Many educational, behavioural and emotional problems can be dealt with in such settings, perhaps with some help from school psychologists and remedial teachers. In *Help Starts Here* Kolvin and his colleagues (1981) describe studies of various methods of intervening in ordinary schools to provide help for disturbed children. These were:

- a 'behaviour modification' approach;
- a nurturing approach, employing 'teacher-aides';
- parent counselling-teacher education;
- group therapy for children.

The progress of children treated using each of these approaches was compared with that of a control group of untreated 'at risk' children. All the approaches proved to be of some value, though short-term results often differed from long-term outcome, the latter being better in some instances. This book is essential reading for anyone planning intervention in schools with the objective of treating or forestalling psychiatric problems in the pupils.

Speech and language therapy

Speech and language disorders are often associated with psychiatric disorders, so that comprehensive treatment plans frequently include speech therapy. Speech therapists, sometimes known as speech pathologists, have major roles in the treatment of children with developmental language disorders. Improved speech and language skills can often contribute to the resolution of other psychiatric problems in children.

Removal from parental care

Some disturbed children are found to be living in severely dysfunctional families which are failing to meet their basic emotional and even physical needs. There may be physical or sexual abuse or severe neglect, as discussed in Chapter 18. While we should first endeavour to help the family acquire the skills and obtain access to the resources necessary to care adequately for its children, sometimes this proves impossible. The motivation of some parents to make the needed changes may be lacking. In others the marital relationship is grossly unstable, or there may be problems of alcohol and drug abuse. In all developed countries there are child welfare agencies which exist to provide help and, if necessary, alternative homes for such children. Many of them are government-run but some are non-governmental charitable organizations. In Great Britain the main non-governmental agencies are the National Society for the Prevention of Cruelty to Children, the National Children's Home and Dr Barnardo's; Dr Barnardo's also has branches in other countries, including some African ones.

Legal aspects of the removal of children from parental care have been discussed in Chapter 17, but it is desirable to have the consent of the parents or other next-of-kin to what is proposed. Some parents realize that they cannot care properly for their children and accept the need for the children's placement elsewhere. Unfortunately adversarial legal proceedings prove necessary in other cases.

Many children who have had to be removed from their families have experienced unstable, rejecting, abusive or neglectful parenting, so that their psychological development has been retarded or distorted. They may show major behaviour problems, emotional difficulties, developmental disorders or educational difficulties. Many are angry and insecure. Child welfare agencies have the often difficult task of meeting these children's needs for love, security and the fostering of their shattered self-esteem. Child welfare staff may seek psychiatric help in their efforts to do this.

The substitute environment provided for these children usually consists of either a foster home or a group home (often called in Britain a 'children's home'). The large impersonal orphanages, which were sometimes also called 'children's homes', of the past have now been mostly replaced by much smaller homes; these usually consist of ordinary houses in which the children are cared for in much the same way as in ordinary families. Nowadays many group homes are run by married couples, one of whom goes out to work as in other families while the other looks after the home, often with the help of one or two other staff who may be full-time or part-time, and resident or nonresident. Unfortunately many mentally handicapped children are still cared for in large, impersonal and understaffed institutions, the drawbacks of which were well described by King and his colleagues (1971).

Children removed from parental care require skilled and patient management; they may also need other treatment measures, including any of those described in this chapter. Multidisciplinary assessment, which may involve social workers, psychiatrists, psychologists, teachers and other specialists, often assists in determining such children's needs and in following their progress.

Many countries also have 'training' or 'correctional' schools and institutions for delinquent children. In Great Britain these are nowadays called 'community homes with education on the premises' and are run by the social services departments of local authorities. The environments and the therapy they offer their residents vary greatly. In some, progressive and humane therapeutic programmes exist, while others are primarily custodial and/or punitive.

Child psychiatric consultation and liaison

It is clear from the prevalence figures quoted earlier that there are many more disturbed children than can be treated by the available numbers of psychiatrists and other child mental health professionals. Much can, however, be done to help these children by the provision of consultation to those caring for them. Such consultation is an important part of the work of child psychiatrists and their colleagues. Psychiatrists may assess these children, determine their needs and give guidance to the staffs of group homes, institutions and schools, and also to foster parents and child welfare social workers, as to how these needs may best be met.

Programme consultation and liaison work with the staffs of agencies dealing with disturbed, deprived and abused children may also lead to the provision of better and more appropriately focused work with the children. This process, which also has applications in the prevention of psychiatric disorders, is discussed further in Chapter 20.

Chapter 20

Prevention of Child Psychiatric Disorders

It is better to prevent child psychiatric disorders than to treat them once they are established, though prevention tends to receive less attention than treatment. Caplan (1964) distinguished three types of prevention:

(1) *Primary prevention*. This comprises planned measures designed to reduce the incidence of specific pathological conditions in a population not currently suffering from those conditions. In our field this would include both psychiatric disorders and mental retardation.

(2) *Secondary prevention*. This aims at early diagnosis and case finding, followed by intervention to bring the disorder rapidly under control so that there is minimal impact on those affected.

(3) *Tertiary prevention*. This consists of measures taken once a disorder is established. It aims to limit the effects of the disorder, to prevent it from getting worse and to give support to afflicted individuals and/or their families.

Definitions

(1) *Epidemiology*. This is concerned with the incidence, prevalence and distribution of disorders in communities. It is a basic tool in the development of primary prevention measures. By means of epidemiological studies it is possible both to establish a baseline so that the effectiveness of primary prevention measures can be judged, and to identify risk factors.

(2) *Risk factors*. These are circumstances that make the development of a disorder more likely.

(3) *Incidence*. This is the number of new cases occurring in a defined population during a specified time period.

(4) *Duration*. This is the length of time a disorder persists, that is the period from the time of onset until recovery or death.

(5) *Prevalence* is a measure of the number of cases of a disorder present

at a given time in a specified population. It is a function of two independent variables – incidence and duration.

(6) *Intervening variables*, in the present context, are the factors that determine whether individuals at risk do or do not develop the disorder in question. No risk factor leads to the disorder in 100 per cent of individuals; in any epidemic some individuals will escape. Primary prevention aims to alter the environment so that more individuals escape.

Primary prevention

The publication of *Principles of Primary Prevention* (Caplan, 1964) was a landmark in the development of preventive psychiatry. Caplan (1980) has also provided an account of methods of primary prevention which may be applicable in child psychiatry.

Risk factors and primary prevention

(a) *Genetic factors*. The role of genetic factors in causing child psychiatric disorders was discussed in Chapter 2. Genetic counselling of parents who have had a child with a genetically caused disorder, and for those in whose families there is history of such disorders, may help reduce the incidence of the conditions concerned. It has also been possible to reduce the incidence of phenylketonuria by the routine testing of the urine of newborn infants, followed by the provision of appropriate diets to those who are afflicted.

(b) *Pregnancy risk factors*. These include toxaemia of pregnancy and various infections which the mother may pass on to the fetus – for example rubella, syphilis, toxoplasmosis and acquired immune deficiency syndrome (AIDS). Good antenatal care can prevent most of these disasters. Congenital syphilis and the mental retardation and other consequences of rubella in early pregnancy are now rare where good antenatal care is practised. The risk of a woman with HIV antibodies (who may not be ill with AIDS) infecting her child is about 50 per cent; such women should therefore be advised against becoming pregnant. Amniocentesis, the prenatal examination of a pregnant woman's amniotic fluid, enables certain congenital conditions to be detected before birth. In some circumstances termination of the pregnancy may be decided upon as a result.

(c) *Birth trauma*. This can cause damage to the brain as well as to other parts of the infant. Good obstetric care reduces this and is an important element in primary prevention.

(d) *Prematurity and other neonatal medical disorders*. These may cause brain damage and they may have indirect effects resulting from the prolonged separation of parents and child which occurs when a newborn child is treated for a long period in a special care unit. This may disrupt the parent-child bonding process.

(e) *Accidents in and outside the home*. These are common causes of neurological and other injuries which in turn may lead to psychiatric disorder or mental retardation.

(f) *Poisons*. The most important is lead (see Chapter 6). Ensuring that children's environments are free of lead is a useful preventive measure.

(g) *Physical illnesses*, especially of the central nervous system, may place children at risk of developing psychiatric disorders. The risks are particularly great when the illnesses are prolonged and lead to repeated admissions to hospital.

(h) *Cultural deprivation*. The rates of psychiatric disorders, mental retardation and learning failure at school have all been found to be higher in culturally deprived homes than in better endowed ones.

(i) *Family disruption and disharmony*. Children from dysfunctional families generally have higher rates of emotional and behavioural disorders than those from better functioning families.

(j) *Parental mental illness*. This is a particularly serious risk factor when both parents suffer from mental illness; also when the parental disorders are serious and prolonged.

(k) *Early school failure*. This is often associated with specific learning disorders, hyperkinesis and neurological problems.

(l) *The experience of being in the care of a child welfare agency*. This is discussed further below.

(m) *Large family size*.

(n) *Father absence*.

This list of risk factors is not exhaustive but in the case of each of those mentioned there is evidence to support the listing. Other risk factors certainly exist. In some cases there is suspicion but no proof; others are no doubt as yet unsuspected.

Protective factors and primary prevention

Protective factors are the converse of risk factors. They reduce the likelihood of a disorder appearing. The World Health Organization (1977b) listed the following:

(a) *Sex*. For little understood reasons girls seem to be less susceptible to psychosocial stress in childhood than boys.

(b) *Temperament*. An adaptable temperament, or an 'easy' one as described by Thomas and Chess (1977), seems to protect against the effects of deprivation and disadvantage.

(c) *Isolated nature of the stress.* Even chronic stresses, if isolated, tend to cause little damage but multiple stresses interact to potentiate the adverse results of each.

(d) *Coping skills.* There is evidence that children can acquire the skills to cope with various stresses. For example, children who are used to brief, happy separation experiences such as short stays with friends or relatives cope better with hospital admission.

(e) *A good relationship with one parent.* This helps protect against the adverse effects which may result when a child is brought up in a discordant, unhappy home.

(f) *Success or good experiences outside the home.* Good schooling can help mitigate the effects of a bad home environment.

(g) *Improved family circumstances.* Later years spent in a harmonious family setting seem to lessen the effects of earlier adverse circumstances.

The concept of invulnerability

It has been observed, for example by Rutter (1979), that some children are able to survive gross deprivation and severe psychosocial stress without developing psychiatric disorders. Precisely what makes some children strikingly less vulnerable than others is not fully understood, though genetic factors may be involved. An important study of children's resilience and invulnerability was reported in *Vulnerable but Invincible* (Werner and Smith, 1982). This book describes the results of a longitudinal study of 698 children living on the Hawaiian island of Kanaii. The authors point out that:

> 'From an epidemiological point of view, these children were at high risk, since they were born and reared in chronic poverty, exposed to higher than average rates of prematurity and perinatal stress, and reared by mothers with little formal education'. (Werner and Smith, 1982, page 153.)

The children were followed from before birth into adult life, with less than a 10 per cent drop-out rate. Some of them triumphed strikingly over adversity, becoming competent and autonomous young adults.

What distinguished the resilient high-risk children? They:

- had few serious illnesses in their first two decades, and recovered quickly from those they had;
- were perceived to be 'very active' and 'socially responsive' as infants;

- showed advanced self-help skills and adequate sensorimotor and language development in the second year of life;
- had adequate problem-solving and communication skills and age-appropriate perceptual-motor development in middle childhood;
- as late adolescents had a more internal locus of control, a better self-concept, and a more nurturant, responsible, achievement-orientated attitude towards life than their less successful peers.

Environmental factors associated with resiliency and stress resistance included:

- the age of the opposite sex parent (younger mothers for resilient boys and older fathers for resilient girls);
- four or fewer children in the family;
- a spacing of more than 2 years between the child and the next-born sibling;
- the presence and number of 'alternate caretakers' (father, grandparents, older siblings) available to the mother within the household;
- the amount of attention given to the child by the primary caretaker(s) in infancy;
- the availability of a sibling as caretaker or confidant in childhood;
- the cumulative number of chronic stressful life events experienced in childhood and adolescence.

Other factors that emerged included the mother's workload; the cohesiveness of the family; and whether there was an informal multigenerational network of kin and friends in adolescence.

Although these families were materially poor, a strong emotional bond was typically forged between infant and primary caregiver in the first year of life.

'The physical robustness of the resilient children, their high activity level, and their social responsiveness were recognized by the caregivers and elicited a great deal of attention. There was little prolonged separation of the infants from their mothers and no prolonged bond disruption during the first year of life. The strong attachment that resulted appears to have been a secure base for the development of the advanced self-help skills and autonomy noted among these children in their second year of life.

Though many of their mothers worked for extended periods and were major contributors to family subsistence, the children had support from alternate caretakers, such as grandmothers or older sisters, to whom they became attached.' (Werner and Smith, 1982, pages 155/6.)

Primary prevention methods

Offord (1987) divides primary prevention programmes into:

- milestone programmes, which restrict their efforts to children at particular ages or developmental levels;
- high-risk programmes, which aim to prevent disorders in groups believed to be at increased risk for disorder;
- community-wide programmes.

Epidemiological data, together with evidence concerning risk factors, intervening variables and protective factors, enable rational primary prevention plans to be made. Some of these were mentioned in the section on risk factors.

Milestone programmes

Good examples of these are the 'Head Start' centres which were established in the USA in the mid-1960s. By the mid-1980s there were over 9,400 of these centres serving some 500,000 children in the USA, supported by federal funding of about one $1 billion (Parker *et al.*, 1987). They aim to provide intensive cognitive and emotional stimulation for preschool children and their families. The programmes resulted in initial spurts in the children's cognitive development, but it was found that after a few years the cognitive functioning of the children was much the same of that of children who had not participated in Head Start. Later studies have, however, suggested that there are longer-term benefits in other areas of the children's lives (Darlington *et al.*, 1980; Consortium for Longitudinal Studies, 1983). It seems also that the help provided at the centres may be of benefit to the families. A study of one centre suggested that a number of benefits accrued to the mothers who participated in the supportive activities offered. These included decreased psychological symptoms, increased feelings of mastery and increased satisfaction with the quality of life. Parker and her colleagues observe:

> 'For some of these mothers, burdened by having to care for a number of small children, living in poor quality housing, and unable to further their own career aspirations, Head Start seemed to be a haven. The benefits they received from their involvement appeared to have alleviated the symptoms of distress they were experiencing.' (Parker *et al.*, 1987, pages 230-231).

Offord (1987) reviews 'milestone' prevention measures which have been suggested for school-age children. 'Affective education' aims to promote awareness and acceptance in children of the ways in which feelings, attitudes and behaviours influence interpersonal behaviour (Baskin and Hess, 1980). Offord (1987) concludes, however, that the results have been disappointing. His conclusions regarding the value of teaching children problem-solving skills, another proposed means of promoting better emotional and social adjustment, are similar. More hopeful may be measures to prevent unwanted pregnancies in teenagers. These often occur in adolescents living in disadvantaged circumstances and carry increased risk of psychosocial disadvantage for both the teenagers and their progeny.

High-risk programmes

Offord (1987) lists as children who may be specially at risk those who are admitted to hospital; those who suffer from chronic physical illnesses; those who have experienced a death in the family. Others are babies with very low birthweights, those treated in special care units in the neonatal period and children admitted to the care of child welfare agencies.

Preventive measures have been suggested for all the above groups. For example, Caplan (1980) suggests that positive steps can be taken to help children cope with crises such as admission to hospital. He advocates 'anticipatory guidance' and 'preventive intervention'. The former consists of explaining and discussing the upcoming crisis and the feelings and experiences the subjects are likely to encounter. This is best done in groups. 'Preventive intervention' consists of guidance given to children and their families, focused on the here-and-now. The subjects are helped to understand what is happening, to find solutions to problems, to counter blame of self and others, and to maintain hope and find outside help – from extended family members, friends and professional caregivers. These measures may enhance children's coping skills, so that what might have been an emotionally damaging experience may become a growth-promoting one. There is evidence that measures such as the above may be effective in reducing the adverse effects of admission to hospital (Byrne and Cadman, 1987).

Children with chronic physical illnesses are a high-risk group, though how best to reduce the risk is not entirely clear. A good review of this difficult field is that of Cadman *et al.* (1987)

Children who are or have been in the care of child welfare agencies are an important group. Many have experienced poor care before being removed from their own families. After they are removed they may be moved from placement to placement, since it can be difficult to provide satisfactory alternative living situations for these often difficult and insecure young people. Another hazard is that of being shuffled between the care of their parents and that of the agency as court proceedings occur, new information comes to light and the parents are given further opportunities to learn and practise the skills needed to care for their children. Psychiatrists can assist child welfare agencies by offering advice as to the needs of particular children and by providing input in the planning of services, with the aim of ensuring that these best meet these children's many needs.

Children whose parents are admitted to hospital for psychiatric reasons are a high-risk group (Shachnow, 1987). In addition to the stress of losing a parent for a time, they may already have been in an unstable environment because of their parents' psychiatric problems. Attention to their emotional needs at this time may prevent them developing disorders of their own.

Steinhauer (1984) provides an excellent summary of the problems of children admitted to the care of child welfare services, and suggests various ways in which these may be mitigated. He suggests ways of preventing 'drift' (the all-too-common process whereby children admitted to care languish in 'temporary' placements for extended periods); minimizing emergency placements; and providing effective casework for the children and their families.

Many self-help groups provide support for individuals and families faced with particular problems. They range from groups for the familes of children with cystic fibrosis or diabetes to organizations such as 'Alateen', which assist teenagers who have alcoholic parents.

The concept of 'high risk' has also been applied to communities. In Britain, attempts have been made to work at the community level in areas of high risk before disorders appear in the children by means of 'intermediate treatment'. This involves the use of various social work techniques, but especially 'community work'. This seeks to promote 'the participation of the parents and adults of the neighbourhood in the planning of services to children and youth, while fostering the involvement of the youngsters in the life of their community' (Leissner *et al.*, 1977). The idea is to apply these methods in 'areas of deprivation', with the objective of achieving both primary and secondary prevention.

Few of the preventive measures mentioned in this section have been subject to rigorous scientific study, so that we cannot be sure how effective they are. Fortunately the study of preventive measures seems to be increasing, and the establishment of journals such as the *Journal of Preventive Psychiatry* and the *Journal of Primary Prevention* is encouraging.

Community-wide measures

These include good obstetric and neonatal care and measures to make homes, vehicles and houses safer for children – for example the use of child car seats. The removal of lead from children's environments and the control of infectious diseases, especially those that affect the nervous system, are also rational preventive measures.

Factors such as cultural deprivation, family disharmony and parental mental illness present difficult challenges, though social change can lead to the lessening of psychiatric morbidity in communities. In a classical study, Leighton (1965) described changes in a rural community over a 10-year period. Initially the community was impoverished materially, culturally and socially, with a high prevalence of broken marriages, interparental strife and child neglect. As a result of changes in the community, notably group action and the emergence of local leadership, there were great improvements in these areas over the 10 years. Factors that contributed were activities of the official responsible for adult education and those of the local teacher. Some external factors, such as the electrification of the village, seemed to help but for the most part the changes in the community came from within. Outside people and agencies did, however, act as catalysts. The role of the 'consolidated school' in a town several miles away seemed important. The village children started going to this school during the course of the study. The influence of this school, through the ideas, concepts, values and standards of behaviour brought home by the children, seemed helpful.

Leighton (1965) reported a great lowering of the prevalence of psychiatric disorders over the 10-year period. By contrast, other communities which had been equally disintegrated when the study started, remained so 10 years later and showed no comparable decline in the prevalence of psychiatric disorders.

Studies by Rutter and his colleagues (1979) have confirmed the important role of the school, as a social institution, in the psychosocial development of children.

Secondary prevention

Secondary prevention involves early diagnosis and case finding, followed by intervention to bring the disorder under control as rapidly as possible. The screening of populations to detect disorders early in their development is a first step.

In most school systems the academic progress of children is assessed from time to time, either by regular administration of tests of educational attainment, or more informally by teachers' observations, supplemented by the use of tests on an *ad hoc* basis. The screening of child populations for behavioural, emotional and other psychiatric disorders is less widespread and systematic, though perceptive teachers are often able to spot children with early signs of such disorders. Various screening questionnaires are available for this purpose. These include Rutter's (1967b) questionnaire and the Bristol Social Adjustment Guide (Stott, 1966).

Academic failure often accompanies psychiatric disorders of various types. Not only is there an association between antisocial behaviour and school failure but children suffering from depression, neurotic disorders, psychotic conditions and other psychiatric problems may also present with academic failure. Vigilance by school staff can pay dividends in the early detection of problems other than primary learning disorders.

When disorders are detected in their early stages, the treatment methods described in the relevant chapters elsewhere in this book are generally indicated. Many schools and school systems have psychological and remedial services which are designed to help children with academic problems, including those associated with other problems. Nowadays many schools have school counsellors, sometimes called guidance counsellors, as members of their staffs. These are usually teachers with special training in dealing with children's emotional and social problems. They offer support and counselling to children in difficulty and, in many cases, also to the families of such children. Children with behavioural, emotional or learning problems may be brought to their attention by other teachers or by parents or others. Some seek help of their own accord. They are very much in the front line of the mental health services for disturbed children.

Most communities also have services which provide support and other help for families containing young children, especially those who have not yet started school. In Britain this service is provided mainly by health visitors, specialized nurses who have statutory duties which include visiting the families of all children soon after birth and at intervals thereafter. In North America nurses with similar functions are usually called public health nurses. These nurses are able to carry out both primary preventive work, by advising parents on the care and management of their children, and secondary prevention, by detecting problems early and either intervening themselves or referring the families for assessment and treatment (Barker, 1967).

Tertiary prevention

Tertiary prevention comprises measures taken once a disorder is established. It aims to limit the effect of the disorder, to prevent it getting worse and to give support to affected individuals or families. It requires active involvement and usually a lot of work on the part of the professionals concerned, but it may be vital, for example with families in which there has been serious abuse and neglect of children. Primary and secondary prevention are to be preferred, but cases often come to attention which are already fully established.

Various agencies provide tertiary prevention services, usually for families at high risk. These include community services for abusive and other dysfunctional families; and hospital 'child abuse' programmes which also provide specialized treatment. There are many services offering treatment for abused children and their families; these aim to restore the families to better functioning, so that further abuse does not occur and the children's healthy development is promoted.

Other points concerning prevention

One of the problems confronting those who want to promote primary prevention is that, as Kessler and Albee (1977) pointed out, 'practically every effort aimed at improving child rearing, increasing effective communication, building inner control and self-esteem, reducing stress and pollution and such like – in short everything aimed at improving the human condition – may be considered to be part of primary prevention of mental or emotional disturbance'. It is therefore important to consider the likely cost effectiveness of proposed measures and to build into programmes measures to assess their effectiveness.

What preventive measures prove feasible depends largely on community attitudes and especially the attitudes of community leaders. Extravagant claims concerning expected results, programme failures and excessively expensive schemes do not endear professionals to the communities they serve. It is the collective motivation of communities that determines whether preventive programmes are implemented and community education is therefore important.

Some believe that modern western society fails to provide a good environment for the raising of emotionally healthy children. Such people point to rising crime rates and the increase in divorce and the break-up of families as evidence of this. Goldsmith (1977) sees modern urban society as undermining the essential functions of the family; the family, in turn, is undermined as the basis of our social system. He believes that the educative, economic, welfare and social control functions of the family have all largely been taken away by the modern industrial state. At the same time, increasing numbers of poor, dispossessed, alienated people struggle to bring up children in deteriorating inner city areas. Economic and social problems make this increasingly difficult. Goldsmith's solution is 'de-urbanization', that is the settlement of people in smaller, ecologically balanced societies.

Bronfenbrenner (1977) has suggested that, 'in recent decades the American family has been falling apart'. He asserts that children's needs are being met less and less effectively and he too sees this as due to changing social standards. How is it, he asks, that we can deliver men and survival systems to the moon but not health care to the neighbourhood? He believes that it is the self-centredness of people in today's society, and their failure to contribute adequately to the communities in which they live, that are at the root of these problems.

It seems clear that social changes, for example a decline in the family break-up rate (Shamsie, 1985), would be helpful; it is less clear what steps should be taken, and by whom, to achieve such changes. Spiritual values seem to be changing and Bronfenbrenner (1977) suggests that a self-seeking materialism is increasingly preferred to a philosophy which puts helping others first. As he puts it, 'doing your own thing (is) our undoing'. The accumulation of material possessions seems to be the main aim of many in today's society. This has its limitations as a background for family life, the rearing of children and the creation of a functional social system.

The above issues are philosophical, moral, social and political, rather than clinical ones. They concern all of society, not just those concerned with mental health. Yet those of us who are professionally involved in the mental health field should be specially aware of them and should constantly bring them to the notice of society as a whole. We ought also to play a major part in the work which must be done to address them.

References

Achenbach, T.M. and Edelbrock, C.S. (1983). *Manual for Child Behaviour Checklist and Revised Child Behaviour Profile*. Burlington: Department of Psychiatry, University of Vermont.

Adams, P.L. (1973). *Obsessive Children*. London; Butterworth; New York: Brunner/Mazel.

Adams, P.L. (1982). *A Primer of Child Psychotherapy*, 2nd edn. Boston: Little, Brown.

Ainsworth, M.D.S., Blehar, M.C., Waters, E. Wall, S. (1978). *Patterns of Attachment: A Psychological Study of Strange Situations*. Hillsdale, N. J.: Lawrence Erlbaum.

Allen, F. H. (1942). *Psychotherapy with Children*. New York: Norton.

Allen, R. and Wasserman, G.A. (1985). 'Origins of language delay in abused infants'. *Child Abuse & Neglect*, **9**, 335–340.

American Psychiatric Association. (1980). *Diagnostic and Statistical Manual of Mental Disorders (DSM–III)*, 3rd edn. Washington, DC: A.P.A.

American Psychiatric Association. (1987). *Diagnostic and Statistical Manual of Mental Disorders (DSM–III–R)*, 3rd edn – revised. Washington, DC: APA.

Amini, F., Salasnek, S. and Burke, E.L. (1976). 'Adolescent drug abuse: etiological and treatment considerations'. *Adolescence*, **11**, 281–299.

Anastasi, A. (1982). *Psychological Testing*, 5th edn. New York: Macmillan.

Andrews, K. and Harris, M. (1964). *The Syndrome of Stuttering*. London: Heinemann.

Anthony, E.J. (1957). 'An experimental approach to the psychopathology of childhood: encopresis'. *British Journal of Medical Psychology*, **30**, 146–175.

Aponte, H. (1976). 'The family-school interview'. *Family Process*, **15**, 303–311.

Araoz, D.L. (1985). *The New Hypnosis*. New York: Brunner/Mazel.

Ash, P. and Guyer, M. (1986). 'The functions of psychiatric evaluation in contested child custody and visitation cases'. *Journal of the American Academy of Child Psychiatry*, **25**, 554–561.

Asperger, H. (1944). 'Die autistichen psychopathen in kindersalter'. *Archiv für Psychiatrie und Nervankrankheiten (Berlin)*, **117**, 76–137.

August, G. J., Stewart, M.A. and Tsai, L. (1981). 'The incidence of cognitive disabilities in the siblings of autistic children'. *British Journal of Psychiatry*, **138**, 416–422.

Bagley, C. (1971). *The Social Psychology of the Child with Epilepsy*. London: Routledge & Kegan Paul.

Baker, E.L. and Nash, M.R. (1987). 'Applications of hypnosis in the treatment of anorexia nervosa'. *American Journal of Clinical Hypnosis*, **29**, 185–193.

Bakwin, H. (1971). 'Enuresis in twins'. *American Journal of Diseases of Children*, **121**, 222–225.

Balbernie, R. (1974). 'Unintegration, integration and level of ego functioning as the determinants of planned 'cover therapy', of unit task and of placement'. *Journal of the Association of Workers for Maladjusted Children*, **2**, 6–46.

Baldwin, J.A. and Oliver, J.E. (1975). 'Epidemiology and family characteristics of severely abused children'. *British Journal of Preventive and Social Medicine*, **29**, 205–221.

Bandler, R. and Grinder, J. (1979). *Frogs into Princes*. Moab, Utah: Real People Press.

Bandler, R. Grinder, J. and Satir, V. (1976). *Changing with Families*. Palo Alto: Science & Behavior Books.

Barker, P. (1967). 'Child psychiatry and the health visitor'. *Nursing Mirror*, **124**, 549–551.

Barker, P. (1968). 'The inpatient treatment of school refusal'. *British Journal of Medical Psychology*, **41**, 381–387.

Barker, P. (1974a). 'History'. In: *The Residential Psychiatric Treatment of Children*, Ed. P Barker. London: Crosby Lockwood Staples.

Barker, P. (Ed) (1974b). *The Residential Psychiatric Treatment of Children*. London: Crosby Lockwood Staples.

Barker, P. (1981). 'Paradoxical techniques in psychotherapy'. In: *Treating Families with Special Needs*, Eds. D.S. Freeman and B. Trute. Ottawa: Canadian Association of Social Workers.

Barker, P. (1982). 'Residential treatment for disturbed children: its place in the '80s'. *Canadian Journal of Psychiatry*, **27**, 634–639.

Barker, P. (1984). 'Recognition and treatment of anxiety in children by means of psychiatric interview'. In: *Anxiety in Children*, Ed. V.P. Varma. London: Croom Helm; New York: Methuen.

Barker, P. (1985). *Using Metaphors in Psychotherapy*. New York: Brunner/Mazel.

Barker, P. (1986). *Basic Family Therapy*, 2nd edn. Oxford: Blackwell, Scientific Publications; New York: Oxford University Press.

Barker, P. (In press). 'The future of residential treatment for children'. In: *Children in Residential Care: Critical Issues In Treatment*, Eds. C.E. Schaefer and A.J. Swanson. New York: Van Nostrand Reinhold.

Barker, P., Buffe, C. and Zaretsky, R. (1978). 'Providing a family alternative for the disturbed child'. *Child Welfare*, **57**, 373–379.

Barnes, D.M. (1986). 'Brain function decline in children with AIDS' *Science*, **232**, 1196.

Barnhill, L. H., and Longo, D. (1978). 'Fixation and regression in the family life cycle' *Family Process*, **17**, 469–478.

Bartak, L., Rutter, M. and Cox, A. (1975). 'A comparative study of infantile autism and specific developmental receptive language disorder'. *British Journal of Psychiatry*, **126**, 127–145.

Baskin, E.J. and Hess, R.D. (1980). 'Does affective education work? A review of seven programs'. *Journal of School Psychology*, **18**, 40–50.

Beard, R.M. (1969). *An Outline of Piaget's Developmental Psychology*. London: Routledge and Kegan Paul.

Bietchman, J.H. (1983). 'Childhood schizophrenia: a review and comparison with adult onset schizophrenia'. *Psychiatric Journal of the University of Ottawa*, **8**, 25–37.

Bellman, M. (1966). 'Studies on encopresis'. *Acta Paediatrica Scandinavica*, Supplement **170**.

Belsky, J., Rovine, M. and Taylor, D.G. (1984). 'The Pennsylvania infant and family development project'. *Child Development*, **55**, 718–728.

Bender, L. and Schilder, P. (1940). 'Impulsions: a specific disorder of the behaviour of children'. *Archives of Neurology and Psychiatry*, **44**, 990–1008.

Benedek, E. (1983). 'Psychiatry and juvenile law'. *Psychiatric Clinics of North America*, **6**, 695–705.

Bentovim, A. and Boston, M. (1973). 'A day-centre for disturbed young children and their parents'. *Journal of Child Psychotherapy*, **3**, 46–60.

Berecz, J.M. (1968). 'Phobias in childhood: aetiology and treatment' *Psychological Bulletin*, **70**, 694–720.

Berg, I. (1979). 'Day wetting in children'. *Journal of Child Psychology and Psychiatry*, **20**, 167–173.

Berg, I. (1985). 'The management of truancy'. *Journal of Child Psychology & Psychiatry*, **26**, 325–331.

Berg, I., Forsythe, I., Holt, P. and Watta, J. (1983). 'A controlled trial of 'Senokot'in faecal soiling treated by behavioural methods'. *Journal of Child Psychology & Psychiatry*, **24**, 543–549.

Berger, M., Yule, W. and Rutter, M. (1975). 'Attainment and adjustment in two geographical areas'. *British Journl of Psychiatry*, **126**, 510–519.

Berney, T., Kolvin, I., Bhate, S.R., Garside, R.F., Jeans, B., Kay, B. and Scarth L. (1981). 'School phobia: a therapeutic trial with clomipramine and short-term outcome'. *British Journal of Psychiatry*, **138**, 110–118.

Bernstein, G.A. and Garfinkel, B.D. (1986). 'School phobia: the overlap of effective and anxiety disorders'. *Journal of the American Academy of Child Psychiatry*, **25**, 235–241.

Bicknell, J. (1975). *Pica: A Childhood Symptom*. London: Butterworth.

Biller, H.B. (1970). 'Father absence and the personality development of the male child'. *Developmental Psychology*, **2**, 181–201.

Blagg, N.R. and Yule, W. (1984). 'The behavioural treatment of school refusal: a comparative study' *Behaviour Research and Therapy*, **22**, 119–127.

Blehar, M.C. (1974). 'Anxious attachment and defensive reactions associated with day care' *Child Development*, **45**, 683–692.

Blum, K. (1984). *Handbook of Abusable Drugs*. New York: Gardner Press.

Boatman, B., Borkan, E.L. and Schetky, D.H. (1981). 'Treatment of child victims of incest'. *American Journal of Family Therapy*, **9**, 43–51.

Bouchard, T.J. and McGue, M. (1981). 'Familial studies of intelligence: a review'. *Science*, **212**, 1055–1059.

Bowlby, J. (1951). *Maternal Care and Mental Health*. Geneva: World Health Organization.

Bowlby, J. (1969). *Attachment*. London: Hogarth; New York: Basic Books.

Bowlby, J. (1977). 'The making and breaking of emotional bonds'. *British Journal of Psychiatry*, **130**, 201–210 and 421–431.

Bowlby, J. (1979). *The Making and Breaking of Affectional Bonds*. London: Tavistock.

Bowlby, J. (1980). *Attachment and Loss: III. Loss, Sadness and Depression*. London: Hogarth; New York: Basic Books.

Boyle, M.H. and Offord, D.R. (1986). 'Smoking, drinking and the use of illicit drugs among adolescents in Ontario'. *Canadian Medical Association Journal*, **135**, 1113–1121.

Boyle, M.H., Offord, D.R., Hofman, H.G., Catlin, G.P., Byles, J.A., Cadman, D.T., Crawford, J.W., Links, P.S., Rae-Grant, N.I. and Szatmari, P. (1987). 'Ontario child health study: methodology'. *Archives of General Psychiatry*, **44**, 826–831.

Bradford, J. and Dimock, J. (1986). 'A comparative study of adolescents and adults who wilfully set fires'. *Psychiatric Journal of the University of Ottawa*, **11**, 228–234.

Bradley, S.J., Doering, R.W., Zucker, K.F., Finegan, J.K. and Gonda, G.M. (1980). 'Assessment of the gender–disturbed child: a comparison to sibling and psychiatric controls'. In: *Childhood and Sexuality*, Ed. J Samson. Montreal: Éditions Études Vivantes.

Bradley, S. and Sloman, L. (1975). 'Elective mutism in immigrant families'. *Journal of the American Academy of Child Psychiatry.* **14**, 510–514.

Brent, D.A., Kalas, R., Edelbrock, C., Costello, A.J., Dulcan, M.K. and Conover, N. (1986). 'Psychopathology and its relationship to suicidal ideation in childhood and adolescence'. *Journal of the American Academy of Child Psychiatry*, **25**, 666–673.

Bridgland, M. (1971). *Pioneer Work with Maladjusted Children*. London: Crosby Lockwood Staples.

British Medical Journal. (1977). 'Enuresis' (editorial) **1**, 4.

Broderick, C.B. and Rowe, P. (1968). 'A scale of pre-adolescent heterosexual development'. *Journal of Marriage & the Family*, **30**, 97–101.

Brofenbrenner, U. (1977). 'Doing your own thing – our undoing'. *Child Psychiatry and Human Development*, **8**, 3–10.

Brown, B., Fuller, J. and Gericke, C. (1975). 'Elective mutism: a review and a report of an unsuccessfully treated case.' *Journal of the Association of Workers for Maladjusted Children*, **3**, 27–37.

Brown, B. and Lloyd, H. (1975). A controlled study of children not speaking at school' *Journal of the Association of Workers for Maladjusted Children*, **3**, 49–63.

Brown, B.D. and Fromm, E. (1986). *Hypnotherapy and Hypnoanalysis*. Hillsdale, NJ: Lawrence Erlbaum.

Brown, G.W., Chadwick, O., Shaffer, D., Rutter, M. and Traub, M. (1981). 'A prospective study of children with head injuries: III. Psychiatric sequelae'. *Psychological Medicine*, **11**, 63–78.

Bruch, H. (1974). 'Obesity' (part II). In: *Eating Disorders, Obesity, Anorexia Nervosa and the Person Within*. London: Routledge and Kegan Paul.

Bullard, D. M., Glaser, H.H., Hagerty, M.C. and Pivchik, E.C. (1967). 'Failure to thrive in the "neglected" child' *American Journal of Orthopsychiatry*, **37**, 680–690.

Burquest, B. (1979). 'Severe female delinquency: when to involve the family in treatment'. In: *Adolescent Psychiatry*, Vol 7 Ed. S.C. Feinstein and P.L. Giovacchini. University of Chicago Press.

Busch, F., Nagero, H., McKnight, J. and Pezzarossi, G. (1973). 'Primary transitional objects'. *Journal of the American Academy of Child Psychiatry*, **12**, 193–214.

Byrne, C.M. and Cadman, D. (1987). 'Prevention of the adverse effects of hospitalization in children'. *Journal of Preventive Psychiatry* **3**, 167–190.

Cade, B. (1980). 'Strategic therapy'. *Journal of Family Therapy*, **2**, 89–99.

Cadman, D., Rosenbaum, P. and Pettinghill, P. (1987). 'Prevention of emotional, behavioural, and family problems of children with chronic medical illness'. *Journal of Preventive Psychiatry*, **3**, 147–165.

Caffey, J. (1946). 'Multiple fractures in the long bones of infants suffering from chronic subdural haematoma'. *American Journal of Roentgenology*, **56** 163–173.

Call, J.D., Galenson, E. and Tyson, R.L. (Eds) (1983). *Frontiers of Infant Psychiatry* Vol I. New York: Basic Books.

Call, J.D., Galenson, E. and Tyson, R.L. (Eds) (1985). *Frontiers of Infant Psychiatry* Vol II. New York: Basic Books.

Cameron, J.R. (1977). 'Parental treatment, children's temperament and the risk of childhood behavioural problems'. *American Journal of Orthopsychiatry*, **47**, 568–576.

Campbell, M., Small, A.M., Green, W.H., Jennings, S.J., Perry, R., Bennett, W.G. and

Anderson, L. (1984). 'Behavioural efficacy of haloperidol and lithium carbonate'. *Archives of General Psychiatry*, **41** 650–656.

Cantor, S. and Kestenbaum, C. (1986). 'Psychotherapy with schizophrenic children'. *Journal of the American Academy of Child Psychiatry*. **25**, 623–630.

Cantwell, D.P. and Baker, L. (1985). 'Speech and Language: Development and Disorders'. In: *Child & Adolescent Psychiatry: Modern Approaches*, 2nd edn, Ed. M. Rutter and L. Hersov. Oxford: Blackwell Scientific Publications.

Caplan, G. (1964). *Principles of Preventive Psychiatry*. New York: Basic Books.

Caplan, G. (1980). 'An approach to preventive intervention in child psychiatry'. *Canadian Journal of Psychiatry*, **25**, 671–682.

Carter, E.A. and McGoldrick M. (1980). *The Family Life Cycle*. New York: Gardner.

Chamberlain, C. and Awad, G. (1979). 'Clinical consultation in custody and access disputes'. In: *New Directions in Children's Mental Health*, Ed. S.J. Shamsie. New York: SP. Medical and Scientific Books.

Chess, S. (1977). 'Follow-up report on autism in congenital rubella'. *Journal of Autism & Childhood Schizophrenia*, **7**, 69–81.

Chess, S. and Thomas, A. (1984). *Origins and Evolution of Behavior Disorders from Infancy to Early Adult Life*. New York: Brunner Mazel.

Chiles, J., Miller, M. and Cox G. (1980). 'Depression in an adolescent delinquent population'. *Archives of General Psychiatry* **37**, 179–183.

Coates, S. and Person, E.S. (1985). 'Extreme boyhood femininity: isolated behavior or pervasive disorder?'. *Journal of the American Academy of Child Psychiatry*, **24**, 702–709.

Cohen, D.J. (1980). 'The pathology of the self in primary childhood autism and Gilles de la Tourette syndrome'. *Psychiatric Clinics of North America*, 3, 383–402.

Cohen, D.J., Volkmar, F.R. and Paul, R.(1986). 'Issues in the classification of pervasive developmental disorders'. *Journal of the American Academy of Child Psychiatry*, **25**, 158–161.

Conners, C.K. (1969). 'A teacher rating scale for use in drug-studies with children'. *American Journal of Psychiatry*, **126**, 884–888.

Conners, C.K. (1980). *Food Additives and Hyperactive Children*. New York: Plenum.

Consortium for Longitudinal Studies. (1983). *As The Twig Is Bent: Lasting Effects of Preschool Programs*. Hillsdale, NJ: Lawrence Erlbaum.

Cooper, S. (1987). 'The fetal alcohol syndrome'. *Journal of Child Psychology & Psychiatry*, **28**, 223–227.

Coopersmith, S. (1967). *The Antecedents of Self-Esteem*. San Francisco: W.H. Freeman.

Coppersmith, E.I. (1985). 'Teaching trainees to think in triads'. *Journal of Marital & Family Therapy*, **11**, 61–66.

Corbett, J.A. (1979). 'Psychiatric morbidity and mental retardation'. In: *Psychiatric Illness and Mental Handicap*, Ed. F.E. James and R.P. Snaith. London: Gaskell Press.

Corbett, J., Harris, R., Taylor, E. and Trimble, M. (1977). 'Progressive disintegrative psychosis of childhood'. *Journal of Child Psychology & Psychiatry*, **18**, 211–219.

Corbett, J.A., Matthews, A.M., Connell, P.H. and Shapiro, D.A. (1969). 'Tics and Gilles de la Tourette's syndrome: a follow-up study and critical review'. *British Journal of Psychiatry*, **115**, 1229–1241.

Corbett, J.A. and Turpin, G. (1985). 'Tics & Tourette's syndrome'. In: *Child and Adolescent Psychiatry: Modern Approaches* 2nd edn, Eds. M. Rutter and L. Hersov. Oxford: Blackwell Scientific Publications.

Costello, A.J. (1986). 'Assessment and diagnosis of affective disorders in children'. *Journal of Child Psychology & Psychiatry*, **27**, 565–574.

344   *Basic Child Psychiatry*

Cotton, N.S. (1983). 'The development of self-esteem and self-esteem regulation'. In: *The Development and Sustenance of Self-Esteem*, Eds. J.E. Mack and S.L. Ablon. New York: International Universities Press.

Covitz, J. (1986). *Emotional Child Abuse: The Family Curse*. Boston: Sigo Press.

Cox, A., Hopkinson, K. and Rutter, M. (1981). 'Psychiatric interviewing techniques II. Naturalistic study'. *British Journal of Psychiatry*, **138**, 283–291.

Cox, A., Holbrook, D. and Rutter, M. (1981). 'Psychiatric interviewing techniques VI. Experimental study: eliciting feelings'. *British Journal of Psychiatry*, **139**, 144–152.

Cox, A., Rutter, M. and Holbrook, D. (1981). 'Psychiatric interviewing techniques V. Experimental study: eliciting factual information'. *British Journal of Psychiatry*, **139**, 29–37.

Crasilneck, H.B. and Hall, J.A. (1985). *Clinical Hypnosis: Principles and Applications* 2nd edn. Orlando, F.L: Grune & Stratton.

Cravioto, J. and Arrieta R. (1983). 'Malnutrition in childhood'. In: *Developmental Neuropsychiatry*, Ed. M. Rutter. New York: Guilford.

Creak, M. (1963). 'Childhood psychosis: a review of 100 cases'. *British Journal of Psychiatry*, **109**, 84–89.

Creighton S.J. (1985). 'An epidemiological study of abused children and their families in the United Kingdom between 1977 and 1982'. *Child Abuse & Neglect*, **9**, 441–448.

Crisp, A. (1977). 'Diagnosis and outcome of anorexia nervosa'. *Proceedings of the Royal Society of Medicine*, **70**, 464–470.

Crisp, A.H., Palmer, R.L. and Kalucy, R.S. (1976). 'How common is anorexia nervosa? A prevalence study'. *British Journal of Psychiatry*, **128**, 549–554.

Cunningham, L., Cadoret, R., Loftus, R. and Edwards, J.E. (1975). 'Studies of adoptees from psychiatrically disturbed biological parents'. *British Journal of Psychiatry*, **126**, 217–224.

Currie, K.H. and Brannigan, C. (1970). 'Behaviour analysis and modification with an autistic child'. In: *Behaviour Studies in Psychiatry* Eds. C. Hutt and S.J. Hutt. Oxford: Pergamon.

Cytryn, L., McKnew, D.H., Zahn-Waxler, C. and Gershon, E.S. (1986). 'Developmental issues in risk research: the offspring of affectively ill parents'. In: *Depression in Young People*, Eds. M. Rutter, C.E. Izard and P.B. Read. New York: Guilford.

Dale, P.S. (1976). *Language Development: Structure and Function*, 2nd edn. Hindsdale, Ill: Dryden Press.

Darlington, R.B., Royce, J.M., Snipper, A.S., Murray, H.W. and Lazar, I. (1980). 'Preschool programs and later school competence of the children from low-income families'. *Science*, **208**, 202–204.

Davidson, S. (1960). 'School phobia as a manifestation of family disturbance'. *Journal of Child Psychology and Psychiatry*, **1**, 270–287.

Davie, R., Butler, N. and Goldstein, H. (1972). *From Birth to Seven*. London: Longman.

DeJonge, G.A. (1973). 'Epidemiology of enuresis: a survey of the literature'. In: *Bladder Control & Enuresis* (Clinics in Developmental Medicine, nos 48/49), Ed. I. Kolvin, R.C. MacKeith, and S.R. Meadow. London: Heinemann.

Devinsky, O. (1983). Neuroanatomy of Gilles de la Tourette's syndrome'. *Archives of Neurology*, **40**, 508–514.

Deykin, E.Y. and MacMahon, B. (1979). 'The incidence of seizures among autistic children'. *American Journal of Psychiatry*, **136**, 1310–1312.

DiLeo, J.H. (1983). *Interpreting Children's Drawings*. New York: Brunner/Mazel.

Dilts, R., Grinder, J., Bandler, R., Bandler, L.C. and DeLozier, J. (1980). *Neuro-Linquistic Programming: Volume 1.* Cupertino, CA: Meta Publications.

Dische, S., Yule, W., Corbett, J. and Hand, D. (1983). 'Childhood nocturnal enuresis: factors associated with outcome of treatment with an enuresis alarm'. *Developmental Medicine & Child Neurology,* **25,** 67–80.

Dobbing, J., Clarke, A.D.B., Corbett, J.A., Hogg, J. and Robinson, R.O. (Eds) (1984). *Scientific Studies in Mental Retardation.* London: Royal Society of Medicine & Macmillan.

Dockar-Drysdale, B. (1968). *Therapy in Child Care* (collected papers). London: Longman Green.

Dockar-Drysdale, B. (1973). *Consultation in Child Care.* London: Longman.

Dorenbaum, D., Mencel, E., Blume, W.T. and Fisman, S. (1987). 'EEG findings and language in autistic children: clinical correlations'. *Canadian Journal of Psychiatry,* **32,** 31–34.

Douglas, V.I., Barr, R.G., O'Neill, M.E. and Britton, B.G. (1986). 'Short term effects of methylphenidate on the cognitive, learning and academic performance of children with attention deficit disorder in the laboratory and classroom'. *Journal of Child Psychology & Psychiatry,* **27,** 191–211.

Driscoll, J.M., Driscoll, Y.T., Steir, M.E., Stark, R.I., Dangman, B.C., Perez, A., Wung, J-T. and Kritz, P., (1982). 'Mortality and morbidity in infants less than 1,001 grams birth weight' *Pediatrics,* **69,** 21–26.

Duvall, E.M. and Miller, B.C. (1985). *Marriage and Family Development,* 6th edn. New York: Harper & Row.

Earls, F. (1980). 'The prevalence of behaviour problems in three-year-old children'. *Archives of General Psychiatry,* **37,** 1153-1157.

Earls, F., Jacobs, G., Goldfein, R., Silbert, A., Beardslee, W. and Rivinus, T. (1982). 'Concurrent validation of a behaviour problems scale to use with 3-year-olds'. *Journal of the American Academy of Child Psychiatry,* **21,** 47–57.

Earls, F. and Richman, N. (1980a). 'The prevalence of behaviour problems in three-year-old children of West Indian-born parents' *Journal of Child Psychology and Psychiatry,* **21,** 99–106.

Earls, F. and Richman, N. (1980b). Behaviour problems in pre-school children of West Indian-born parents: a re-examination of family and social factors'. *Journal of Child Psychology and Psychiatry,* **21,** 107–117.

Edelbrock, C., Costello A.J. and Kessler, M.D. (1984). 'Empirical corroboration of attention deficit disorder'. *Journal of the American Academy of Child Psychiatry,* **23,** 285–290.

Edwards, S.D. and van der Spuy, H.I.J. (1985). 'Hypnotherapy as a treatment for enuresis'. *Journal of Child Psychology & Psychiatry,* **26,** 161–170.

Egger, J., Carter, C.M., Graham, P.J., Gumley, D. and Soothill J.F. (1985). 'Controlled trial of oligoantigenic diet in the hyperkinetic syndrome'. *Lancet,* **1,** 540–545.

Elmer, E. (1986). 'Outcome of residential treatment for abused and high-risk infants.' *Child Abuse & Neglect,* **10,** 351–360.

Emde, R.N. (1984). 'The affective self: continuities and transformations from infancy'. In: *Frontiers of Infant Psychiatry Vol. II,* Ed. J.D. Call, E. Galenson and R.L. Tyson. New York: Basic Books.

Emde, R.N. (1985). 'Assessment of infancy disorders'. In: *Child and Adolescent Psychiatry: Modern Approaches,* 2nd edn, Eds. M Rutter and L. Hersov. Oxford: Blackwell Scientific Publications.

Emde, R.N. and Sorce, J.F. (1983). 'The rewards of infancy: emotional availability and maternal referencing'. In: *Frontiers of Infant Psychiatry Vol I*, Ed. J.D. Call, E. Galenson and R.L. Tyson. New York: Basic Books.

Emler, N., Reichler, S. and Ross, A. (1987). 'The social context of delinquent conduct'. *Journal of Child Psychology & Psychiatry*, **28**, 99–109.

Erickson, M.H., Hersman, S. and Secter, I.I. (1961). *The Practical Application of Medical and Dental Hypnosis*. Chicago: Seminars on Hypnosis Publishing Co.

Erikson, E.H. (1965). *Childhood and Society*. London: Penguin.

Erikson, E.H. (1968). *Identity and the Life Cycle*. London: Faber.

Evans-Jones, L.G. and Rosenbloom, L. (1978). Disintegrative psychosis in childhood'. *Developmental Medicine & Child Neurology*, **20**, 462–470.

Eysenck, H.J. (1959). 'Learning theory and behaviour therapy'. *Journal of Mental Science*, **105**, 61–95.

Falconer, D.S. (1981). *Introduction to Quantitative Genetics*, 2nd edn. London: Longman.

Farber, E.D., Kinast, C., McCoard, W.D. and Falkner, D. (1984). 'Violence in families of adolescent runaways'. *Child Abuse & Neglect*, **8**, 295–299.

Farrell, C. and Kellaher, L. (1978). *My Mother Said: The Way Young People Learn about Sex and Birth Control*. London: Routledge & Kegan Paul.

Farrington, D.P. (1978). 'The family background of aggressive youths'. In: *Aggression and Anti-social Behaviour in Childhood and Adolescence*, Ed. L. Hersov, M. Berger and D. Shaffer. Oxford: Pergamon.

Feingold, B.F. (1975). 'Hyperkinesis and learning disabilities linked to artificial food flavors and colors'. *American Journal of Nursing*, **75**, 797–903.

Ferguson, B.G. (1986). 'Kleine-Levin syndrome: a case report'. *Journal of Child Psychology & Psychiatry*, **27**, 275–278.

Ferrari, M. (1986). 'Fears and phobias in childhood: some clinical and developmental considerations'. *Child Psychiatry & Human Development*, **17**, 75–87.

Field, E. (1967). *A Validation of Hewitt and Jenkins' Hypothesis*. Home Office Research Study in the Causes of Delinquency and the Treatment of Offenders. London: HMSO.

Fisch, G.S., Cohen, I.L., Wolf, E.G., Brown, W.T. Jenkins, E.C. and Gross, A. (1986) 'Autism and the fragile X syndrome'. *American Journal of Psychiatry*, **143**, 71–73.

Fish, B. (1977). 'Neurobiologic antecedents of schizophrenia in children'. *Archives of General Psychiatry*, **34**, 1297–1313.

Fish, B. (1986). 'Antecedents of an acute schizophrenic break' *Journal of the American Academy of Child Psychiatry*, **25**, 595–600.

Flament, M., Rapoport, J., Berg. C., Screey, W., Kilts, C., Mellstromm, B. and Linnoila, M. (1985). 'Clomipramine treatment of childhood obsessive compulsive disorder'. *Archives of General Psychiatry*, **42**, 977–983.

Flavell, J.H., (1963). *The Developmental Psychology of Jean Piaget*. Princeton: van Nostrand.

Folstein, S. and Rutter, M. (1977). 'Genetic influences and infantile autism'. *Nature*, **265**, 726–728.

Fossen, A., Knibbs, J., Bryant-Waugh, R. and Lask, B. (1987). 'Early onset anorexia nervosa'. *Archives of Disease in Childhood*, **62**, 114–118.

Frankl, V.E. (1960). 'Paradoxical intention: a logotherapeutic technique'. *American Journal of Psychotherapy*, **14**, 520–535.

Freud, A. (1966). *Normality and Pathology in Childhood*. New York: International Universities Press; and London: Hogarth

Freud, A. (1970). 'The symptomatology of childhood: a preliminary attempt at classification'. *The Psychoanalytic Study of the Child*, **25**, 19–41.

Freud, A. (1972). *A Short History of Child Analysis*. London: Hogarth Press.

Freud, S. (1905). 'Three essays on the theory of sexuality'. *Standard Edition*. **7**, London: Hogarth (1953).

Friedman, A.S. Utada, A. and Morrissey, M.R. (1987). 'Families of adolescent drug abusers are 'rigid': are these families either 'disengaged' or 'enmeshed', or both?' *Family Process*, **26**, 131–148.

Fundudis, T. (1986). 'Anorexia nervosa in a pre-adolescent girl: a multimodal behaviour therapy approach'. *Journal of Child Psychology & Psychiatry*, **27**, 261–273.

Gabel, S. and Hsu, L.K.G. (1986). 'Routine laboratory tests in adolescent inpatients'. *Journal of the American Academy of Child Psychiatry* **25**, 113–119.

Gaensbauer, T.J. and Harmon, R.J. (1981). 'Clinical assessment in infancy utilizing structured playroom situations'. *Journal of the American Academy of Child Psychiatry*, **20**, 264–280.

Garbarino, J., Guttman, E. and Seeley, J.W. (1986). *The Psychologically Battered Child*. San Francisco: Jossey-Bass.

Gardner, G.G., and Olness, K. (1981). *Hypnosis and Hypnotherapy with Children*. New York: Grune & Stratton.

Garfinkel, P.E. and Garner, D.M. (1982). *Anorexia Nervosa: A Multidimensional Perspective*. New York: Brunner/Mazel.

Garmezy, N. (1986). 'Children under severe stress: critique and commentary'. *Journal of the American Academy of Child Psychiatry*, **384–392**.

Garner, D.M. and Garfinkel. P.E. (1980). 'Sociocultural factors in the development of anorexia nervosa'. *Psychological Medicine*, **10**, 647–656.

Gath, A. (1985). 'Chromosomal abnormalities'. In: *Child & Adolescent Psychiatry: Modern Approaches*, 2nd edn, Eds. M. Rutter and L. Hersov. Oxford: Blackwell Scientific Publications.

Gaynor, J. and Hatcher, C. (1987). *The Psychology of Child Firesetting*. New York: Brunner/Mazel.

Geller, E., Ritvo E.R. Freeman, B.J. and Yuwiter, A. (1982). 'Preliminary observations of the effect of fenfluramine on blood serotonin and symptoms in three autistic boys'. *New England Journal of Medicine*, **307**, 335–342.

German, G.A. (1972). 'Aspects of clinical psychiatry in Sub-Saharan Africa'. *British Journal of Psychiatry*, **121**, 461–479.

Ghent, W.R. Da Sylva, N.P. and Farren, M.E. (1985). 'Family violence; guidelines for recognition and management'. *Canadian Medical Association Journal*, **132**, 541–548.

Gil, D.G. (1975). 'Unravelling child abuse'. *American Journal of Orthopsychiatry*, **45**, 346–356.

Gilberg, C. and Wahlstrom, J. (1985). 'Chomosome abnormalities in infantile autism and other childhood psychosis'. *Developmental Medicine and Child Neurology*, **27**, 293–304.

Ginott, H.G. (1961). *Group Psychotherapy with Children*. New York: McGraw-Hill.

Gittelman, R. (1985). 'Controlled trials of remedial approaches to reading disability'. *Journal of Child Psychology & Psychiatry*, **26**, 843–836.

Gittelman, R. (1986). (Ed.) *Anxiety Disorders of Childhood*. New York: Guilford.

Goldsmith, E. (1977). 'The future of an affluent society: the case of Canada'. *Ecologist*, **7**, 160–194.

348   *Basic Child Psychiatry*

Goldsmith, H.H. (1983). 'Genetic influences on personality from infancy to adulthood'. *Child Development*. **54**, 331–355.

Gomez, M.R. and Klass, D.W. (1983). 'Epilepsies of infancy and childhood'. *Annals of Neurology*, **13**, 113–124.

Goodman, J.D. and Sours, J.A. (1967). *The Child Mental Status Examination*. New York: Basic Books.

Goodyer, I.M. (1985). 'Epileptic and pseudoepileptic seizures in childhood and adolescence'. *Journal of the American Academy of Child Psychiatry*, **24**,3–9.

Government of Alberta. (1984) *Child Welfare Act*. Edmonton: Queen's Printer.

Graham, P.J. (1985). 'Psychosomatic relationships'. In: *Child & Adolescent Psychiatry: Modern Approaches*, 2nd edn, Eds. M. Rutter and L. Hersov, Oxford: Blackwell Scientific Publications.

Graham, P. and Rutter, M. (1985). 'Adolescent disorders'. In: *Child & Adolescent Psychiatry: Modern Approaches* 2nd edn, Eds. M. Rutter and L. Hersov. Oxford: Blackwell, Scientific Publications.

Green, R. (1974). *Sexual Identity Conflict in Children and Adults*. New York: Basic Books.

Green, R. (1985a). 'A typical psychosexual development'. In: *Child & Adolescent Psychiatry: Modern Approaches*, 2nd edn, Eds. M. Rutter and L. Hersov. Oxford: Blackwell Scientific Publications.

Green, R. (1985b). 'Gender identity in childhood and later sexual orientation: follow-up of 78 males'. *American Journal of Psychiatry*, **142**, 339–341.

Green, W.H., Campbell, M., Hardesty, A.S., Grega, D.M., Padron-Gayol, M. Shell, J. and Erlenmeyer-Kimling, L. (1984). 'A comparison of schizophrenic and autistic children'. *Journal of the American Academy of Child Psychiatry*, **23**, 399–409.

Greenberg, L.M. and Stephans, J.H. (1977). 'Use of drugs in special syndromes'. In: *Psychopharmacology in Childhood & Adolescence*, Ed. J.M. Wiener. New York: Basic Books.

Greiner, J.R., Fitzgerald, H.E., Cooke P.A. and Djurdjic, S.D. (1985). 'Assessment of sensitivity to interpersonal stress in stutterers and non-stutterers'. *Journal of Communication Disorders*, **18**, 215–225.

Grinker, J.A. (1981). 'Behavioral and metabolic factors in childhood obesity'. In: *The Uncommon Child*, Eds. M. Lewis and L.A. Rosenblum. New York: Plenum.

Gross, M. (1983). 'Hypnosis in the treatment of anorexia nervosa'. *American Journal of Clinical Hypnosis*, **26**, 175–181.

Group for the Advancement of Psychiatry. (1968). *Normal Adolescence: Its Dynamics and Impact*. New York: GAP. (Also London: Crosby Lockwood Staples, 1974.)

Gualtieri, C.T., Wargin, W., Kanoy, P., Patrick, K., Shen, C.D., Youngblood W. Mueller, R.A. and Breese, G.R. (1982). 'Clinical studies of methylphenidate serum levels in children and adults'. *Journal of the American Academy of Child Psychiatry*, **21**, 19–26.

Gubbay, S.S. (1975). *The Clumsy Child*. London: Saunders.

Guilleminault, C., Eldridge, F.L. Simmons, F.B. and Dement, W.C. (1976). 'Sleep apnoea in eight children', *Pediatrics*, **58**, 23–30.

Guinness, E. (1986). 'Social origins of a neurosis: the African brain fag syndrome'. Paper presented at the meeting of the African Psychiatric Association, Nairobi, Kenya, August, 1986.

Guyer, M.J. (1982). 'Child abuse and neglect statutes: legal and clinical implications'. *American Journal of Orthopsychiatry*, **52**, 73–81.

Hack, M., Fanaroff, A.A. and Merkatz, I.R. (1979). 'The low birth-weight infant: evolution of a changing outlook'. *New England Journal of Medicine*, **301**, 1162–1165.

Haley, J., (1976). *Problem-Solving Therapy*. San Francisco: Jossey-Bass.

Haley, J. (1980). *Leaving Home*. New York: McGraw-Hill.

Halliday, S., Meadow, S.R. and Berg, I. (1987). 'Successful management of daytime enuresis using alarm procedures: a randomly controlled trial'. *Archives of Disease in Childhood*, **62**, 132–137.

Halmi, K.A. (1974) 'Anorexia nervosa: demographic and clinical features in 94 cases'. *Psychosomatic Medicine*, **36**, 18–26.

Harlow, H.F. (1958). 'The nature of love'. *American Journal of Psychology* **13**, 673–685.

Hassanyeh, F. and Davison, K. (1980). 'Bipolar affective psychosis with onset before age 16 years: report of 10 Cases'. *British Journal of Psychiatry*, **137**, 530–537.

Hawton, K., O'Grady, J., Osborn, M. and Cole, D. (1982). 'Adolescents who take overdoses: their characteristics, problems and contacts with helping agencies'. *British Journal of Psychiatry*, **140**, 118–123.

Hayden, T.L. (1980). 'Classification of elective mutism'. *Journal of the American Academy of Child Psychiatry*, **19**, 118–113.

Hazel, N. (1977). 'How family placements can combat delinquency' *Social Work Today*, **8**, 6–7.

Heard, D. H. (1981). 'The relevance of attachment theory to child psychiatric practice'. *Journal of Child Psychology & Psychiatry*, **22**, 89–96

Heard, D. (1982). 'Family systems and the attachment dynamic'. *Journal of Family Therapy*, **4**, 99–116.

Heard, D. (1987). 'The relevance of attachment theory to child psychiatric practice: an update'. *Journal of Child Psychology & Psychiatry*, **28**, 25–28.

Heaton-Ward, W.A. and Wiley, Y. (1984). *Mental Handicap*. Bristol: Wright.

Heller, T. (1954). 'About dementia infantilis' (translation). *Journal of Nervous & Mental Disease*, **119**, 471–477.

Hensey, O., Williams, J.K. and Rosenbloom, L. (1983). 'Intervention in child abuse: experience in Liverpool'. *Developmental Medicine & Child Neurology*, **25**, 606–611.

Hersov, L. (1960a). 'Persistent non-attendance at school'. *Journal of Child Psychology & Psychiatry*, **1**, 130–136.

Hersov, L. (1960b). 'Refusal to go to school'. *Journal of Child Psychology & Psychiatry*, **1**, 137–145.

Hersov, L. (1980). 'Hospital inpatient and daypatient treatment of school refusal'. In: *Out of School – Modern Perspectives in School Refusal and Truancy*, Eds. L. Hersov and I. Berg. Chichester: Wiley.

Hersov, L. (1985a). 'Emotional disorders'. In: *Child & Adolescent Psychiatry: Modern Approaches* 2nd edn, Eds. M. Rutter and L. Hersov. Oxford: Blackwell Scientific Publications.

Hersov, L. (1985b) 'School refusal' In: *Child and Adolescent Psychiatry: Modern Approaches* 2nd edn, Eds M. Rutter and L. Hersov. Oxford: Blackwell Scientific Publications.

Hersov, L. and Bentovim, A. (1985). 'In-patient and day-hospital units'. In: *Child & Adolescent Psychiatry: Modern Approaches*, 2nd edn, Eds. M. Rutter and L. Hersov. Oxford: Blackwell Scientific Publications.

Hetherington, E.M., Cox, M. and Cox, R. (1982). 'Family interaction and the social, emotional and cognitive development of children following divorce'. In: *The Family – Setting Priorities*, Ed. V. Vaughan and T. Brazelton. New York: Science and Medicine.

Hewitt, L.E. and Jenkins, R.L. (1946). *Fundamental Patterns of Maladjustment*. Illinois: Michigan Child Guidance Institute.

Hoag, J.M., Norriss, N.G., Himeno, E.J. and Jacobs, J. (1971. 'The encopretic child & his family'. *Journal of the American Academy of Child Psychiatry*, **10**, 242–256.

Hobson, R.P. (1985). 'Piaget: on ways of knowing in childhood'. In: *Child & Adolescent Psychiatry: Modern Approaches*, 2nd edn, Eds. M Rutter and L Hersov. Oxford: Blackwell Scientific Publications.

Hoefler, S.A. and Bornstein, P.H. (1975). 'Achievement place: an evaluative review'. *Criminal Justice & Behaviour*, **2**, 146–168.

Holland, A.J., Hall, A., Murray, R., Russell, G.F.M. and Crisp, A.H. (1984). 'Anorexia nervosa: a study of 34 twin pairs and one set of triplets'. *British Journal of Psychiatry*, **145**, 414–419.

Hong, K. (1978). 'The transitional phenomena'. *Psychoanalytic Study of the Child*, **3**, 47–49.

Hopkinson, K., Cox, A. and Rutter, M. (1981). 'Psychiatric interviewing techniques III. Naturalistic study: eliciting feelings'. *British Journal of Psychiatry*, **138**, 406–415.

Howells, J.G. (Ed.) (1979). *Modern Perspectives in the Psychiatry of Infants*. New York: Brunner/Mazel.

Hunt, R.D., Minderaa, R.B. and Cohen, D.J. (1985). 'Clonidine benefits children with attention deficit disorder and hyperactivity'. *Journal of the American Academy of Child Psychiatry*, **24**, 617–639.

Irving, H. (1981). 'Family mediation: a method for helping families resolve legal disputes'. In: *Treating Families with Special Needs*, Eds. D.S. Freeman and B. Trute. Ottawa: Canadian Association of Social Workers.

Jacobs, B.W. and Isaacs, S. (1986). 'Prepubertal anorexia nervosa: a retrospective controlled study'. *Journal of Child Psychology & Psychiatry*, **27**, 237–250.

Jacobs, P.A., Mayer, M., Matsuura, M., Rhoads, F. and Yee, S.C. (1983). 'A cytogenic study of a popualtion of mentally retarded males with special reference to the marker (X) syndrome'. *Human Genetics*, **63**, 139–148.

Jacobson, R.R. (1985a). 'Child firesetters: a clinical investigation'. *Journal of Child Psychology & Psychiatry*, **26**, 759–768.

Jacobson, R.R. (1985b). 'The subclassification of child firesetters'. *Journal of Child Psychology & Psychiatry*, **26**, 769–775.

Jalali, B., Jalali, M.D., Crocetti, G. and Turner, F. (1981). 'Adolescents and drug use: toward a more comprehensive approach' *American Journal of Orthopsychiatry*, **51**, 120–130.

Jenkins, R.L. (1973). *Behaviour Disorders of Childhood and Adolescence*. Springfield, Ill: Charles C. Thomas.

Jones, D.J. Fox, M.M. Babigian, H.M. and Hutton, H.E. (1980). 'Epidemiology of anorexia nervosa in Monroe County, New York'. *Psychosomatic Medicine*, **42**, 551–558.

Jones, D.P.H. (1986). 'Individual psychotherapy for the sexually abused child'. *Child Abuse & Neglect*, **10**, 377–385.

Kandel, D.B. and Logan, J.A. (1984). 'Patterns of drug use from adolescence to young adulthood: I. Periods of risk for initiation, continued use and discontinuation'. *American Journal of Public Health*, **74**, 660–666.

Kanner, L. (1943). 'Autistic disturbance of affective contact' *Nervous Child*, **2**, 217–250.

Kanner, L. (1944). 'Early infantile autism' *Journal of Pediatrics*, **25**, 211–217.

Karpel, M.A. and Strauss, E.S. (1983). *Family Evaluation*. New York: Gardener Press.

Kashani, J.H., McGee, R.D. Clarkson, S.E. Anderson, J.C., Walton, L.A., Williams, S., Silva, P.A., Robins, A.L., Cytryn, L. and McKnew, D.H. (1983) 'Depression in a sample of nine year old children'. *Archives of General Psychiatry*, **40**, 1217–1227.

Kaslow, F.W. (1984). 'Divorce mediation and its emotional impact on the couple and their children'. *American Journal of Family Therapy*, **12**(3), 58–66.

Kaufman, E. and Kaufman, P.N. (1979). 'From a psychodynamic orientation to a structural family therapy approach in the treatment of drug dependency'. In: *Family Therapy of Drug and Alcohol Abuse*, Ed. E. Kaufman and P.N. Kaufman. New York: Gardner Press.

Kaufman, J. and Zigler, E. (1987). 'Do abused children become abusive parents?' *American Journal of Orthopsychiatry*, **57**, 186–192.

Keat, D.B. (1979). *Multimodal Therapy with Children*. New York: Pergamon.

Keith, P.R. (1975). 'Night terrors' *Journal of the American Academy of Child Psychiatry*, **14**, 477–489.

Kempe, C.H., Silverman, F.N., Steele, B.F., Droegemueller, W. and Silver, H.K. (1962) 'The battered child syndrome' *Journal of the American Medical Association*, **191**, 17, 23.

Kendall, P.C. and Braswell, L. (1985). *Cognitive-Behavioral Therapy for Impulsive Children*. New York: Guilford.

Kennedy, W.A. (1965). 'School phobia: rapid treatment of fifty cases'. *Journal of Abnormal Psychology*, **70**, 285–289.

Kessler, M. and Albee, G.W. (1977). 'An overview of the literature of primary prevention'. In: *Primary Prevention of Psychopathology Volume 1*, Ed. W. Albee and J.M. Jolle. Hanover, New Hampshire: University Press of New England.

Kidd, K.K., Kidd, J.R. and Records, M.A. (1978). 'The possible cause of the sex ratio in stuttering and its implications.' *Journal of Fluency Disorders*, **3**, 13–23.

Kiernan, C. (1983). 'The use of nonvocal communication techniques with autistic individuals'. *Journal of Child Psychology & Psychiatry*, **24**, 339–375.

King, C. and Young, R.D. (1982). 'Attentional deficits with and without hyperactivity'. *Journal of Abnormal Psychology*, **10**, 483–495.

King, R.D., Raynes, N.V. and Tizard, J. (1971). *Patterns of Residential Care*. London: Routledge & Kegan Paul.

Kirschner, D.A. and Kirschner, S. (1986). *Comprehensive Family Therapy*. New York: Brunner/Mazel

Klein, M. (1932). *The Psychoanalysis of Children*. London: Hogarth.

Klein, M. (1948). *Contributions to Psychoanalysis 1921–1945*. London: Hogarth.

Kolvin, *et al.* (1971). 'Studies in the childhood psychoses'. *British Journal of Psychiatry*, **118**, 381–419.

Kolvin, I. and Fundudis, T. (1981). 'Electively mute children: psychological development & background factors'. *Journal of Child Psychology & Psychiatry*, **22**, 219–232.

Kolvin, I., Garside, R.F., Nicol, A.R., MacMillan, A., Wolstenholme, F. and Leitch, I.M. (1981). *Help Starts Here: The Maladjusted Child in the Ordinary School*. London: Tavistock.

Kolvin, I., MacKeith, R.C. and Meadow, S.R. (Eds) (1973). *Bladder Control and Enuresis* (Clinics in Development Medicine, nos 48/49). London: Heinemann.

Kovach, J.A. and Glickman, N.W. (1986). 'Levels and psychosocial correlates of adolescent drug use'. *Journal of Youth & Adolescence*. **15**, 61–77.

Kraemer, S. (1987). 'Working with parents: casework or psychotherapy?' *Journal of Child Psychology & Psychiatry*, **28**, 207–213.

Krupinski, J., Baikie, A.G., Stoller, A., Graves, J., O'Day, D.M. and Polke, P. (1967) 'A community mental health survey of Heyfield, Victoria'. *Medical Journal of Australia*, **1**, 1204–1211.

Kuperman, S., Beeghly, J.H.L., Burns, T.L. and Tsai, L.Y (1985). 'Serotonin relationships of autistic probands and their first-degree relatives'. *Journal of the American Academy of Child Psychiatry*, **24**, 186–190.

Kurita, H. (1985). 'Infantile autism with speech loss before the age of thirty months'. *Journal of the American Academy of Child Pschiatry*, **24**, 191–196.

Kushlick, A. (1972). 'The need for residential care of the mentally handicapped'. *British Journal of Hospital Medicine*, **8**, 161–167.

Lahey, B. B., Schaughency, E.A., Strauss, C.C. and Frame, C.L. (1984) 'Are attention deficit disorders with and without hyperactivity similar or similar disorders?' *Journal of the American Academy of Child Psychiatry*, **23**, 302–329.

Lahey, B.B., Schaughency, E.A., Frame, C.L. and Strauss, C.C. (1985). 'Teacher ratings of attention problems in children'. *Journal of the American Academy of Child Psychiatry*, **24**, 613–616.

Lahey M. and Bloom, L. (1977). 'Planning a first lexicon: which words to teach first'. *Journal of Speech & Hearing Disorders*, **42**, 340–369.

Lamb, D. (1986). *Psychotherapy with Adolescent Girls*, 2nd edn. New York: Plenum.

Landreth, G.L. (Ed) (1982). *Play Therapy.* Springfield, Ill: Charles C. Thomas.

Lansdown, R. (1978). 'Retardation in mathematics; a consideration of multi-factorial determination'. *Journal of Child Psychology & Psychiatry*, **19**, 181–185.

Larson, G., Allison, J. and Johnston, E. (1978). 'Alberta Parent Counsellors: a community treatment programme for disturbed youths'. *Child Welfare*, **57**, 47–52.

Leff, J.P., Kuipers, L. and Berkowitz, R. (1983). 'Intervention in families of schizophrenics and its effect on relapse rates'. In: *Family Therapy in Schizophrenia*, Ed. W.R. McFarlane. New York: Guilford.

Leff, J.P. and Vaughn, C. (1985). *Expressed Emotion in Families.* New York: Guilford.

Leighton, A. (1965). 'Poverty and social change'. *Scientific American*, **212**, No 5, 21 27.

Leissner, A., Powley, T. and Evans, D. (1977). *Intermediate Treatment.* London: National Children's Bureau.

Lerner, J.A., Inui, T.S., Trupin, E.W. and Douglas, E. (1985). 'Preschool behaviour can predict future psychiatric disorders'. *Journal of the American Academy of Child Psychiatry*, **24**, 42–48.

Leslie, S.A. (1974). 'Psychiatric disorders in the young adolescents of an industrial town'. *British Journal of Psychiatry*, **125**, 113–124.

Levin, S., Rubenstein, J.S. and Streiner, D.C. (1976). 'The parent-therapist program: an innovative approach to treating emotionally disturbed children'. *Hospital & Community Psychiatry*, **27**, 407–410.

Liebman, R., Minuchin, S. and Baker, L. (1974). An integrated treatment program for anorexia nervosa.' *American Journal of Psychiatry*, **131**, 432–436.

Litt, C.J. (1981). 'Children's attachment to transitional objects'. *American Journal of Orthopsychiatry*, **51**, 131–139.

Little, R.E. and Streissgath, A.P. (1981). 'Effects of alcohol on the fetus'. *Canadian Medical Association Journal*, **125**, 159–163.

Livingstone, S. (1972). 'Epilepsy in infancy, childhood & adolescence'. In: *Manual of Child Psychopathology*, Ed. B.J. Wolman. New York: McGraw-Hill.

Lord, C., Schopler, E. and Revick, D. (1982). 'Sex differences in autism'. *Journal of Autism & Developmental Disorders*, **12**, 317–330.

Lotter, V. (1966). 'Epidemiology of autistic conditions in young children. I Prevalence'. *Social Psychiatry*, **1**, 124–137.

Lotter, V. (1978a). 'Childhood autism in Africa'. *Journal of Child Psychology & Psychiatry*, **19**, 231–244.

Lotter, V. (1978b). 'Follow-up studies'. In: *Autism: A Reappraisal of Concepts & Treatment*. New York: Plenum.

Lovaas, O.I., Koegel, R., Simmons, J.Q. and Long, J.S. (1973). 'Some generalisations and follow-up measures on autistic children in behaviour therapy'. *Journal of Applied Behavioural Analysis*, **6**, 131–166.

Lowe, T.L. and Cohen, D.J. (1980). 'Mania in childhood and adolescence'. In: *Mania: An Evolving Concept*, Ed. R.H. Belmaker and H.M. van Praag. New York: Spectrum.

Lynch, M.A. (1978). 'The prognosis of child abuse'. *Journal of Child Psychology & Psychiatry*, **19**, 175–180.

Lynch, M.A. (1985). 'Child abuse before Kempe: an historical literature review'. *Child Abuse & Neglect*, **9**, 7–15.

Maccoby, E.E. and Martin, J.A. (1983). 'Socialization in the context of the family: parent-child interaction'. In: *Socialization, Personality and Social Development* (Volume IV, Handbook of Child Psychology, 4th edn), Ed. E.M. Hetherington. New York: Wiley.

Mack, J.E. and Ablon, S.L. (1983). *The Development and Sustenance of Self-Esteem in Childhood*. New York: International Universities Press.

Maclay, D. (1970). *Treatment for Children in Child Guidance*. New York: Science House.

Maier, S.F., Seligman M.E.P. and Solomon, R.L. (1969). 'Pavlovian fear conditioning and learned helplessness'. In: *Punishment*, Ed. B.A. Campbell and R.M. Church. New York: Appleton-Century-Crofts.

Manning, D.J. and Rosenbloom, L. (1987). 'Non-convulsive status epilepticus'. *Archives of Disease in Childhood*, **62**, 37–40.

Marmor, J. (1983): 'Systems thinking in psychiatry: some theoretical and clinical implications'. *American Journal of Psychiatry*, **140**, 833–838.

Marriage, K., Fine, S, Moretti, M. and Haley, G. (1986) 'Relationship between depression and conduct disorder in children and adolescents'. *Journal of the American Academy of Child Psychiatry*, **25**, 687–691.

Martin, H.P. and Beezley, P. (1977). 'The emotional development of abused children'. *Developmental Medicine and Child Neurology*, **19**, 373–387.

Martin, J.A.M. (1980). 'Syndrome delineation in communication disorders'. In: *Language and Language Disorders in Children*, Ed. L.A. Hersov, M. Berger and A.R. Nicol. Oxford and New York: Pergamon.

Martin, P.R. and Lefebvre, A.M. (1981). 'Surgical treatment of sleep-apnoea-associated psychosis'. *Canadian Medical Association Journal*, **124**, 978–980.

Masterson, J.S. (1972). *Treatment of the Borderline Adolescent: Developmental Approach*. New York: Wiley-Inter-Science.

Maughan, B., Gray, G. and Rutter, M. (1985). 'Reading retardation and antisocial behaviour'. *Journal of Child Psychology & Psychiatry*, **26**, 741–758.

Mbanefo, S.E. (1966). 'Heat in the body as a psychiatric symptom'. *Journal of the College of General Practitioners*, **11**, 234–240.

McCormack, A., Janus, M.D. and Burgess, A.W. (1986). 'Runaway youths and sexual victimization: gender differences in an adolescent runaway population' *Child Abuse & Neglect*, **10**, 281–285.

McFarlane, W.R. (1983a) 'Introduction'. In: *Family Therapy in Schizophrenia*, Ed. W.R. McFarlane. New York: Guilford.

McFarlane, W.R. (Ed) (1983b). *Family Therapy in Schizophrenia*. New York: Guilford.

McGee, R., Williams, S., Share, D.L., Anderson, J. and Silva, P.A. (1986). 'The relationship between specific reading retardation, general reading backwardness and behavioural problems in a large sample of Dunedin boys'. *Journal of Child Psychology & Psychiatry*, **27**, 597–610.

McGoldrick, M. and Carter, E.A. (1982). 'The family life cycle'. In: *Normal Family Processes*, Ed. F. Walsh. New York: Guildford.

McGoldrick, M. and Gerson, R. (1985). *Genograms in Family Assessment*. New York: Norton.

McGuffin, P. and Gottesman, I.I. (1985). 'Genetic influences on normal and abnormal development'. In: *Child and Adolescent Psychiatry: Modern Approaches*, 2nd edn, Ed. M. Rutter and L. Hersov. Oxford: Blackwell Scientific Publications.

McGuire, J. and Richman, N. (1986). 'Screening for behaviour problems in nurseries: the reliability and validity of the preschool behaviour checklist'. *Journal of Child Psychology & Psychiatry*, **27**, 7–32.

Mian, M., Wehrspan, W., Klajner-Diamond, H., LeBaron, D. and Winder, C. (1986). 'Review of 125 children 6 years of age and under who were sexually abused'. *Child Abuse & Neglect*, **10**, 223–229.

Mikkelsen, M. (1981) 'Epidemiology of trisomy 21'. In: *Trisomy 21*, Ed. G. Burgio, M. Fraccaro, L. Tiepolo and U. Wolf. Berlin: Springer-Verlag.

Miller, L.C., Barrett, C.C. and Hampe, E. (1974). 'Phobias of childhood in a pre-scientific era'. In: *Child Personality and Psychopathology: Current Topics*, Ed. A. Davids. New York: Wiley.

Mills, J.C. and Crowley, R.J. (1986). *Therapeutic Metaphors for Children and the Child Within*. New York: Brunner/Mazel.

Minde, K. (1974). 'Study problems in Ugandan secondary school students: a controlled evaluation'. *British Journal of Psychiatry*, **125**, 131–137.

Minde, K. and Minde, R. (1981). 'Psychiatric intervention in infancy'. *Journal of the American Academy of Child Psychiatry*, **20**, 217–238.

Minde, K., Schosenberg, N., Marton, P., Thompson, J., Ripley, J. and Burns, S. (1980). 'Self-help groups in a premature nursery'. *Journal of Pediatrics*, **96**, 933–940.

Minuchin, S. (1974). *Families and Family Therapy*. Cambridge, Mass: Harvard University Press.

Minuchin, S. and Fishman, H.C. (1981). *Family Therapy Techniques*. Cambridge, Mass: Harvard University Press.

Minuchin, S., Baker, L., Rosman, B.L., Liebman, R., Milman, L. and Todd, T.C., (1975) 'A conceptual model of psychosomatic illness in children'. *Archives of General Psychiatry*, **32**, 1031–1038.

Minuchin, S., Rosman, B.L. and Baker, L. (1978). *Psychosomatic Families: Anorexia Nervosa in Context*. Cambridge, Mass: Harvard University Press.

Moretti, M.M., Fine, S., Haley, G. and Marriage, K. (1985). 'Childhood and adolescent depression: child-report versus parent-report information'. *Journal of the American Academy of Child Psychiatry*, **24**, 298–302.

Morrison, J. and Stewart, M. (1973). 'The psychiatric status of the legal families of adopted hyperactive children'. *Archives of General Psychiatry*, **28**, 888–891.

Mrazek, D.A. (1986). 'Childhood asthma: two central questions for child psychiatry'. *Journal of Child Psychology & Psychiatry*, **27**, 1–5.

Mulvey, E.P. and LaRosa, J.F. (1986). 'Delinquency cessation and adolescent development.' *American Journal of Orthopsychiatry*, **56**, 211–224.

Mundy, P., Sigman, M., Ungerer, J. and Sherman, T. (1986). 'Defining the social deficits of autism'. *Journal of Child Psychology & Psychiatry*, **27**, 657–669.

Murray, I. (1986). 'Looking back: reminiscences from childhood and adolescence'. In: *Hyperactive Children Grown Up* by G. Weiss and L.T. Hechtman. New York: Guilford.

Myers, K.M., Burke, P. and McCauley, E. (1985). 'Suicidal behaviour by hospitalized preadolescent children on a psychiatric unit'. *Journal of the American Academy of Child Psychiatry*, **24**, 474–480.

National Centre on Child Abuse & Neglect. (1981). *Child Sexual Abuse: A Follow-Up Study* (DHHS Publication No. (OHDS) 81-30166). Washington, DC: US Government Printing Office.

Newson, J. and Newson, E. (1968). *Four Years Old in an Urban Community*. London: Allen & Unwin.

Ney, P.G. and Mulvihill, D.L. (1985). *Child Psychiatric Treatment: A Practical Guide*. Beckenham, Kent: Croom Helm.

Nielson, J. and Christensen, A.L. (1974). 'Thirty-five males with double Y chromosome'. *Psychological Medicine*, **4**, 28–37.

Nuechterlein, K.H. (1986). 'Childhood precursors of adult schizophrenia.' *Journal of Child Psychology & Psychiatry*, **27**, 133–144.

Nurcombe, B. (1986) 'The child as witness: competency and credibility'. *Journal of the American Academy of Child Psychiatry*, **25**, 473–480.

Oates, R.K. (1984). 'Personality development after physical abuse'. *Archives of Disease in Childhood*, **59**, 147–150.

Oates, R.K., Forrest, D. and Peacock, A. (1985). 'Self-esteem of abused children'. *Child Abuse & Neglect*, **9**, 159–163.

Oates, R.K. and Forrest, D. (1986). 'Self-esteem and early background of abusive mothers'. *Child Abuse & Neglect*, **9**, 89–93.

O'Connor, D.J. (1979). 'A profile of solvent abuse in school children'. *Journal of Child Psychology & Psychiatry*, **20**, 365–368.

Offord, D.R. (1987). 'Prevention of behavioural and emotional disorders in children'. *Journal of Child Psychology & Psychiatry*, **28**, 9–19.

Offord, D.R., Boyle, M.H., Szatmari, P., Rae-Grant, N.I., Links, P.S., Cadman, D.T., Byles, J.A. Crawford, J.W., Blum, H.M., Byrne, C., Thomas, H. and Woodward, C.A. (1987). 'Ontario child health study: prevalence of disorder and rates of service utilization'. *Archives of General Psychiatry*, **44**, 832–836.

Oliver, J.E. and Buchanan, A.H. (1979). 'Generations of maltreated children and multiagency care in one kindred'. *British Journal of Psychiatry*, **135**, 289–303.

Opinion Research Corporation. (1976) *National Statistical Survey of Runaway Youth*. Princeton NJ.

Orlosky, M.L. (1982). 'The Kleine-Levin syndrome: a review' *Psychosomatics*, **23**, 609–621.

Osofsky, J.D. (Ed) (1979). *Handbook of Infant Development*. New York: Wiley.

Palazzoli, M.S., Boscolo, L., Cecchin, G. and Prata, G. (1980). 'Hypothesizing –

circularity – neutrality: three guidelines for the conductor of the session'. *Family Process*, **19**, 3–12.

Parker, F.L., Piotrkowski, C.S. and Peay, L. (1987). 'Head Start as a social support for mothers'. *American Journal of Orthopsychiatry*, **57**, 220–233.

Parkinson, C.E., Scrivener, R., Graves, L., Bunton, J. and Harvey, D. (1986) 'Behavioural differences of school-age children who were small-for-dates babies'. *Developmental Medicine and Child Neurology*, **28**, 498–505.

Patterson, G.R. (1971). *Families: Application of Social Learning to Family Life*. Champaign, Illinois: Research Press.

Patterson, G.R. (1976). 'The aggressive child: victim or architect of a coercive system'. In: *Behaviour Modification and Families* Ed. E.J. Mash, L.A. Hamerlynck and L.C. Handy. New York; Brunner/Mazel.

Patterson, G.R. (1982). *Coercive Family Processes*. Eugene, Oregon: Castalia.

Patterson, G.R. and Gullion, M.E. (1968). *Living with Families: New Methods for Parents and Teachers*. Champaign, Illinois: Research Press.

Pauls, D.L. and Leckman, J.F. (1986). 'The inheritance of Gilles de la Tourette's syndrome and associated behaviors'. *New England Journal of Medicine*, **315**, 993–997.

Pfeffer, C.R., Zuckerman, S., Plutchkin, R. and Mizruchi, M.S. (1984). 'Suicidal behaviour in normal school children'. *Journal of the American Academy of Child Psychiatry*, **23**, 416–423.

Philipp, R. (1979). 'Conducting Parent Training Groups: Approaches and Strategies'. In: *New Directions in Children's Mental Health*, Ed. S.J. Shamsie. New York: SP Medical and Scientific Books.

Pinkerton, P. (1958). 'Psychogenic megacolon in children; the implications of bowel negativism'. *Archives of Disease in Childhood*, **33**, 371–380.

Pinkerton, P. (1974). 'Inpatient treatment of children with psychosomatic disorders'. In: *The Residential Psychiatric Treatment of Children*, Ed. P. Barker. London: Crosby Lockwood Staples; New York: Halsted Press.

Platt, J.E., Campbell, M., Green, W.H. and Grega, D.M. (1984). 'Cognitive effects of lithium carbonate and haloperidol in treatment-resistant aggressive children'. *Archives of General Psychiatry*, **41**, 657–662.

Pollack, S. (1974). 'The role of psychiatry in the rule of law'. *Psychiatric Annals*, 4, 816–831.

Powell, G.F., Brasel, J.A. and Blizzard, R.M. (1967). 'Emotional deprivation and growth retardation simualting idiopathic hypopituitarism'. *New England Journal of Medicine*, **276**, 1271–1283.

Pratt, G.J., Wood, D.P. and Alman, B.M. (1984). *A Clinical Hypnosis Primer*. La Jolla, CA: Psychology & Consulting Associates.

Preskorn, S., Weller, E.B. and Weller, R.A. (1982). 'Depression in children: relationship between plasma imipramine levels and response'. *Journal of Clinical Psychiatry*, **43**, 450–453.

Prince, R. (1960). 'The 'brain fag' syndrome in Nigerian students' *Journal of Mental Science*, **106**, 559–570.

Prior, M. and Sanson, A. (1986). 'Attention deficit disorder with hyperactivity: a critique'. *Journal of Child Psychology & Psychiatry*, **27**, 307–319.

Prior, M. Sanson, A., Freethy, C. and Geffen, G. (1985). 'Auditory attentional abilities in hyperactive children'. *Journal of Child Psychology & Psychiatry*, **26**, 289–304.

Provence, S. and Lipton, R. (1962). *Infants in Institutions*. New York: International Universities Press.

Puig-Antich, J. (1980). 'Affective disorders in childhood'. *Psychiatric Clinics of North America*, **3**, 403 424.

Puig-Antich, J. (1981). 'Antidepressant treatment in children: current state of the evidence'. In: *Depression and Antidepressants* Ed. E. Friedman and S. Gershon. New York: Raven.

Puig-Antich, J. (1982). 'Major depression and conduct disorder in prepuberty'. *Journal of the American Academy of Child Psychiatry*, **21**, 118–128.

Puig-Antich, J. (1986). 'Psychobiological markers: effects of age and puberty'. In: *Depression in Young People*, Ed. M. Rutter, C.E. Izard and P.B. Read. New York: Guilford.

Quay, H.C. (1979). 'Classification'. In: *Psychopathological Disorders of Childhood*, 2nd edn, Ed. H.C. Quay and J.S. Werry. New York: Wiley.

Quinn, D.M.P., (1986). 'Prevalence of psychoactive medications in children and adolescents'. *Canadian Journal of Psychiatry*, **31**, 575–580.

Rachelefsky, G.S., Wo, J., Adelson, J., Mickey, M.R., Spector, S.L., Katz, R.M., Siegel, S.C. and Rohr, A.S. (1986). 'Behaviour abnormalities and poor school performance due to oral theophylline use'. *Pediatrics*, **78**, 1133–1138.

Rapoport, J. (1986). 'Childhood obsessive compulsive disorder.' *Journal of Child Psychology & Psychiatry*, **27**, 289–295.

Rapoport, J., Buchsbaum, M.S., Zahn, T.P. *et al.* (1978). 'Dextroamphetamine: cognitive and behavioural effects in normal prepubertal boys'. *Science*, **199**, 560–562.

Ratcliffe, S. (1982). 'Speech and learning difficulties in children with sex chromosomal abnormalities'. *Developmental Medicine and Child Neurology*, **24**, 80–84.

Ratcliffe, S., Bancroft, J., Axworthy, D. and McLaren, W. (1982). 'Klinefelter's syndrome in adolescence'. *Archives of Disease in Childhood*, **57**, 6–12.

Ratcliffe, S.G. and Field, M.A.S. (1982). 'Emotional disorder in XXY children: four case reports'. *Journal of Child Psychology & Psychiatry*, **23**, 401–406.

Reid, K. (1985). *Truancy and School Absenteeism*. London: Hodder & Stoughton.

Reid, K. (1986). 'Truancy and school absenteeism: the state of the art'. *Maladjustment & Therapeutic Education*, **4**(3), 4–17.

Reilly, D.M. (1984). 'Family therapy with adolescent drug abusers and their families: defying gravity and achieving escape velocity'. *Journal of Drug Issues*, **14**, 381–391.

Reynolds, C.R. and Gutkin, T.B. (1982). *The Handbook of School Psychology*. New York; Wiley.

Richman, N. (1981a). 'A community survey of characteristics of one- to two-year-olds with sleep disruptions'. *Journal of the American Academy of Child Psychiatry*, **20**, 281–291.

Richman,N. (1981b). 'Sleep problems in young children'. *Archives of Disease in Childhood* **56**, 491–493.

Richman, N. (1985). 'A double-blind drug trial of treatment of sleep disorders – a pilot study'. *Journal of Child Psychology & Psychiatry*, **26**, 591–598.

Richman, N. and Graham, P.J. (1971). 'A behavioural screening questionnaire for use with 3-year-old children; preliminary findings'. *Journal of Child Psychology & Psychiatry*, **12**, 5–33.

Richman, N., Stevenson, J.E. and Graham, P.J. (1975). 'Prevalence of behaviour problems in 3-year-old children: an epidemiological study in a London borough'. *Journal of Child Psychology and Psychiatry*, **16**, 277–287.

Richman, N., Douglas, J., Hunt, H., Lansdown, R. and Levere, R. (1985) 'Behavioural methods in the treatment of sleep disorders – a pilot study'. *Journal of Child Psychology & Psychiatry*, **26**, 581–590.

Rivinus, T.M., Jamison, D.L. and Graham, P.J. (1975). 'Childhood organic neurological disease presenting as psychiatric disorder'. *Archives of Disease in Childhood*, **50**, 115–119.

Robins, L.N. (1966). *Deviant Children Grown Up*. Baltimore: Williams & Wilkins.

Robins, L. (1978). 'Sturdy childhood predictors of adult antisocial behaviour: replications from longitudinal studies'. *Psychological Medicine*, **8**, 611–622.

Robinson, H.B. (1981). 'The uncommonly bright child'. In: *The Uncommon Child*, Ed. M. Lewis and L.A. Rosenblum. New York: Plenum.

Romig, D.A. (1978). *Justice for Our Children*. Lexington: DC Heath.

Rosenthal, N.E., Carpenter, C.J., James, S.P., Parry, B.L., Rogers, S.L.B. and Wehr T.A. (1986). 'Seasonal affective disorder in children and adolescents'. *American Journal of Psychiatry*, **143**, 356–358.

Rossi, E. (1986a). *The Psychobiology of Mind-Body Healing*. New York: Norton.

Rossi, E. (1986b). 'The state-dependent memory and learning theory of therapeutic hypnosis'. In: *Mind-Body Communication in Hypnosis*, by M.H. Erickson, Ed. E.L. Rossi and M.O. Ryan. New York: Irvington.

Rossman, P.G. (1985). 'The aftermath of abuse and abandonment: a treatment approach for ego disturbance in female adolescence'. *Journal of the American Academy of Child Psychiatry*, **24**, 345–352.

Rubinstein, J.S. (1977). 'Institutions without walls for emotionally disturbed children'. *Hospital & Community Psychiatry*, **28**, 849–851

Rumsey, J.M., Rapoport, J.L. and Sceery, W.R. (1985). 'Autistic children as adults'. *Journal of the American Academy of Child Psychiatry*, **24**, 465–473.

Russell, D.H. (1981). 'On running away'. In: *Self-Destructive Behaviour in Children & Adolescents*, Ed. C.F. Wells and L.R. Stuart. New York: Van Nostrand Reinhold.

Russell, G.F.M. (1985). 'Anorexia and bulimia nervosa'. In: *Child and Adolescent Psychiatry: Modern Approaches*, 2nd edn, Ed. M. Rutter and L. Hersov. Oxford: Blackwell Scientific Publications.

Rutter, M. (1967a). 'Psychotic disorders in early childhood'. In: *Recent Developments in Schizophrenia*, Ed. A. Coppen and A. Walk. Ashford, Kent: Headley Bros.

Rutter, M. (1976b). 'A children's behaviour questionnaire for completion by teachers: preliminary findings'. *Journal of Child Psychology and Psychiatry*, **8**, 1–11.

Rutter, M. (1970). 'Autistic children: infancy to adulthood'. *Seminars in Psychiatry*, **2**, 435–450.

Rutter, M. (1971). 'Normal psychosexual development'. *Journal of Child Psychology & Psychiatry*, **11**, 359–383.

Rutter, M. (1979). 'Invulnerability or why some children are not damaged by stress'. In: *New Directions in Children's Mental Health*, Ed. S.J. Shamsie. New York: SP Medical and Scientific Books.

Rutter, M. (1980a) 'School influences on children's behaviour and development'. *Pediatrics*, **65**, 208–220.

Rutter, M. (1980b). *Changing Youth in a Changing Society*. Cambridge, Mass.: Harvard University Press.

Rutter, M. (1981). 'The city and the child'. *American Journal of Orthopsychiatry*, **51**, 610–625.

Rutter, M. (1983a). 'Cognitive defects in the pathogenesis of autism', *Journal of Child Psychology & Psychiatry*, **24**, 513–531.

Rutter, M. (Ed) (1983b). *Developmental Neuropsychiatry*. New York: Guilford.

Rutter, M. (1985a). 'Infantile autism and other pervasive developmental disorders'. In: *Child & Adolescent Psychiatry; Modern Approaches*, 2nd edn, Ed. M. Rutter and L. Hersov. Oxford: Blackwell Scientific Publications.

Rutter, M. (1985b). 'The treatment of autistic children'. *Journal of Child Psychology & Psychiatry*, **26**, 193–214.

Rutter, M.(1986). 'The developmental psychopathology of depression: issues and perspectives'. In: *Depression in Young People*, Ed. M. Rutter, C.E. Izard and P.B. Read. New York: Guilford.

Rutter, M., Chadwick, O., Shaffer, D. and Brown, G. (1980). 'A prospective study of children with head injuries: I. Design and methods' *Psychological Medicine*, **10**, 633–644.

Rutter, M. and Cox, A. (1981). 'Psychiatric interviewing techniques: 1. methods and measures'. *British Journal of Psychiatry*, **138**, 273–282.

Rutter, M., Cox, A., Egert, S., Holbrook, D. and Everitt, B. (1981). 'Psychiatric interviewing techniques. IV. Experimental study: four contrasting styles'. *British Journal of Psychiatry*, **138**, 456–465.

Rutter, M., Cox, A., Tupling, G., Berger, M. and Yule, W. (1975). 'Attainment and adjustment in two geographical areas. I. The prevalence of psychiatric disorder'. *British Journal of Psychiatry*, **126**, 493–501.

Rutter, M. and Garmezy, N. (1983). 'Developmental psychopathology'. In: *Socialization, Personality & Social Development, Vol 4. Handbook of Child Psychology*, 4th edn, Ed. E.M. Hetherington. New York: Wiley.

Rutter, M. and Gould, M. (1985). 'Classification'. In: *Child & Adolescent Psychiatry: Modern Approaches*, 2nd edn, Ed. M. Rutter and L. Hersov. Oxford: Blackwell Scientific Publications.

Rutter, M. and Graham, P. (1967). 'The reliability and validity of the psychiatric assessment of the child: 1. Interview with the child'. *British Journal of Psychiatry*, **114**, 563–579.

Rutter, M., Graham, P., Chadwick, O. and Yule, W. (1976). 'Adolescent turmoil: fact or fiction?'. *Journal of Child Psychology & Psychiatry*, **17**, 35–56.

Rutter, M., Graham, P, and Yule, W.A. (1970). *A Neuropsychiatric Study in Childhood*. London: Heinemann.

Rutter, M., Izard, L.E. and Read, P.B. (Eds) (1986). *Depression in Young People: Developmental and Clinical Perspectives*. New York: Guilford.

Rutter, M. and Lockyer, L. (1967). 'A 5- to 15-year follow-up of infantile autism and specific developmental receptive language disorder'. *British Journal of Psychiatry*, **126**, 127–145.

Rutter, M., Maughan, N., Mortimore, P. and Ouston, J. (1979). *Fifteen Thousand Hours*. London: Open Books.

Rutter, M., Shaffer, D. and Sturge, C. (1975). *A Guide to a Multi-Axial Classification Scheme for Psychiatric Disorders in Childhood and Adolescence* Dept. of Child & Adolescent Psychiatry, Institute of Psychiatry, London, SE8 8AF.

Rutter, M., Tizard, J. and Whitmore, K. (1970). *Education, Health and Behaviour*. London: Longman.

Rutter, M. and Yule, W. (1975). 'The concept of specific reading retardation'. *Journal of Child Psychology & Psychiatry*, **16**, 181–197.

Safer, D.J. and Allen, R.P. (1976). *Hyperactive Children: Diagnosis and Management.* Baltimore: University Park Press.

Savicki, V. and Brown, R. (1981). *Working with Troubled Children.* New York: Human Sciences Press.

Schaefer, C.E. and Swanson, A. J. (Eds) (In press) *Children in Residential Care: Critical Issues in Treatment.* New York: Van Nostrand Reinhold.

Schmitt, B. D. (1975). 'The minimal brain dysfunction myth'. *American Journal of Diseases of Children,* **129,** 1313–1319.

Schmidt, E. and Eldridge, A. (1986). 'The attachment relationship and child maltreatment'. *Infant Mental Health Journal,* **7,** 264–273.

Schoettle, U.C. (1984). 'Termination of parental rights – ethical issues and role conflicts'. *Journal of the American Academy of Child Psychiatry,* **23,** 629–632.

Scott, P.D. (1977). 'Non-accidental injury in children'.*British Journal of Psychiatry,* **131,** 366–380.

Seligman, M.E.P. and Peterson, C. (1986). 'A learned helplessness perspective in childhood depression'. In: *Depression in Young People,* Ed. M. Rutter, C.E. Izard and P.B. Read. New York: Guilford.

Shachnow, J. (1987). 'Preventive intervention with children of hospitalized psychiatric patients'. *American Journal of Orthopsychiatry,* **57,** 66–77.

Shaffer, D. (1974). 'Suicide in childhood and adolescence'. *Journal of Child Psychology & Psychiatry,* **15,** 275–291.

Shaffer, D. (1985a). 'Brain damage'. In: *Child and Adolescent Psychiatry: Modern Approaches,* 2nd edn, Ed. M. Rutter and L. Hersov. Oxford: Blackwell Scientific Publications.

Shaffer, D. (1985b). 'Depression, mania and suicidal acts'. In: *Child and Adolescent Psychaitry: Modern Approaches,* 2nd edn, Ed. M. Rutter and L. Hersov. Oxford: Blackwell Scientific Publications.

Shaffer, D. (1986). 'Development factors in child and adolescent suicide'. In: *Depression in Young People,* Ed. M. Rutter, C.E. Izard and P.B. Read. New York: Guilford.

Shaffer, D. and Fisher, P. (1981). 'The epidemiology of suicide in children and adolescents'. *Journal of the American Academy of Child Psychiatry,* **20,** 513–565.

Shaffer, D., Gardner, A. and Hedge, B. (1984). 'Behaviour and bladder disturbance of enuretic children: a rational classification of a common disorder'. *Developmental Medicine & Child Neurology,* **26,** 781–792.

Shaffer, D. and Greenhill, L. (1979). 'A critical note on the predictive validity of "the hyperkinetic syndrome". *Journal of Child Psychology & Psychiatry,* **18,** 61–72.

Shaffer, D., O'Connor, P.A., Shafer, S.Q. and Prupis, S. (1983). 'Neurological 'soft signs': their origins and significance for behaviour'. In: *Developmental Neuropsychiatry,* Ed. M. Rutter. New York: Guilford.

Shafii, T. (1986). 'The prevalence and use of transitional objects: a study of 230 adolescents'. *Journal of the American Academy of Child Psychiatry,* **25,** 805–808.

Shamsie, S.J. (1981). 'Antisocial adolescents; our treatments do not work – where do we go from here?' *Canadian Journal of Psychiatry,* **26,** 357–364.

Shamsie, S.J. (1985). 'Family breakdown and its effects on emotional disorders in children'. *Canadian Journal of Psychiatry,* **30,** 281–287.

Shapiro, S.K. and Garfinkel, B.D. (1986). 'The occurrence of behaviour disorders in children: the interdependence of attention deficit disorder and conduct disorder'. *Journal of the American Academy of Child Psychiatry,* **25,** 809–819.

Shapland, L.M. (1978). 'Self-reported delinquency in boys aged 11 to 14'. *British Journal of Criminology,* **18,** 255–266.

Shaywitz, S.E., Shaywitz, B.A., Cohen, D.J. and Young, J.G. (1983). 'Monoaminergic mechanisms in hyperactivity'. In: *Developmental Neuropsychiatry*, Ed. M. Rutter. New York: Guilford.

Shekim, W.O., Kashani, J., Beck, N., Cantwell, D.P. Martin, J., Rosenberg, J. and Costello, A. (1985). 'The prevalence of attention deficit disorders in a rural midwestern community sample of nine-year-old children'. *Journal of the American Academy of Child Psychiatry*, **24**, 765–770.

Shepherd, M., Oppenheim, B. and Mitchell, S. (1971). *Child Behaviour and Mental Health*. University of London Press.

Sigman, M., Mundy, P., Sherman, T. and Ungerer, J. (1986). 'Social interactions of autistic, mentally retarded and normal children and their caregivers'. *Journal of Child Psychology & Psychiatry*, **27**, 647–656.

Silva, P.A., McGee, R. and Williams, S. (1985). 'Some characteristics of 9-year-old boys with general reading backwardness or specific reading retardation'. *Journal of Child Psychology & Psychiatry*, **26**, 407–421.

Silver, H.K. and Finkelstein, M. (1967). 'Deprivation dwarfism'. *Journal of Pediatrics*, **70**, 317–324.

Simmons, J.E. (1987). *Psychiatric Examination of Children*, 4th edn. Philadelphia: Lea & Febiger.

Simon, G.B. (Ed) (1980). *The Modern Management of Mental Handicap*. Lancaster: MTP Press.

Singer, M.T., Wynne, L.C. and Toohey, M. (1978). 'Communication deviance and the families of schizophrenics'. In: *The Nature of Schizophrenia*, Ed. L.C. Wynne, R.L. Cromwell and S. Matthysse. New York: Wiley.

Skynner, A.C.R. (1975). *One Flesh: Separate Persons*. London: Constable. (Published in the USA as *Systems of Family & Marital Psychotherapy*. New York: Brunner/Mazel.)

Slade, P.D. and Russell, G.F.R. (1971). 'Developmental dyscalculia: a brief report on 4 cases'. *Psychological Medicine*, **1**, 292–298.

Sluckin, A. (1975). 'Encopresis: a behavioural approach described' *Social Work Today*, **5**, 643–646.

Spitz, R.A. (1946). 'Anaclitic depression'. *Psychoanalytic Study of the Child*, **2**, 113–117.

Sreenivasan, U. (1985). 'Effeminate boys in a child psychiatric clinic: prevalence and associated factors'. *Journal of the American Academy of Child Psychiatry*, **24**, 689–694.

Stanley, L. (1980). 'Treatment of ritualistic behaviour in an eight-year-old girl by response prevention'. *Journal of Child Psychology & Psychiatry*, **21**, 85–90.

Stanton, M.D. and Todd, T.C. (1982). *The Family Therapy of Drug Abuse and Addiction*. New York: Guilford.

Starfield, B. (1967). 'Functional bladder capacity in enuretic and non-enuretic children'. *Journal of Pediatrics*. **70**, 777–781.

Stein, M.D. and Davis, J.K. (1982). *Therapies for Adolescents*. San Francisco: Jossey-Bass.

Steinberg, D. (1987). *Basic Adolescent Psychiatry*. Oxford: Blackwell Scientific Publications.

Steinberg, D. (In Press) *Inter-professional Consultation*. Oxford: Blackwell Scientific Publications.

Steinberg, D. (1983). *The Clinical Psychiatry of Adolescence*. Chichester: Wiley.

Steinhauer, P.D. (1984). 'The management of children admitted to child welfare services in Ontario'. *Canadian Journal of Psychiatry*, **29**, 473–484.

Steinhauer, P.D., Santa-Barbara, J. and Skinner, H. (1984). 'The process model of family functioning'. *Canadian Journal of Psychiatry*, **29**, 77–88.

Stevenson, J., Graham, P., Fredman, G. and McLoughlin, V. (1987). 'A twin study of genetic influences on reading and spelling ability and disability'. *Journal of Child Psychology & Psychiatry*, **28**, 229–247.

Stevenson, J. and Richman, N. (1978). 'Behaviour, language and development in three-year-old children'. *Journal of Autism & Childhood Schizophrenia*, **8**, 299–313.

Stevenson, J., Richman, N. and Graham, G. (1985). 'Behaviour problems and language abilities at 3 years and behavioural deviance at 8 years'. *Journal of Child Psychology & Psychiatry*, **26**, 215–120.

Stores, G. (1985). 'Clinical and EEG evaluation of seizures and seizure-like disorders'. *Journal of the American Academy of Child Psychiatry*, **24**, 10–16.

Stores, G. (1987). 'Pitfalls in the management of epilepsy, *Archives of Disease in Childhood* **62**, 88–90.

Stott, D.H. (1966). *The Social Adjustment of Children*, 3rd edn. University of London Press.

Stubbs, E.G., Ritvo, E.R. and Mason-Brothers, A. (1985). 'Autism and shared parental HLA antigens'. *Journal of the American Academy of Child Psychiatry*, **24**, 182–185.

Sturge, C. (1982). 'Reading retardation and antisocial behaviour'. *Journal of Child Psychology & Psychiatry*, **23**, 21–31.

Swirsky-Sacchetti, T. and Margolis C.G. (1986). 'The effect of a comprehensive self-hypnosis training program on the use of factor VIII in severe haemophilia'. *International Journal of Clinical & Experimental Hypnosis*, **34**, 71–83.

Tallal, P. (1980). 'Auditory temporal perception, phonics and reading disabilities in children'. *Brain & Language*, **9**, 182–198.

Tanguay, P.E (1984). 'Toward a new classification of serious psychopathology in children'. *Journal of the American Academy of Child Psychiatry*, **23**, 373–384.

Tanguay, P.E. and Cantor, S.L. (1986). 'Schizophrenia in children: introduction'. *Journal of the American Academy of Child Psychiatry*, **25**, 591–594.

Taylor, E. (1980). 'Development of attention'. In: *Scientific Foundations of Developmental Psychiatry*, Ed. M. Rutter. London: Heinemann.

Taylor, E. (1985). 'Drug treatment'. In: *Child and Adolescent Psychiatry: Modern Approaches*, 2nd edn, Ed. M. Rutter and L. Hersov. Oxford: Blackwell Scientific Publications.

Taylor, E.A. (Ed). (1986a). *The Overactive Child* (Clinics in Developmental Medicine, No. 97). Oxford: Blackwell Scientific Publications; Philadelphia: Lippincott.

Taylor, E.A. (Ed) (1986b). 'The basis of drug treatment'. In: *The Overactive Child* (Clinics in Developmental Medicine, No. 97), Ed. E.A. Taylor. Oxford: Blackwell Scientific Publications; Philadelphia: Lippincott.

Terr, L. (1986). 'The child psychiatrist and the child witness'. *Journal of the American Academy of Child Psychiatry*, **25**, 463–472.

Thomas, A. and Chess, S. (1977). *Temperament and Development*. New York: Brunner/Mazel.

Thompson, T.R. (1987). 'Childhood and adolescent suicide in Manitoba: a demographic study'. *Canadian Journal of Psychiatry*, **32**, 264–269.

Tisher, M. (1983). 'School refusal: a depressive equivalent'. In: *Affective Disorders in Childhood & Adolescence: An Update*, Ed. D.P. Cantwell and G.A. Carlson. New York: Spectrum.

Tizard, B. and Hodges, J. (1978). 'The effect of early institutional rearing on the development of eight year old children'. *Journal of Child Psychology & Psychiatry*, **19**, 99–118.

Tonge, W.L., James, D.S. and Hillam, S.M. (1975). *Families Without Hope* (British Journal of Psychiatry Special Publication No. 11). Ashford, Kent: Headley Brothers.

Torgerson, A.M. (1981). 'Genetic factors in temperamental individuality'. *Journal of the American Academy of Child Psychiatry*, **20**, 702–711.

Torgerson, A.M. and Kringlen, E. (1978). 'Genetic aspects of temperamental differences in infants'. *Journal of the American Academy of Child Psychiatry*, **17**, 433–444.

Tramontana, M.G. and Sherrets S.D. (1985). 'Brain impairment in child psychiatric disorders: correspondencies between neuropsychological and CT scan results'. *Journal of the American Academy of Child Psychiatry*, **24**, 590–596.

Trites, R.L. and Laprade, K. (1983). 'Evidence for an independent syndrome of hyperactivity'. *Journal of Child Psychiatry*, **24**, 573–586.

Tsai, L., Stewart, M.A. and August, G. (1981). 'Implication of sex differences in the familial transmission of infantile autism'. *Journal of Autism & Developmental Disorders*, **11**, 165–173.

Turgay, A. (1980). 'Conversion reactions in children'. *Psychiatric Journal of the University of Ottawa*, **5**, 287–294.

Turpin, G. (1983). 'The behavioural management of tic disorders: a critical review'. *Advances in Behaviour Research & Therapy*. **5**, 203–245.

Vandenberg, S.G. Singer, S.M. and Pauls, D.L. (1986). *The Heredity of Behaviour Disorders in Adults and Children*. New York: Plenum.

van der Hart, O. (1983). *Rituals in Psychotherapy*. New York: Irvington.

Vandersall, A. and Wiener, J.M. (1970). 'Children who set fires'. *Archives of General Psychiatry*, **22**, 63–71.

van Krevelen, D.A. (1971). 'Early infantile autism and autistic psychopathy'. *Journal of Autism & Childhood Schizophrenia*, **1**, 82–86.

Van Koor-Lambo, G. (1987). 'The reliability of axis V of the multiaxial classification scheme.' *Journal of Child Psychology and Psychiatry*. **28**, 597–612.

Varma, V. (Ed.) (1984). *Anxiety in Children*. London: Croom Helm; New York: Methuen.

Verhulst, J.H.L., Akkerhuis, G.W., Sanders-Woudstra, J.A.R., Timmer, F.C. and Donkhorst, I.D. (1985). 'The prevalence of nocturnal enuresis'. *Journal of Child Psychology & Pschiatry*, **26**, 989–993.

Vicary, J.R. and Lerner, J.V. (1986). 'Parental attributes and adolescent drug use'. *Journal of Adolescence*, **9**, 115–122.

von Bertalanffy, L. (1968). *General Systems Theory*. New York: Braziller.

Vorrath, H.H., and Brendthro, L.K. (1985). *Positive Peer Culture*, 2nd edn. New York: Aldine.

Wagner, B.R. and Breitmeyer, R.G. (1975). 'PACE: a residential, community oriented behaviour modification programme for adolescents'. *Adolescence*, **10**, 277–286.

Wallas, L. (1985). *Stories for the Third Ear*. New York: Norton.

Wallerstein, J.S. (1983). 'Children of divorce: stress and developmental tasks'. In: *Stress, Coping and Development in Children*, Ed. N. Garmezy and M. Rutter. New York: McGraw-Hill.

Wallerstein, J.S. and Kelly, J.B. (1980). *Surviving the Breakup: How Children and Parents Cope with Divorce*. London: Grant McIntyre.

Walsh, F. (Ed) (1982). *Normal Family Processes*. New York: Guilford.

Walton, J.N. Ellis, E. and Court, S.D.M. (1962). 'Clumsy children: developmental apraxia and agnosia'. *Brain*, **85**, 603–612.

Walzer, S. (1985). 'X chromosome abnormalities and cognitive development'. *Journal of Child Psychology & Psychiatry*, **26**, 177–184.

Wardle, C.J. (1961). 'Two generations of broken homes in the genesis of conduct and behaviour disorders in children'. *British Medical Journal*, **2**, 349–354.

Washington, J., Minde, K. and Goldberg, S. (1986). 'Temperament in preterm infants: style and stability'. *Journal of the American Academy of Child Psychiatry*, **25**, 493–502.

Weeks, G.R. and L'Abate, L. (1982). *Paradoxical Psychotherapy*. New York: Brunner/Mazel.

Weiner, I.B. (1982). *Child and Adolescent Psychopathology*. New York: Wiley.

Weiss, G. (1981). 'Controversial issues of the pharmacotherapy of the hyperactive child'. *Canadian Journal of Psychiatry*, **26**, 385–392.

Weiss, G. and Hechtman, L.T. (1986). *Hyperactive Children Grown Up*. New York: Guilford.

Weissman, M.M., Gershon, E.S., Kidd, K.K., Prusoff, B.A., Leckman, J.F., Dibble, E., Hamovit, J., Thompson, W.D., Pauls, D.L. and Guroff J.J. (1984) 'Psychiatric disorders in the relatives of probands with affective disorders'. *Archives of General Psychiatry*, **41**, 13–21.

Werner, E.E. and Smith, R.S. (1982). *Vulnerable but Invincible: A Longitudinal Study of Resilient Children and Youth*. New York: McGraw-Hill.

White, R., Benedict, M.I., Wulff, L. and Kelley, M. (1987). 'Physical disabilities as risk factors for child maltreatment'. *American Journal of Orthopsychiatry*, **57**, 93–101.

White, S., Strom, G.A., Santilli, G. and Halpin, B.M. (1986). 'Interviewing young sexual abuse victims with anatomically correct dolls'. *Child Abuse & Neglect*, **10**, 519–529.

Willerman, L. (1973). 'Activity level and hyperactivity in twins'. *Child Development*, **44**, 288–293.

Williams, K., Goodman, M. and Green, R. (1985). 'Parent-child factors in gender role socialization in girls'. *Journal of the American Academy of Child Psychiatry*, **26**, 720–731.

Wilson, H. (1980). 'Parental supervision: a neglected aspect of delinquency'. *British Journal of Criminology*, **20**, 203–235.

Wing, L. (1980). 'Childhood autism and social class; a question of selection?; *British Journal of Psychiatry*, **137**, 410–417.

Wingate, M.E. (1976). *Stuttering: Theory and Treatment*. New York: Irvington.

Winnicott, D. (1960). *The Maturational Process and the Facilitating Environment*. London: Hogarth.

Winnicott, D.W. (1965). *The Family and Individual Development*. London: Tavistock.

Wolff, S. and Barlow, A. (1979). 'Schizoid personality in childhood: a comparative study of schizoid, autistic and normal children'. *Journal of Child Psychology & Psychiatry*, **20**, 29–46.

Wolff, S. and Chick, J. (1980). 'Schizoid personality in childhood: a controlled follow-up study'. *Psychological Medicine*, **10**, 85–100.

Wolkind, S.N. (1974). 'Sex differences in the aetiology of antisocial disorder in children'. *British Journal of Psychiatry*, **125**, 125–130.

Wolkind, S. (1981). 'Depression in mothers of young children'. *Archives of Disease in Childhood*, **56**, 1–3.

Woodward, J. and Jackson, D. (1961). 'Emotional reactions in burned children and their mothers'. *British Journal of Plastic Surgery*, **13**, 316–324.

World Health Organization (1977a). *International Classification of Diseases*, 1975 Revision. Geneva: WHO.

World Health Organization (1977b). *Child Mental Health and Psychosocial Development*. Geneva: WHO.

Wortis, J. (1986). 'Neuropsychiatry of acquired immune deficiency syndrome'. *Biological Psychiatry*, **21**, 1357–1359.

Wright, H.H., Miller, M.D., Cook, M.A. and Littman, J.R. (1985). 'Early identification and intervention with children who refuse to speak' *Journal of the American Academy of Child Psychiatry*, **24**, 739–746.

Wright, H.H., Young, S.R., Edwards, J.G., Abrahamson, R.K. and Duncan, J. (1986). 'Fragile X syndrome in a population of autistic children'. *Journal of the American Academy of Child Psychiatry*, **25**, 641–644.

Wynn, A. (1974). 'Health care systems for pre-school children'. *Proceedings of the Royal Society of Medicine*, **67**, 340–343.

Wynne, L.C. (1981). 'Current concepts about schizophrenics and family relationships'. *Journal of Nervous & Mental Disease*, **167**, 144–158.

Yalom, I. (1975). *The Theory and Practice of Group Psychotherapy*, 2nd edn. New York: Basic Books.

Yamaguchi, K. and Kandel, D.B. (1984a). 'Patterns of drug use from adolescence to young adulthood: II. Sequences of progression'. *American Journal of Public Health*, **74**, 668–672.

Yamaguchi, K. and Kandel, D.B. (1984b). 'Patterns of drug use from adolescence to young adulthood: III. Predictors of progression'. *American Journal of Public Health*, **74**, 668–672.

Yarnell, H. (1940). 'Fire-setting in children'. *American Journal of Orthopsychiatry*, **10**, 272–286.

Youngerman, J. and Canino, I. (1978). 'Lithium carbonate use in children and adolescents'. *Archives of General Psychiatry*, **35**, 216–224.

Yule, W. (1967). 'Predicting reading ages on Neal's analysis of reading disability'. *British Journal of Educational Psychology*, **37**, 252–255.

Yule, W. and Carr, J. (Eds) (1980). *Behaviour Modification for the Mentally Handicapped*. London: Croom Helm.

Zimet, S.G. and Farley, G.K. (1985). 'Day treatment for children in the United States'. *Journal of the American Academy of Child Psychiatry*, **24**, 732–738.

Zimet, S.G., Farley, G.K. (1986). 'Four perspectives on the competence and self-esteem of emotionally disturbed children beginning day treatment'. *Journal of the American Academy of Child Psychiatry*, **25**, 76–83.

Zucker, K.J., Bradley, S.J., Doering, R.W. Lozinski, J.A. (1985). 'Sex-typed behaviour in cross-gender-identified children: stability and change at one-year follow-up'. *Journal of the American Academy of Child Psychiatry*, **24**, 710–719.

Glossary

This glossary is provided primarily for readers who do not have a medical or psychological background. Certain terms which are explained where they occur in the text have been omitted.

Acquired immune deficiency syndrome (AIDS) A virus disease which damages the body's resistance to infection by invading certain lymphocyte cells. Is often sexually transmitted but other modes of transmission, such as from mother to fetus, occur.

Affect mood. An *affective psychosis* is one in which the primary problem is deviation from normal of the mood.

Agenesis Failure to grow normally.

Allele Genes that have the same relative positions on each of a pair of chromosomes and are responsible for alternative characteristics, for example the presence or absence of a particular metabolic disorder.

Amino acids Organic nitrogen-containing compounds made up of amino and acidic groups. Proteins are more complex compounds composed of amino acids arranged in various patterns.

Amniotic fluid The liquid surrounding the fetus in the uterus. It is enclosed by a membrane, called the amnion.

Anal fissure A longitudinal ulcer in the wall of the anal canal. Often causes severe pain on defecation.

Anorexia Loss of appetite.

Anterior pituitary The anterior lobe of the pituitary gland (see below).

Anti–Parkinsonian drug A drug which controls the symptoms of Parkinsonism (see below).

Apnoea Failure to breath.

Apraxia The inability to carry out purposeful actions despite possession of the ability to perform all the individual movements required. The subject cannot synthesize movements to produce the desired result.

Ataxia Lack of muscular coordination.

Atonic attacks Attacks of loss of muscle tone.

Autistic Behaviour controlled by factors within the individual, rather than by the realities of the person's social situation.

Automatism An action carried out without the subject's conscious awareness of it.

Autonomic nervous system A system of nerves supplying heart muscle, blood vessels and certain glands. Affects heart rate, blood pressure, various glands and other bodily functions. It is not under conscious control.

Autosomal Concerned with those chromosomes not involved in the determination of the individual's sex (namely all except the X and Y chromosomes). An autosomal gene is one carried on any chromosome other than an X or Y chromosome.

Barium enema An X-ray examination in which a barium compound is given as an enema to outline the large intestine.

Benzodiazepine The chemical name of a group of drugs (e.g. diazepam) used to produce a tranquillizing, anxiety-reducing action.

Blood dyscrasia An abnormal condition of the blood, as for example when certain types of cells are not produced normally.

Body image The view a person has of the size, shape and nature of his or her body.

Carbohydrates Organic chemical compounds, for example glucose, made up of carbon, hydrogen and oxygen atoms arranged in a particular way. Important constituents of the body and the diet.

CAT scan An abbreviation for computerized axial tomography, a radiological technique for obtaining images of different plane sections of the brain or other organs.

Cerebral cortex The outer layer of the brain, also known as the grey matter. It is infolded to increase its area and is concerned with many associative mental processes including thinking. Incoming neurological messages are received in the cortex and outgoing ones, including those leading to voluntary movements, originate from it.

Cerebral palsy Weakness of various muscle groups, sometimes widespread, present from early in life. Many forms exist. The muscles are often abnormally stiff and rigid (or 'spastic'), though this is not always the case. Individuals with these disorders are sometimes referred to as 'spastics'.

Cerebrospinal fluid A clear colourless liquid occupying the space surrounding the brain and spinal cord.

Chelating agents Chemical substances which combine with, and thus inactivate, metallic ions. Such agents are used in the treatment of lead poisoning and to remove excess copper from the body in hepato-lenticular degeneration (Wilson's disease).

Chorea A group of conditions in which there are involuntary movements (of face, tongue, limbs etc.) which consist of parts of normal organized movements. They are not under voluntary control and

are fragmented, irregular and purposeless. The movements themselves are called *chloreiform movements*.

Chromosomes Microscopic bodies contained in the nuclei of cells. The
normal human complement is 23 pairs. The chromosomes carry the
genetic material responsible for the development of cells and thus of
the whole organism.

Colon That part of the large intestine immediately before the rectum.
Shorter and of larger diameter than the small intestine which
precedes it.

Conditioning A term derived from learning theory. It describes various
ways in which human beings and animals can be systematically
taught to respond in particular ways to stimuli. In Pavlov's classical
experiment a dog was conditioned to salivate by giving it food at the
same time as a bell was rung; when subsequently the bell was rung
the dog still salivated, even though no food was presented – a
'conditioned response'. In 'operant conditioning' a dog might be
placed in a situation in which it could obtain food by pressing a lever.
Doing this at first by chance, or in response to coaxing, it would
learn how the action was rewarded and thus would be conditioned
to perform the act repeatedly.

Conflict a clash between the demands of reality and those of unconscious drives and feelings. This can lead to anxiety and other forms
of emotional disorder, the cause not being consciously understood
by the subject.

Contingency This term refers to the consequences which follow
particular behaviours. In behaviour therapy these are planned so as
to bring about changes in behaviour.

Control group a group of subjects in an experiment, or the investigation
of a treatment method, who do not receive the treatment under
investigation. They may receive no treatment or a 'placebo', or a
standard treatment. The control group should be matched as closely
as possible to the 'experimental' group in order to provide a
comparison for detecting the effects of the experiment or
treatment.

Correlation A measure of the. degree of correlation between two
variables. A correlation of 1.0 would indicate that the relationship
between them always remains the same; one of zero that they are
totally independent.

Cortisol The principal hormone secreted by the cortex of the adrenal
gland. Also known as hydrocortisone.

Defence The process of dealing with feelings such as anxiety and guilt by
means of mental mechanisms, as described in Chapter 1.

Delirium A state of clouded consciousness with confusion and disorientation for time, place and person. Often due to an acute febrile

illness or to excessive doses of drugs which affect brain function. Also occurs in various forms of acute brain disease.

Delusion A false belief that is held irrationally and despite evidence to the contrary.

Dementia The deterioration of intellectual function, usually due to degeneration of, or damage to, the brain.

Depression A state of morbid sadness or depression of mood.

Desensitization Treating undue sensitivity to a stimulus by carefully graduated, increasing exposure to the stimulus. The latter may be a physical allergen (like pollen in 'hay fever') or an object or situation which arouses fear (as in phobic disorders).

Developmental A term used in a special sense to describe disorders which are considered to be primarily anomalies of the development of certain functions, e.g. speech or motor coordination.

Diabetes In the commonest form of diabetes the blood sugar level is raised and there are thirst, production of excess amounts of urine and other serious symptoms. Responds to diet, insulin and other drugs.

Diuretic A drug that promotes the secretion of urine.

Dominant In genetics a trait which is manifest when the gene concerned is carried on only one of a pair of chromosomes. (Compare *recessive*).

Dysphasia Impaired capacity to speak due to damage to or disease of certain areas of the brain.

Dyspnoea Shortness of breath.

Echolalia The inappropriate repetition of words or phrases spoken to the subject. In 'delayed echolalia' the repetition occurs later, perhaps by hours or even days.

Electroencephalograph (EEG) A record of the variations in electrical potential between different parts of the brain. Normally a number of channels are recorded simultaneously using electrodes placed at different points on the skull.

Electrolytes Chemical ions such as sodium (Na^+), potassium (K^+) or chloride (Cl^-) contained in the blood plasma and other tissues; so called because they can conduct electricity.

Encephalitis Inflammation of the brain; may have various causes.

Encephalopathy Disease of, or affecting, the brain.

Endocrine Endocrine glands are those which produce hormones which circulate in the blood stream to produce various effects on bodily function. Endocrine disorders are those in which the functioning of these glands, or of the hormones they produce, is abnormal.

Enzyme Enzymes are complex chemical substances which enable particular chemical reactions to take place in the body. There are many enzymes, facilitating a vast number of chemical processes needed for normal bodily functioning.

Epicanthic fold A fold of skin over the inner angle of the eye.

Fantasy The production of mental images, often to provide gratification or satisfaction not obtainable in reality. The term 'fantasy' is also used for the images themselves.

Functional bladder volume The effective capacity of the bladder, as opposed to its actual anatomical size.

Gene A unit of heredity occupying a fixed position on a chromosome.

Gene penetrance Refers to the proportion of individuals in whom a gene has its effect. If a dominant gene leads to the production of the relevant characteristic in every individual carrying it, the penetrance is 100 per cent. If only a proportion of the individuals carrying the gene show the characteristic, the penetrance is expressed as the percentage of such individuals who are affected.

Goitre Enlargement of the thyroid gland, which appears as swelling in the neck.

Growth hormone A hormone produced by the pituitary gland. Is necessary for normal growth to occur.

Hallucination The subjective experience of a sensory perception which does not arise in the external world. Thus auditory hallucinations may take the form of hearing voices when no-one is speaking; and visual hallucinations of seeing things which are not there.

Hemiplegia Paralysis, partial or complete, of one side of the body. May be *spastic*, with increased muscle tone, or *flaccid*, with decreased tone.

Heterozygote An individual who has dissimilar alleles (see above) for a particular gene.

Homozygote An individual who has identical alleles (see above) for a particular gene.

Hormone Substance produced by an endocrine gland (see above), to circulate in the bloodstream and have certain effects on the functioning of other parts of the body.

Hyperkinesis Excessive motor activity.

Hypochondriasis Excessive preoccupation with physical symptoms, even in the absence of physical disease, often seen in unduly anxious individuals

Hypoglycaemia Blood sugar level that is below normal.

Hypothalamus An important neural control centre at the base of the brain.

Ideas of reference The belief that things in the subject's environment or experience refer to the subject when this is not so. Chance remarks, glances, gestures, advertisements and statements on radio or television are examples of things that may be misinterpreted in this way.

Identification The adoption of the views, attitudes or behaviours of another person as a result of a close, usually loving or admiring, relationship with that person.

Illusion a false perception of reality, resulting from the misinterpretation of sensory stimuli.

Infection Disease caused by the establishment and multiplication in the body of organisms such as bacteria or viruses.

Institutionalization The effects upon individuals of prolonged periods of living in the impersonal atmosphere of institutions. Characterized by overdependence on staff, loss of initiative and a progressive inability to cope with life in the outside world.

Maladjusted Primarily an administrative, educational term used in the United Kingdom to describe a group of children requiring a certain type of special education. Also sometimes used, loosely, to describe any child who is emotionally disturbed.

Malocclusion The condition that exists when the teeth do not meet in the most effective way.

Metabolic Metabolism is the process whereby substances entering the body are processed and used in various ways, their unwanted breakdown products being excreted from the body. Metabolic processes are those concerned with this; metabolic disorders are those in which some of the processes are not occurring normally.

Micturition The passing of urine.

Mutism Emotionally determined failure to speak, despited the physical ability to do so.

Myelin A substance forming the sheaths of nerves. Loss of their myelin sheaths causes failure of the functioning of the nerves, as in 'demyelinating diseases'.

Neurological Concerned with the nervous system, that is the brain and spinal cord and the nerves connected to them.

Nuclear magnetic resonance (NMR) Also known as magnetic resonance imaging (MRI). The patient is placed inside a powerful electromagnet which lines up the hydrogen atoms in the body water. The apparatus induces these atoms to oscillate; as they do so they give off weak radiofrequency signals which are picked up by coils surrounding the patient and processed by a computer. By this means cross-sectional images of the body are obtained. No ionizing radiation is used. A new and currently expensive procedure only available in certain centres.

Organic Concerned with the physical structures of the body. Thus an 'organic disease' is one in which there is demonstrable physical abnormality of the parts or organs involved.

Palpitation The sensation of rapid beating of the heart.

Parkinsonism A condition in which there is muscular rigidity, tremor which is worse on voluntary movement and weakness of voluntary movements. Facial muscles and those responsible for speech may be affected as well as limb muscles. Usually due to damage to or disease of certain structures at the base of the brain. Can also be a side-effect of certain drugs used in psychiatry.

Peptic ulcer A form of ulceration of the inside surface of the wall of the stomach or duodenum (that part of the gastrointestinal tract into which the stomach leads).

Phenothiazine The generic name of a group of drugs used in certain types of psychotic disorder, notably schizophrenia. They also have other medical uses. The first one introduced was chlorpromazine, but many others are now available.

Phenotype The physical constitition of a person or other organism. It is the result of the interaction of genetic and environmental factors. The *genotype* is the genetic constitution of the organism.

Phenylalanine An amino acid which accumulates in the body in excessive quantities in phenylketonuria.

Phobia An irrational fear.

Pituitary gland An important endocrine gland attached to the base of the brain. Influences the activity of many other glands. Consists of anterior and posterior lobes.

Plasma The clear, yellowish fluid in which the blood cells are suspended.

Polyuria The production of excessive amounts of urine.

Projection A term used for the process whereby ideas arising from within an individual's mind are attributed to some other person or organization.

Psychiatrist A medically qualified practitioner who has specialized in the study and treatment of patients with disorders affecting the mind.

Psychologist A person with training and expertise in the scientific study of behaviour and its modification. Psychologists are non-medical graduates who, after their basic university course, undertake further training in one (or more) special branches of psychology. Clinical and educational psychologists are those who mainly work with psychiatrists in the study and treatment of children's psychiatric disorders.

Psychopathology The abnormalities of the mind, of which the subject is often consciously unaware, responsible for or associated with mental and emotional disorders.

Pyloric stenosis Obstruction at the lower end of the stomach, where it joins the duodenum. Can be a congential disorder requiring surgical treatment in the early days or weeks of life.

Recessive In genetics, a recessive trait is one which is manifest only when the gene is carried on both members of a pair of chromosomes. (Compare *dominant*.)

Regression Reversion to a mode of behaviour and/or an emotional state characteristic of a younger age.

Reliability In statistics, reliability describes the extent to which a measuring device gives the same results when applied more than once under similar conditions. 'Inter-rater' reliability refers to the use of the same device by different persons; 'test-retest' reliability refers to the use of the same device with the same subjects at different times.

Rubella German measles.

Soft (neurological) signs Minor abnormalities of neurological response, often characteristic of children of a younger age than the subject, and not indicative of structural diseases of the nervous system. (See Shaffer *et al.*, 1983, for a fuller discussion.)

Spastic Having increased muscle tone.

Sphincter muscles Circular muscles which serve to regulate the opening and closing of the orifices of hollow organs such as the anus and the bladder.

Standard deviation A measure of the scatter of a series of values round the mean. The amounts by which each of the values differs from the mean are taken and each is squared. The square root of the mean of these squares is the standard deviation. In practice the following formula is used.

$$SD = \sqrt{\frac{\Sigma \ (Y - \bar{Y})^2}{n - 1}}$$

where *n* is the number of values of the measurement, Y; $\bar{Y}$ is the mean of all the values of Y and Σ signifies 'the sum of'.

Stereotypies Actions or thoughts occurring in rigid, repetitive and often meaningless patterns.

Stupor A state of mental unresponsiveness, short of unconsciousness. The subject, although appearing dazed and unresponsive, may hear what is being said and be aware of what is happening

Subarachnoid haemorrhage Bleeding from an artery lying beneath the arachnoid membrane, which covers the surface of the brain. Often due to the rupture of a congenital aneurysm (or saccular swelling) on the artery wall.

Suppository A solid preparation of a drug for rectal administration.

Syphilis A sexually transmitted disease due to the organism *Treponema pallidum*. In its later stages it can affect the nervous system and cause dementia and other symptoms.

Systemic infection a generalized infection involving the whole body.

Tardive dyskinesia A syndrome of rhythmical involuntary movements of the tongue, face mouth or jaw. There may also be involuntary movements of the limbs.

Temporal lobe One of the areas of the cortex of the brain. The temporal
   lobes are situated in the lower, lateral parts of each cerebral
   hemisphere.

Toxaemia The presence in the circulating blood and in the body tissues
   generally of harmful substances (toxins) formed by infective agents,
   or produced in the body as a result of disease, injury or other
   disorder.

Toxoplasmosis A disease due to the protozoon *Toxoplasma gondii*.

Tricylic drug A group of antidepressant drugs, so called because of their
   chemical structure. Imipramine was the first tricyclic drug introduced but it has been joined by many others.

Truancy The wilful avoidance of school.

Urethra The passage leading from the bladder to the exterior. Conveys
   urine and, in the male, semen.

Validity The accuracy with which a measuring device measures that
   which it is supposed to measure. Thus the validity of a rating scale
   designed to measure depression would describe how well the scale
   actually measures the degree to which subjects are depressed.

Variance A statistical term for a measure of the dispersion of values
   around their mean. It is the square of the standard deviation (see
   above).

Subject Index

Author Index